MEDICAL PSYCHIATRY

THEORY AND PRACTICE

MEDICAL PSYCHIATRY

THEORY AND PRACTICE

Vol. 2

Edited by
Enrique S. Garza-Treviño
*Assistant Professor of Psychiatry
and Behavioral Sciences*

*University of Texas
Health Science Center
at Houston*

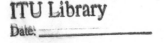

World Scientific
Singapore • New Jersey • London • Hong Kong

Published by

World Scientific Publishing Co. Pte. Ltd.
P O Box 128, Farrer Road, Singapore 9128

USA office: World Scientific Publishing Co., Inc.
687 Hartwell Street, Teaneck, NJ 07666, USA

UK office: World Scientific Publishing Co. Pte. Ltd.
73 Lynton Mead, Totteridge, London N20 8DH, England

Library of Congress Cataloging-in-Publication Data

Medical psychiatry: theory and practice/edited by Enrique S. Garza
-Trevino.
     p.   cm.
    Includes index.
    ISBN 9971507749
    1. Medicine, Psychosomatic. 2. Biological psychiatry. 3. Psychological
manifestations of general diseases. I. Garza-Treviño, Enrique S.
(Enrique Sergio)
    [DNLM: 1. Mental   Disorders.   2. Psychophysiologic   Disorders.
    WM 90 M4888]
RC49.M42 1989
616.08--dc 19
DNLM/DLC
for Library of Congress   89-5473
                                        CIP

Printed in Singapore by JBW Printers & Binders Pte. Ltd.

VOLUME 1

VOLUME 2

PSYCHONEUROENDOCRINOLOGY

Juan Ramon de la Fuente, M.D.
Associate Professor, Psychiatry
Director, Division of Clinical Research
Mexican Institute of Psychiatry

Hector A. Ortega-Soto, M.D.
Associate Professor, Psychiatry
Universidad Nacional Autonoma de Mexico
Mexican Institute of Psychiatry

Enrique S. Garza-Trevino, M.D.
Assistant Professor, Psychiatry
University of Texas
Health Science Center at Houston

M. Dhyanne Warner, Ph.D.
Medical Student
University of Texas
Medical School at Houston

Cecilia A. Peabody, M.D.
Associate Professor, Psychiatry
University of Texas
Medical School at Houston

CONTENTS:

PSYCHONEUROENDOCRINOLOGY

Juan Ramon de la Fuente, M.D

Hector A. Ortega-Soto, M.D.

Enrique S. Garza-Treviño, M.D.

M. Dhyanne Warner, PhD

Cecilia A. Peabody, M.D.

Although the human interest about the relationships between the body "humoral state" and behavior goes back to Greek Hipocratic Medicine, a rigorous scientific approach was not initiated until the end of the past century. Several classic endocrinologists, such as Addison, Cushing, and Graves dedicated much of their work to describe the mental changes associated with adrenal and thyroid diseases (1,2,3). In the last 15 years much progress has been made toward understanding the nature of these relationships. Schally and Guillemin have elucidated the structure of several hypothalamic hormones and their regulation by neurotransmitters are beginning to be understood (4,5). Since some of these same neurotransmitters are believed to be involved in various psychiatric disorders, one may postulate various neuroendocrine changes in these diseases. This chapter describes some of the endocrine pathology in psychiatry as well as psychiatric characteristics of endocrine diseases.

HYPOTHALAMIC-PITUITARY-THYROID AXIS

The importance of the thyroid axis in psychiatry has been appreciated for some time since both hyper- and hypothyroidism are associated with depression and other mental changes. The secretion of the thyroid hormones triiodothyronine (T_3) and thyroxine (T_4) is controlled by the anterior pituitary hormone, thyroid stimulating hormone (TSH, thyrotropin). TSH is regulated by the hypothalamic hormone thyrotropin releasing hormone (TRH), and is also under feedback inhibition by T_3 and T_4. These hormones have been extensively studied in affective disorders.

Psychiatric symptoms of thyroid disease range from mild cognitive impairment and flattened affect to dementia and severe depression (6). Psychiatric presentations are the first signs of hypothyroidism in approximately 2% of cases, with an intellectual impairment being the most frequently reported. Initial manifestions of this impairment are forgetfulness, carelessness in every day activities, and difficulty in concentration. Usually, patients find their cognitive deficit quite frustrating, but eventually may become indifferent to it. The prevalence of cognitive impairment has been reported as high as 93% (7).

An abnormal mood may also be the first manifestation of hypothyroidism. Gold and associates evaluated thyroid function in 250 patients referred to a psychiatric hospital for treatment of depression or anergia (8). Two patients (less than 1%) had overt hypothyroidism ; nine patients (3.6%) had mild hypothyroidism with few clinical signs and normal T_3RU and T_4 levels but elevated baseline TSH. Ten patients (4%) had an exaggerated TSH response to

TRH but normal thyroid tests otherwise. This later group was diagnosed as subclinical hypothyroidism.

The prevalence of depression in overt hypothyroidism has been estimated as high as 80% (9). This high rate of depression suggests that the affective state is more than an adaptive reaction to a chronic illness. One study reported an 83% incidence of depression in hypothyroid patients and only 50% incidence in arthritic patients (10). Both groups were under adequate medical control and were matched for age, sex and chronicity of illness.

Affective disturbances may also present as irritability or mood lability (7). Occasionally, patients may be hyperactive or hypomanic rather than apathetic and withdrawn (11,12). A psychotic state, "myxedema madness", occurs in a small percentage of patients. The symptoms include confusion, memory dysfunction, agitation, and in some instances, paranoia, delusions, and hallucinations resembling schizophrenia or a Capgras' Syndrome (13,14,15).

The diagnosis of hypothyroidism needs to be confirmed by laboratory tests. Subclinical conditions, which occur without classical signs of thyroid failure, and with normal levels of T_3, T_4, and TSH, are characterized by an exaggerated response of TSH to TRH challenge (16,17). The significance of subclinical thyroid disease is controversial.

The response of psychiatric symptoms to thyroid replacement is variable (7,11). Most patients improve as a euthyroid state is achieved, and improvement can continue for months after laboratory tests have returned to normal (18). Cognitive deficits may be irreversible if hypothyroidism is severe and longstanding.

Tonks reports that a better response can be expected if patients are older than 50 years and have less than two years of thyroid deficiency (6). When psychiatric symptoms prove refractory to substitution therapy, psychotropic drugs or electroconvulsive therapy may be used.

Patients with hyperthyroidism are often anxious and emotionally labile. Although they usually feel that their energy is increased, their ability to work productively is decreased owing to a shortened attention span and other cognitive dysfunctions (7). The picture may be confused with an anxiety disorder, but Sachar suggests that the warm dry hands in hyperthyroidism may help to distinguish this disorder from euthyroid anxiety in which the hands may be cold and clammy (19).

Manic symptoms may be associated with hyperthyroidism; however, in the elderly the condition may be expressed as a psychomotor retardation, confusion, and apathy suggesting a major depressive disorder. The differential diagnosis is very important because administration of antidepressants could exacerbate the cardiovascular disease associated with a hyperthyroid state (11). Occasionally, one may find hyperthyroid patients with suspiciousness and paranoid ideas, although truly paranoid psychotic states are rare.

The reports regarding a high rate of depression among hypothyroid patients, and of a T_3 potentiation of tricyclic antidepressant therapy (20), suggest that there may be an inverse relationship between affect and hypothyroidism. However, multiple studies have demonstrated that 25-30% of patients with major depression have a blunted TSH response to TRH challenge, a response pattern which is found in hyperthyroidism. The physiological meaning of this neuroendocrine abnormality is not clear.

It has been proposed that the blunted TSH response may be due to a hyposensitivity of the TRH pituitary receptors which could be developed gradually as a consequence of a hypothalamic increased TRH secretion. Although the quantifications of the peptide in the cerebrospinal fluid (CSF) of depressed patients has been reported to be increased, these alterations have not been found to correlate with TRH-test results (21). The hypothesis of an elevated TRH release is congruent with both the indolaminergic (22) and the modified catecolaminergic theories of depression (23).

The physiological meaning of this neuroendocrine abnormality is not clear. Other hormonal parameters have not been helpful in understanding this since they have been inconsistent. For example, the blood levels of T_4 and reverse T_3 (an inactive triiodothyronine) have been reported increased, while T_3 levels are within the normal range, or slightly diminished, in depressed patients (24,25,26,27). Moreover, the normal increment of TSH levels during the night may not be present in subjects with depression (28); in consequence the total 24 hour levels of TSH are decreased (29).

It has been proposed that the blunted TSH response may be due to a hyposensitivity of the TRH pituitary receptors which could be developed gradually by some depressed subjects as a consequence of a hypothalamic increased TRH secretion. Although the quantifications of the peptide in the cerebrospinal fluid (CSF) of depressed patients has been reported to be increased, these alterations do not correlate with TRH-test results (21). The hypothesis of an elevated TRH release could be associated with abnormalities in either the indolaminergic or the catecolaminergic CNS systems. Both of these systems have been postulated to be dysfunctional in depression. Since serotonin (5-HT) decreases, and norepinephrine (NE) increases TRH release from the hypothalamus, the occurrence of one or even both processes may be involved in the neuroendocrine abnormality. However, there is no substantial evidence to link these endocrine and neurotransmitter abnormalities in depressed patients. Multiple other neurotransmitters and neuromodulators are involved in the regulation of the thyroid axis, such as dopamine, somatostatin and neurotensin. Multiple investigators have attempted to demonstrate a relationship between thyroid and cortisol abnormalities in depression but there does not appear to be any correlation. A blunted response to a TRH challenge is a non-specific finding. In addition to hyperthyroidism it has been reported in patients with alcoholism and schizophrenia.

Recently, Joffe et al (30) proposed that depression may be associated with a true hyperthyroid state at the CNS level. According to them, depressed subjects have an increased intraneuronal conversion of T_4 to T_3, and antidepressant treatments, particularly lithium and carbamazepine, restore HPT equilibrium by producing a decrement of T_4 blood levels. They argue that adding T_3 to a tricyclic antidepressant drug has the same effect, i.e., it decreases T_4 release by means of the negative pituitary feedback system. Although highly speculative, the hypothesis can explain the hyperthyroid-like TSH response to TRH, the normalization of the test with treatment and the enhancement of antidepressant response to tricyclic drugs in spite of the abnormality of TRH test results resembling the hyperthyroid state.

HYPOTHALAMIC-PITUITARY-ADRENAL AXIS

The hormones released by the hypothalamic-pituitary- adrenal axis (HPA) have been extensively studied in psychiatry. Corticotropin releasing factor (CRF) is released from the hypothalamus and stimulates the pituitary hormone corticotropin (ACTH). ACTH stimulates the secretion of cortisol from the adrenal glands. Both hyper- and hypofunction conditions of the axis are associated with psychiatric syndromes, especially affective disorders (31).

Depressive symptomatology is as common in patients suffering from Addison's disease as in patients with endogenous Cushing's disease (31,32). However, iatrogenic Cushing is more frequently associated with manic symptoms (33). In an attempt to explain this fact, Sachar proposed that ACTH could have a "depressogenic" effect while corticosteroids could have the opposite effect (34), since ACTH is increased both in Addison's and in endogenous Cushing's syndromes, but decreased in iatrogenic hypercortisolism. However, in patients with endogenous Cushing's disease treated with drugs that block the synthesis of cortisol without decreasing ACTH blood levels, improvement in depression correlates significantly with the free cortisol level decrements and not with ACTH changes (35). These findings suggest that cortisol, and not ACTH, may influence mood regulation.

There is consistent evidence that a significant proportion of depressed patients show a moderate hypercortisolism without structural abnormalities of the HPA axis (36,37,38). The increase in cortisol release leads not only to elevated blood levels, but also to CSF and urine increments. In addition, it has been demonstrated that the circadian rhythm of cortisol secretion is abnormal, and that depressed patients show an active secretion of cortisol during the night, regardless of whether they are asleep (39). The study of the circadian pattern of cortisol release in depressive patients suggests that their hypercortisolemia is different from normal subjects under stress (40).

Abnormal circadian pattern of cortisol release is characterized by an increment in the magnitude of the pulses secreted, and by what is known as a "phase-advancement" pattern. The last, in conjunction with the reported (39,41) shortened latency to the first period of rapid eye movement (REM) sleep has led some authors to claim that this depressive syndrome (with short REM latency and phase-advancement pattern of cortisol release) must be catalogued as a primary chronobiological rhythmopathy (42).

Multiple research groups have tested the HPA response to dexamethasone challenge among depressed patients (43,44,45,46). The dexamethasone suppression test (DST) is performed by administrating 1 mg of the synthetic steroid by oral route at 2300 hr and quantifying plasma cortisol levels at 2 points during the next day, usually at 0800 and 1600 hrs. Approximately 50% of patients with major depressive disorder fail to suppress cortisol levels as normal controls do.

The adequate performance of the DST in psychiatry is influenced by several technical and methodological factors that have been reviewed elsewhere (43,47). When all these factors are adequately controlled, the test is highly specific (>90%) and reasonably sensitive (>50%). If the test is performed at an institution with a high prevalence rate of depression, the DST has a diagnostic accuracy similar to that of other laboratory tests used in clinical medicine.

Although DST seems not to be a good predictive parameter regarding therapeutic response to specific antidepressant treatments (48), it is clear that abnormal results tend to normalize when the symptoms improve (43,44,46). Figure 1 shows the typical pattern of a depressed patient before and after a tricyclic drug trial.

Frequently, what is found in depression is an "early escape" rather than a true non-suppression to dexamethasone (44). In other words, some patients show a diminution in cortisol levels, after dexamethasone administration, lasting several hours, but thereafter cortisol levels rise. This pattern can be present among patients with Cushing's disease; however, the response to CRF infusion is different between these two groups (49,50). Depressed subjects do not respond with a rise of ACTH levels, but their cortisol levels rise as in normals. In contrast, patients with Cushing's disease have exaggerated ACTH and cortisol responses (51). Furthermore, it has been reported that CRF concentration is higher in the CSF of depressed subjects than in the CSF of subjects suffering from Cushing's disease, and that cortisol response to ACTH exogenous administration is also increased among affective patients (51). All these data suggest that there is a hypersensitivity state of the adrenal glands to ACTH actions in depressive disorder.

Recently, two independent research groups (52,53) have reported that the density of glucocorticoid receptors is decreased in the lymphocytes of depressed patients. If this phenomena also occurs at the hypothalamic level it may explain the lack of response to dexamethasone; however, this has not been demonstrated. The report that antidepressant drugs provoke an increment of the glucocorticoid receptor density in the hippocampus (54) may suggest the mechanism by which antidepressant treatment restores the HPA function in depressed patients.

The pathophysiology of the HPA alterations in depression is unknown, but some evidence seems to indicate that the processes may be initiated by a disinhibition of the axis secondary to an altered noradrenergic transmission (43,47). It is possible that in these conditions the glucocorticoid receptors at the hypothalamus desensitize, thus maintaining a high rate of CRF release. In these instances the corticotropes initially release large quantities of ACTH but, eventually, they become hyposensitive reducing their capability of response to CRF. Finally, the adrenals may develop hypertrophy leading to an excessive release of cortisol in spite of the small ACTH concentrations (50).

HYPOTHALAMIC-PITUITARY-GONADAL AXIS

It is well recognized that the hypothalamic-pituitary-gonadal

(HGP) axis is associated with mood changes. The hypothalamic hormone, gonadotropin releasing hormone (GnRH), stimulates the release of leutinizing hormone (LH) and folicle stimulating hormone (FSH) from the anterior pituitary. LH and FSH release the gonadal hormones such as the androgens and estrogens from the target organs. There is much evidence to suggest an interaction of these hormones and affective disorders. Decreased libido and impotence are prominent features of major depression. In women depression is frequently associated with cessation of the menstrual cycle. When rhesus monkeys are removed from a free environment to a confined one, the menstrual cycle ceases. These observations suggest the existence of an inherent central mechanism to prevent reproduction in unfavorable circumstances.

Clinically, some women experience significant emotional changes associated with the menstrual cycle, and the incidence of depressive disorders after menopause, and during the puerperium, is high (55,56,38). Moreover, it has been observed that hormonal contraceptives, particularly those with large progesterone content, produce depressive syndromes (57) post menopausal.

The relationship between the hormonal changes and the affective ones during the menstrual cycle is not clear. A prospective investigation (58) in women without a psychiatric history, reported that depressive symptoms usually appear 4 to 7 days after the progesterone blood peak and that the severity of symptoms correlates significantly with the magnitude of the peak. Paradoxically, severity also correlates positively with the clearance rate of progesterone; i.e., the patients with the largest peaks, that disappear the fastest, were those with the most severe affective disturbances. The authors speculated that these kinds of hormonal stimuli, repetitive and intense, could act along time such as a kindling stimulus and, eventually, may produce a complete major depressive disorder. The hypothesis is of interest because other data also implicate a kindling phenomena in the pathogenesis of affective disorders (59); it may explain some of the inconsistencies about the reported affective syndromes related to the menstrual cycle (60,61).

The levels of gonadotropins and gonadal steroids in depression have been of considerable interest. Several investigators have reported low baseline LH levels and a decreased response to GnRH in about 25% of depressed males (62,63, 64) but others have not found any differences (65, 66, 67). One investigator found decreased total and free mean plasma testosterone levels and increased plasma estradiol in depression (68) but other investigators reported normal plasma testosterone (65,69). Decreased plasma LH levels have been reported in postmenopausal depressed women (70).

In summary, although decreased libido is frequently found in depression it has not been correlated with specific gonadal hormone changes. Several reports suggest a relationship between the HPG axis and mood regulation, but the exact mechanisms have not been clarified.

GROWTH HORMONE

Growth hormone (GH) secretion has been studied in psychiatry since it is regulated by neurotransmitter systems, such as catecholamines which are thought to be implicated in psychiatric disorders. The hypothalamic hormone, growth hormone releasing factor (GHRF) stimulates the secretion of GH from the anterior pituitary and somatostatin inhibits its release. Alpha-2 adrenergic agonists stimulate GH via a direct effect on GHRF and somatostatin. Beta adrenergic agonists inhibit GH via an effect on blood glucose and fatty acids. DA, GABA, 5HT, acetylcholine and estrogens all stimulate GH secretion.

There have been consistent reports of a decreased GH response to clonidine in major depression (36). This has been interpreted as evidence of subsensitive post-synaptic alpha-2-adrenergic receptors and an increased NE release (71). One report suggests a negative correlation between GH response to clonidine and noradrenergic activity (72). Treatment with tricyclic anti-depressants or monoamine oxidase inhibitors had no effect on the suppressed GH response, suggesting that it is a trait marker for depression (73,74).

The release of GH during nocturnal sleep appears to be regulated by cholinergic mechanisms (72). Since depressed patients show several sleep abnormalities, the nocturnal GH release pattern has been postulated to be altered. However, no significant changes have been found as compared with normal controls (72). Nevertheless, a diurnal GH hypersecretion has been reported to be present in some depressed subjects (75); this abnormality may be the result of an increased release of the stimulatory hypothalamic factor (GRH) or to an increment of the pituitary sensitivity to this factor.

It is interesting to note that GH abnormalities in

depression could be related to HPA disturbances. There is evidence that glucocorticoids can enhance the pituitary GH response to the hypothalamic GHRF (76,77); so GH hypersecretion can be secondary to the hypercortisolism. Furthermore, it seems that glucocorticoid administration decreases pituitary GH response to pharmacological challenges thought to act at the hypothalamic level (77). Thus, GH abnormalities of depressive patients could be only an epiphenomenon not reflecting a primary physiopathologic process.

The behavioral and neuroendocrine consequences of abnormal levels of GH or exogenous administration, is not known. Investigations in rats indicate that GH may enhance appetite (78), so it is possible that alterations of eating behavior in depression are related to GH abnormalities.

PROLACTIN

Prolactin is an anterior pituitary hormone which has been studied extensively in schizophrenia. The secretion of prolactin is largely controlled by inhibition from dopamine. Prolactin has a negative feedback on its own secretion. Separate peptide releasing and inhibiting factors have been proposed but never substantiated. TRH is a potent stimulator of prolactin secretion but it is not known whether TRH in portal venous blood is physiologically important.

Schizophrenia is thought to involve a dysregulation of the dopaminergic system in the mesolimbic and mesocortical areas of the brain. The hypothalamic tuberoinfundibular dopamine system has been hypothesized to be involved, and thus multiple investigations have focused on prolactin. Baseline serum prolactin levels in unmedicated acute and chronic schizophrenics have been found to be within normal limits in the majority of studies. Several investigators have attempted to correlate low serum prolactin levels with psychotic symptoms and tardive dyskinesia, hypothesizing that all three conditions may represent supersensitive dopamine receptors. While there has been some preliminary data to suggest such correlations may exist, no firm conclusions can be made (79).

In depressed patients baseline prolactins have been reported to be decreased, increased and normal. Several studies have investigated the prolactin response to TRH and the majority have found a blunted response (80). Other investigators have reported a blunted prolactin response to morphine (81) or methadone (82) in depression. It has been suggested that this reflects an abnormality in the endogenous opiate regulation of prolactin secretion. It may also implicate a serotonergic abnormality since there is evidence that morphine stimulates prolactin by promoting the release of 5HT.

CONCLUSIONS

It is evident that the endocrine system and psychiatric disorders are strongly interrelated although the exact nature of their interactions have not been clarified. Major depresssion is associated with a large number of functional pituitary abnormalities , which may reflect the interaction of the hypothalamus and CNS neurotransmitters. The abnormalities of the HPA axis is the area which has received the most attention in depression. In spite of the extensive investigations in neuro-endocrine measures, none have proven to have significant clinical utility.

The dexamethasone suppression test and the TRH stimulation test have consistently been demonstrated to be abnormal in depression but do not appear to correlate with each other. This is consistent with the theory that depression may have multiple etiologies and hence more than one neurotransmitter may be involved. This heterogeneity of depression makes it more difficult to demonstrate consistent abnormalities. Clearly more work is needed before neuroendocrine strategies can truly provide a window into the brain.

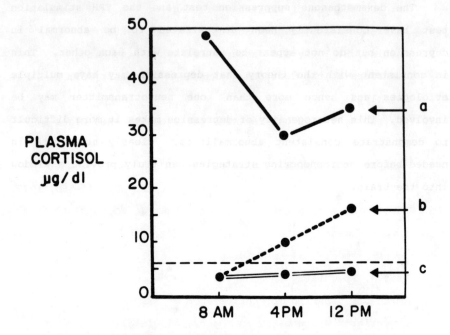

Figure 1.   Results of a Dexamethasone Suppression Test in a
depressed   patient.

a. Pretreatment.   Cortisol level is high and it
is not suppressed by dexamethasone.

b. Partial Remission.   After 3 weeks of treatment
there is a suppression at 8 am but it does not
persist

c. Total Remission. After 8 weeks of treatment
the suppressive response shows a normal pattern.

Suppression Criteria: 6 μg/dl.

REFERENCES

1. Addison, T. Diseases of the supra-renal capsules.
   In: Collection of Published Writings of the late Thomas
   Addison. New Syndenham Society, London, 1968.

2. Cushing, H. Psychic disturbances associated with
   disorders of the ductless glands. Am J Insanity 69:
   965, 1913.

3. Graves, R.J. Clinical letters, Lecture XII. Med Class 5:
   25-43, 1940.

4. Schally, A.V., Arimura, A., Kastin, A.J.
   Hypothalamic regulatory hormones. Science 179:341-350, 1973.

5. Guillemin, R. & Burgus, R. The hormones of the
   hypothalamus. Sci Am, 227:29-33, 1972.

6. Tonks J. Mental illness in hypothyroid patients.
   Brit J. Psychiatry 110:706-710;1964

7. Smith C.K., Barish J., Correa J., et al.
   Psychiatric disturbance in endocrinologic disease.
   Psychosom Med 34:69-86, 1972.

8. Gold M.S., Pottash A.L.C., Extein I. Hypothyroidism
   and depression. JAMA 245:1919-1922;1981

9. Whybrow, P.C. Mental changes accompanying
   thyroid gland dysfunction. Arch Gen Psychiatry
   20:48-63, 1969

10. Mezquita-Orozco, R.I. Depression in hypothyroid patients.
    Salud Mental 8:90-93, 1985

11. Wilson W.H., Jefferson J.W. Thyroid disease, behavior

and psychopharmacology. Psychosomatics 26:481-492, 1985.

12. Stasiek C., Zetin M. Organic manic disorders.
    Psychosomatics 26:394-402;1985

13. Pitts F.N., Guze S.B. Psychiatric disorders and
    myxedema. AM J Psychiatry 118:142-147;1961.

14. Esson W.M. Myxedema with psychosis. Arch Gen
    Psychiatry 14:277-283, 1966.

15. Madakusira S., Hall T.B. Capgras syndrome in a patient
    with myxedema. Am J Psychiatry 138:1506-1508;1981.

16. Jurney, T.H. & Wartotsky, L. Thyrotropin-
    releasing hormone test in an out-patient clinic.
    South Med J 78:774-781, 1985.

17. Extein, K., Gold, M.S. Psychiatric applications
    of thyroid tests. J Clin Psychiatry 47(supl 1):13-16, 1986.

18. De Fine-Oliverius B., Boder E. Reversible psychosis
    and dementia in myxedema. Acta Psychiat Scand 46:12;
    1970.

19. Sachar E.J. Psychiatric disturbances associated with
    endocrine disorders. In American Handbook of
    Psychiatry, IV, Organic Disorders and Psychosomatic
    Medicine. (Arietis, Reiser M.F. ed). Basic Books, Inc.
    New York, 1975.

20. Goodwin, F.K., Prange, A.J., Post, R.M., et al.
    Potentiation of antidepressant effects of L-triiodothyronine
    in tricyclic non responders. Am J Psychiatry 139:34-38, 1982.

21. Kirkegaard, C., Barber, J., Hummer, et al.
    Increased levels of TRH in cerebrospinal fluid from
    patients with endogenous depression. Psychoneuro-
    endocrinol 4:275-286, 1979.

22. Coppen, A.J., Prange, A. J., Whybrow, P.C.
    Abnormalities of indolamines in affective disorders.
    Arch Gen Psychiatry 26:474-478, 1972.

23. Stahl, S.M. & Palazidou, L. The pharmacology
    of depression: studies of neurotransmitter receptors
    lead the search for biochemical lesions and new drug
    therapies. TIPS 7:349-354, 1986.

24. Kirkegaard, C., Faber, J. Altered serum levels
    of thyroxine, triiodothyronines, and diiodothyronines
    in endogenous depression. Acta Endocrinol 96:199, 1981.

25. Linnoila, M., Lamberg, B.A. Potter, W.Z., et al.
    High reverse T_3 in manic and unipolar depressed women.
    Psychiat Res 6:271-276, 1982.

26. Sternbach, H.A., Gwirtsman, H.E., Gerner, R.H.
    The TRH stimulation test and reverse T_3 in depression.
    J Affect Dis 8:267-270, 1985.

27. Joffe, R.T., Blank, D.W., Post, R.M., et al.
    Decreased triiodothyronines in depression: a preliminary
    report. Biol Psychiat 20:922-925, 1985.

28. Kjellman, B.F., Beck-Friis, J., Ljunggren, J.G.,
    et al. Twenty-four hour serum levels of
    TSH in affective disorders. Acta Psychiat
    Scand 69:491-502, 1984.

29. Unden, F., Ljunggren, J.G., Kjellman, V.F., et al. Twenty-four hour serum levels of T_4 and T_3 in relation to decreased TSH serum levels and decreased TSH response to TRH in affective disorders. Acta Psychiat Scand 73:358-365, 1986.

30. Joffe, R.T., Roy-Byrne, P.P., Uhde, T.W., et al. Thyroid function in affective illness: A reappraisal. Biol Psychiat 19:1685-1691, 1984.

31. Hall, C.W., Stickney, S., Beresford, T.P. Endocrine disease and behavior. Integ Psychiatry 4:122-135, 1986.

32. Starkman, M.N. & Scheintgard, D.E. Neuropsychiatric manifestations of patients with Cushing's Syndrome. Arch Intern Med 141:215-219, 1981.

33. Kaufmann, H.E., Casadonte, R.E., Peselow, E.D. Steroid Psychosis. NY St J Med 81:1795-1797, 1981.

34. Sachar, E.J. Hormonal changes in stress and mental illness. Hosp Pract 10:49-55, 1975.

35. Starkman, M.N., Scheintgard, D.E. & Schrok, M.A. Cushing's Syndrome after treatment: changes in cortisol and ACTH levels, and amelioration of the depressive syndrome. Psychiat Res 19:177-188, 1986.

36. de la Fuente, J.R., Salin-Pascual, R.J., Berlanga, C.A., et al. In search of biological markers in affective disorders. Acta Psiquiat Psicol Amer Lat 31:17-24, 1985.

37. Linkowsky, P., Mendlewicz, J., Lecleroq, R., et al. The 24 hour profile of adrenocorticotropin and cortisol in

Medicine, 41:203-208, 1979.

68. Vogel, W , Klarber, E.L., and Broveıman, O.H. Gonadal
Function in Depression, Progress in Neuropsychopharmacology,
2:487-503, 1978.

69. Sachar, E.J., et al. Prasma and Urinary Testosterone Levels
in Depressed Men, Arch Gen Psych, 28:15-18, 1973.

70. Altman, N., Sachar, E.J., Gruen, P.H., et al. Reduced Plasma
LH concentration in postmenopausal depressed women. Psychosom
Med 37:274-276, 19,5.

71. de la Fuente, J.R. & Rosenbaum, A.H. Psychoendocrinology.
Mayo Clin Proc 54:109-118. 19,9.

72. de la Fuente, J.R., & Wells, L.A. Human Growth Hormone in
Psychiatric Disorders. J. Clin Psychiatry 42:270-274, 1981.

73. Charney, D.S., Heninger. G.R., Sternberg, D.E. "Alpha-2
Adrenergic Receptor Sensitivity and the Mechanism of Action
of Antidepressant Therapy. The Effect of Long-Term
Amitriptyline Treatment," Br J Psych, 142:265-275, ı983.

74. Siever, L.J., et al. "Growth Hormone Response to Clonidine
Unchanged by Chronic Clorgyline Treatment". Psychiatry
Research 7:139-144, 1982.

75. Mendlewicz, J., Linkowski, P., Kerhofs, M., et al. Diurnal
hypersecretion of growth hormone in depression. J Clin
Endocrinol Metab 60:505-511, 1985.

76. Wehrenberg, W.B, Baird, A., Ling, N. Potent interaction
between glucocorticoids and growth hormone-releasing factor

in vivo. Science 221:556-558, 1983.

77. Seifert, H., Perrin, M., Rivier, J., et al. Growth hormone-releasing factor binding sites in rat anterior pituitary membrane homogenates modulation by glucocoricoids. Endocrinol 117:424-236, 1985.

78. Vaccarino, F.J., Bloom, F.E., Rivier, J., et al. Stimulation of food intake in rats by centrally administered hypothalamic growth hormone-releasing factor. Nature 314:167-168, 1985.

79. Csernansky, J.G., Prosser, E., Kaplan, J., et al. Possible associations among plasma prolactin levels, tardive dyskinesia and paranoia in treated male schizophrenics. Biol Psychiatry 21:632-642, 1986.

80. Loosen, R.T., Prange, A.J. Serum thyrotropin response to thyrotropin-releasing hormone in psychiatric patients: a review. Am J Psychiatry 139:405-416, 1982.

81. Extein, I., et al. Deficient Prolactin Response to Morphine in Depressed Patients. Am J Psychiatry 137:845-846, 1980.

82. Judd, L.L., et al. Blunted Prolactin Response. A Neuroendocrine Abnormality Manifested by Depressed Patients. Arch Gen Psychiatry 39:1413-1416, 1982.

PSYCHOSOMATIC CONSIDERATIONS OF INFERTILITY

Diane Martinez, M.D.*

Contents:

1. Emotional Impact of Infertility

2. Psychological Considerations of Current Therapies for Infertility

    a) Hormonal
    b) Artificial Insemination
    c) In Vitro Fertilization and Embryo Transfer
    d) Genetic Intrafallopian Transfer
    e) Surrogate Motherhood

3. Psychological Aspects of Infertility and the Infertility Specialist

4. Role of the Psychiatrist and Other Mental Health Professionals

5. Ethics of Reproductive Intervention

6. Conclusion

7. References

* Clinical Assistant Professor
University of Texas Health Science Center
at San Antonio

PSYCHOSOMATIC CONSIDERATIONS OF INFERTILITY

Diane Martinez, M.D.

Infertility is typically defined as failure to successfully conceive after twelve consecutive months of unprotected intercourse. This definition derives from the fact that 95 percent of normal couples will conceive within that time. As recently as twenty years ago, 40 to 50 percent of infertility cases were attributed to emotional factors (1); this determination was made by process of elimination, when no organic cause could be found. Disturbances in neuroendocrine balance as a result of altered emotional states was thought to be the basis of this phenomena. Concentrations of endogenous opiate peptides, dopamine, epinephrine, norepinephrine, prolactin, oxytocin, and prostaglandins are all affected by psychological stress. Although the mechanisms could not be demonstrated empirically, it was assumed these stress-related biochemical alterations could influence ovulation, sperm production, uterotubal transport, and conception, initiation or maintainence of pregnancy . Such assumptions were then "validated" by studies that looked at the emotional state of infertile women. Multiple studies demonstrated infertile women to be more dependent, anxious, and neurotic than fertile women (1). Cases of resolution of infertility by psychotherapy (2) or adoption were also regarded as validating, despite their anecdotal nature.

Obviously, the state of the psyche bears upon reproduction. Vaginismus, tubal spasm, psychogenic failure to ovulate for women, and psychologically-based erectile or ejaculatory problems, and perhaps oligospermia for men, do occur; however, these are not common causes of infertility. In fact, there is no evidence that patients with infertility have a higher incidence of diagnosable sexual dysfunction or psychiatric disorder than occurs in the general population (3,4). The faulty structure of previous studies is obvious in that the focus is solely on infertile women, despite the fact that the organic cause of infertility lies with the male at least 35% of the time (5). Perspective is also gained on this matter by keeping in mind that a lack of desire for pregnancy is an inadequate barrier for most people.

The prevalence of infertility has increased over the past ten years, due to delayed child rearing and sexually transmitted diseases (6). There is a 30 per cent lower pregnancy rate in women over thirty and increasing infertility among women in their twenties. The problem is now more pressing as 90 percent of single mothers keep their babies rather than give them up for adoption. At least 15% (7) of married couples, a minimum of some 4½ million couples, will experience some degree of problem with fertility. Approximately 35% of infertility is a problem solely of the female and another 35% is a problem solely with the male. In about 25% of cases there is a problem found in both members of the couple (5,7).

Of the 25% of couples whose identifiable organic cause(s) for problems with conception is found, more than 50-60% can be successfully treated with medical or surgical techniques (7). Also, approximately 50% of couples with unexplained infertility will conceive (6). Secondary infertility is the term used for the inability to achieve pregnancy after at least one successful pregnancy; the rate of cure for secondary infertility is the same as the rate for primary infertility, approximately 50%.

Advances in reproductive physiology have reduced the number of cases of infertility currently attributed to emotional factors to less than 5% (1). Parallel to this determination, has come an increasing sensitivity to the emotional stress inherent to the infertile state and in undergoing infertility treatment for both members of the couple. It is now suggested that the humbler term "unexplained infertility" be used when no physical cause can be identified (8). From looking at emotional factors as a cause of infertility, we have come full circle to looking at infertility as the cause of emotional problems.

EMOTIONAL IMPACT OF INFERTILITY

Information about the emotional impact of infertility is almost entirely drawn from experience with couples undergoing infertility treatment. No information is available on couples who do not seek treatment. In that couples who seek treatment for their infertility are only a subset of infertile couples, it is not surprising that they have certain common personality characteristics. Typically they are high-functioning individuals who are well equipped psychologically to handle the hope and disappointment that infertility treatment entails. This is particularly true for those who have made it to the more extensive treatments like In Vitro Fertilization and Embryo Transfer (IVF-ET) or Gamete Intra-Fallopian Transfer (GIFT). Women undergoing treatment for infertility have been found to significantly differ from the norm in several ways (9). Most pronounced are tendencies to approach things cognitively, to value clear and thorough information, and to avoid changes in the environment. This same study found these women in general to be persevering, ambitious, goal-directed, challenged by competition, and to have high standards for performance. Men of infertile couples undergoing more radical therapies (IVF-ET, GIFT) differ from husbands of couples undergoing general infertility treatment in that they are more ambitious, creative, and independent (10). The women of these couples showed the same profile, except the female IVF-ET patients were in addition more upwardly mobile and ambitious than the non-IVF-ET woman patient.

These characteristics are not surprising. People who would choose to do something about their infertility would be those who see obstacles as something to overcome, who have the perseverance to work for a long-term goal, who want what they want and will try to achieve it through their own efforts. They would also be people to whom a scientifically based approach has appeal, as opposed to people who would look to fate or religion to take care of things. The information about the emotional reactions of these couples to infertility and infertility treatment is best understood in the context of these personality characteristics.

The psychological component of infertility begins the moment the couple starts to suspect there is a problem with conception. The emotional responses infertility evokes have common patterns. Barbara Eck Menning describes a sequence of feelings in those who must confront infertility: surprise, denial, anger (rational and irrational), isolation, guilt, and grief (7). Other authors stress the affects of anger and depression which are usually intense enough to make people feel "crazy" (8). For example, women describe extreme mood swings paralleling menstrual cycles with statements like "each period involves grieving a child." Intense feelings of jealousy directed at those for whom childbearing comes easily are commonly described, as are rageful feelings toward people insensitive to the pain of being infertile.

If the emotional impact of infertility can be put into a single category of experience, loss is probably the most accurate. Infertility involves a multiplicity of losses: actual, threatened, and symbolic. Most obviously there is the loss of a child. Parallel to this is the loss of being a parent; having a child is the passage to adulthood and not having this experience is a major loss. Yet rarely are either of these losses clear-cut, certain, or final. As such, there are often no end points to the loss, and certainly there are no rituals to bind the grief or to draw the couple to family and friends for comfort.

To the contrary, the infertility experience often serves to isolate the infertile couple from loved ones and even from each other. Most couples (9) choose not to tell family and friends about their infertility or its treatment. This maneuver, which the couple does to to protect themselves from overly intrusive or unempathic responses, can serve to invite hurt as family and friends respond negatively to the distancing or unknowingly make hurtful comments.

At the same time, the infertility experience can lead to a real or threatened loss of the marital relationship. Many couples have not had to face a crisis prior to their inability to get pregnant, which would have allowed them to develop coping skills. It is not known how often infertility is a primary factor in actual divorce, but it is likely not a rare occurrence. What is common for the infertile couples undergoing treatment is a temporary loss of intimacy as the stress of the experience drives a wedge between them. A typical problem is a wife needing to deal with her feelings of depression, loss, and anger by discussing them with her husband, and the husband feeling frightened or overwhelmed by the intensity of her affects. Often the husband needs to deal with his own feelings by suppression which increases his wife's distress. This scenario is exacerbated if there are issues of blame (whose "fault" is the infertility), ambivalence, or unequal levels of motivation for pursuing treatment. In addition, there is universal agreement that infertility treatment impacts negatively on sexual relations. The focus on making babies instead of making love predictably drains the mystery and romance from the act. This can be a profound loss for the couple, particularly if there is diminished intimacy on other levels. However, about half of couples report that, in the long-run, the experience of infertility and the treatment deepened their relationship and commitment to each other (9).

The inability to produce a child also involves a loss of self-esteem as do aspects of the treatment. Treatment demands almost always interfere with career requirements, and work is a central source of self-validation in our society. There is also a societal status derived from having children. Infertile men and women often see themselves and are, in fact, viewed by others as not having complete lives. The intense negative affects associated with infertility may make the person feel unworthy or less than "human". There is a loss of a positive body image, a feeling of defectiveness deriving from the inability to make one's body perform as one wants. The infertile woman may begin to see herself as sick and may actually begin to be sick from the effects of the infertility treatment. The negative impact of infertility and its treatment on sexual relations also has a self-esteem component. As a response to this, the following recommendation by infertility physician was made to women in a support group many years ago.

"The physician must discreetly emphasize the importance of maintaining or sustaining the male ego. . . wife must never tell her husband that the doctor wants them to have intercourse the night before. Rather she should seduce

him in whatever manner she has found to be most reliable in this respect.

Her husband must never feel that she is having intercourse with him only

because the doctor suggested it or only because she wants to get pregnant. .

Command performances are never conducive to a happy marriage, much less

to a buoyant male ego (11)."

In fact, "sex on demand" not infrequently leads to a temporary sexual dysfunction for the man. Any interference with positive sexual experience is a loss of a source of deep affirmation for both members of the couple.

Infertile couples also report a loss of control over their lives that is multileveled. The intense affects that most infertile couples describe are often a new experience of themselves and can make them feel out of control emotionally. The inability to conceive itself involves being out of control of one's own body. Having children is a major determinant on the shape of a couples life. Not knowing whether or not there will be children puts the couples life plan "on hold." They face a realistic inability to plan ahead. As Mahlstedt (12) says:

....the whole process of trying to conceive takes over ones life, eliminating the

sense of self-confidence, competence, and control which comes from familiarity

with success and in accomplishing a particular challenge.

As is clear from the above, the diagnosis of infertility leads the couple, at least those that we see in treatment, to focus their lives upon it. It becomes a project which can lead to frustration and disappointment but which, in many ways, is helpful to the infertility treatment team.

PSYCHOLOGICAL CONSIDERATIONS OF CURRENT THERAPIES FOR INFERTILITY

There are now some 125 fertility clinics around the country, where an estimated 2 million couples now become pregnant per year. Some couples pay over $20,000 for a chance to have a biologic child. While there are commonalities of the emotional experience for a couple undergoing any type of infertility treatment, each procedure makes unique emotional demands. The current therapies for infertility fall into five categories.

Hormonal:

Various drugs are used to stimulate ovulation in women who have infertility on the basis of an ovulatory problem or in conjunction with more complicated reproductive interventions (GIFT, IVF-ET). These drugs can have significant side effects on mood, most commonly tension, depression, and fatigue. It can be impossible to differentiate the impact of the drug and the impact of the stress of the treatment itself. The extremes of mood the woman experiences while on these drugs can be quite disturbing to her, as well as to her husband and their physician.

Artificial Insemination:

The possibility of artificial insemination was discussed in the Talmud in the 2nd century A.D. However, artificial insemination with husband's sperm (AIH) was not performed until the 1700's, and artificial insemination by a donor (AID) was first recorded in 1884 (13). Although rarely discussed, the procedure has become increasingly common. In 1960, approximately 10,000 babies were born in the United States through AID (13); this number has increased significantly in recent years to close to 20,000 annually. In 1979, the number of people in the United States born as a result of AID was estimated to be around 500,000 (14). There are a variety of reasons for the "low profile" artificial insemination, particularly AID, has had. From a societal perspective, the two major concerns with regard to AID have been the possibility of consanguinous marriage of half-siblings and of threat to the integrity of the family around issues of legitimacy and fidelity.

There are three general indications for artificial insemination: inadequate sperm count, failure to deliver enough sperm to the cervix, and failure of sperm migration in the female genital tract. AIH may be attempted in these situations; if there is no success, AID may be the next recommendation. The overall success rate with AID is approximately 40%. Approximately 20% of women receiving AID conceive each month, and 50-75% of women destined to conceive by the method do so within 3 months. Therefore, there is little reason to extend a trial of AI beyond eight or ten months (13). As would be expected, any pelvic disease or ovulatory problem decreases the chance of success of artificial insemination; also chances for success are somewhat less for a woman over 30.

The evaluation, the diagnosis leading up to the recommendation for AID, the decision to undergo or forego the procedure, the procedure itself, and the outcome are all potentially stressful for the couple involved. About half of men find semen analysis psychologically difficult. Having to produce a semen sample in the hospital can prove impossible. Men describe feelings of shame, embarrassment, and degradation; they feel anxious awaiting the results, as if it is a measure of their manhood. In one study (13), 63% of husbands experienced a period of impotence and depression after receiving a diagnosis of azospermia. In addition, 40% of the wives became significantly angrier at their husbands and severe marital difficulties occurred within three months of the diagnosis. Surprisingly, none of the couples linked these troubles to the diagnosis.

These findings suggest an approach for the physician to convey his determination. The infertile couple should be seen together to be told their diagnosis. Under no circumstances should they be informed over the phone. During the interview, they should be allowed time to react or to ask any questions. Since the couple will often not remember what is discussed immediately after they are given a diagnosis, a followup interview should be scheduled to discuss treatment options. The physician should warn the couple of likely emotional reactions to the information and reassure them of their temporary nature. In the followup interview, the infertile couple for whom AID is a possibility should be presented with all options which would include: adoption, any possible medical or surgical treatment of oligospermia or azospermia, and not having children.

The suggestion of AID may raise a variety of conflicts for a couple. One-third to one-half of couples will choose not to go ahead with the procedure when fully informed (15). Of those who decide to proceed, about twenty-five percent will change their mind or stop before pregnancy occurs (15). Most will do so out of a psychological concern about the procedure; the most common concerns include issues of donor selection, physical characteristics, blood group, intelligence, anonymity, discomfort with the technique itself, and fear of an undesired outcome. However, religious issues may also be significant. The Catholic Church still regards AID as adultery and a child produced by AID as illegitimate. The Vatican issued a document in March, 1987 that states:

"Recourse to the gametes of a third person in order to have sperm or ovum available constitutes a violation of the reciprocal commitment of the spouses and grave lack in regard to that essential property of marriage which is its unity." (16)

Orthodox Judiasm also believes AID is immoral.

The insemination period can be psychologically stressful, particularly for the woman. The emotional nature of AID or AIH can actually speed up or delay ovulation (13). The insemination itself can be as disagreeable or "veterinary" in nature. The possibility of transmission of venereal disease, including AIDS may lead to anxiety which is not altogether unfounded despite stringent safeguards. Some women experience a transfer of affectionate or sexual feelings to their physician which may be disturbing to either or both parties as well as to the husband. Some even suggest making the husband a part of the procedure psychologically by having him present, or actually having him do the procedure.

Despite the stress and uncertainty of the AID process, most studies show good psychological outcomes with couples who have AID, including better marital cohesion (13,14). One study found AID fathers to devote more time to their children than natural fathers (13). One survey indicates that 51% of couples who had a child by AID had a second child and another 34% wanted another child through AID (17). By far, the majority of parents who have a child by AID choose not to tell their child about it. In fact, only 15% of couples tell anyone about the process (13). The medical literature, with one exception recommends maintaining the secret. This plan, of course, has the effect of isolating the couple from support from family or friends.

There are also important legal considerations for the couple contemplating AID and for the physician who performs the procedure. These include the legitimacy of the child, the legality of the artificial insemination process, the status of the birth certificate, the relevance of adoption, and liability for child support in the event of a divorce. Many states have statutes pertaining to one or more of these concerns. It is wise for the physician to get legal consent from both members of the couple as he would for any other important medical procedure.

In Vitro Fertilization and Embryo Transfer (IVF-ET):

In women, blockage of the fallopian tubes may account for 30 to 35% of all infertility. This in itself could account for the intense interest in the IVF-ET procedure developed by Patrick Steptoe and Robert Edwards. The first successful IVF-ET was completed in 1979 in England. Approximately 50 programs offer IVF-ET in the United States at this time (6). The IVF-ET procedure is demanding economically, emotionally, and physically. It is a safe, but invasive, treatment method for infertility.

Realistically, IVF-ET is an option for a relatively small number of infertile couples. Indications for IVF-ET include tubal disease, endometriosis or cervical mucus problems which are unresponsive to therapy, the presence of antisperm antibodies in female, and oligospermia or low sperm motility. IVF-ET is also an option in the case of unexplained, long-term infertility. With IVF-ET, successful treatment outcomes are currently in the 10-20% range. Despite its "end of the line" status as a treatment for infertility, patients should be promptly referred if it is the indicated treatment, as delays decrease the chance of success.

IVF-ET programs require participation in a sequence of medical procedures spanning 30 days per treatment cycle. Technically, IVF-ET is a means of initiating a pregnancy by obtaining mature oocytes surgically, incubating them with sperm, and effecting fertilization in culture; the resultant embryo(s) are then transferred to the uterus where they undergo implantation, from which point the natural progression of pregnancy proceeds. The medical procedures occur in four phases. Phase one consists of stimulation of follicle development. On the third day of her menstrual cycle, the woman begins daily injections of pergonal, a drug which induces the ovaries to produce multiple egg follicles. After day five, the couple may be told to stop sexual relations. On day eight, the woman begins daily serum estrogen levels (rising levels indicate approaching ovulation) and ultrasound tests (to follow size and number of developing ovarian follicles). Retrival and fertilization of the ova is the second phase. When the follicles are sufficiently "ripe", they are harvested by laparoscopy or by trans-abdominal, transvaginal, or transvesical, ultrasound-directed aspiration. Several hours later, the husband collects a semen sample. The follicles and semen are jointly incubated for 48 to 72 hours. Any fertilized ova are then implanted in the third phase of the IVF-ET. The embryo transplant is accomplished via a catheter inserted into the uterus through the vagina. There is no anesthesia for this procedure and it causes some discomfort. Depending upon the position of the woman's uterus, she must either crouch on her hands and knees or lie on her back for the procedure. In any case, she must remain immobile for up to three hours after transplant. The fourth phase of IVF-ET consists of waiting to determine if pregnancy has occurred. For example, some programs do pregnancy tests every three days until a positive result is obtained or menses occurs.

Gamete Intra-Fallopian Transfer (GIFT)

Gamete Intra-Fallopian Transfer (GIFT) was developed by Ricardo Asch at The

University of Texas Health Science Center in San Antonio in 1984. GIFT differs from IVF-ET by relying to a greater degree on the body's natural processes and time table to produce pregnancy. Couples whose infertility results from a severe male factor or from unexplained infertility are the best candidates for a successful pregnancy using GIFT. Women whose infertility stems from cervical factors are also good candidates, as are couples who cannot conceive due to immunological factors.

As with IVF-ET, there are several phases of GIFT. To prepare the woman for the GIFT procedure, hormones are given for 7-10 days to stimulate development of ovarian follicles; this increases the odds of retrieving several ripened eggs. During this time, the woman is monitored with ultrasound to watch the development of the ova. When ovulation is imminent, the patient is admitted to the hospital for the surgical part of the GIFT procedure. This procedure consists of the eggs being removed from the ovary through a laproscope. The retrieved eggs and the sperm (obtained about two hours before the procedure from the husband) are placed in separate laboratory dishes and then sequentially loaded into a catheter. Up to 4 ova and the sperm are transferred to a fallopian tube through the catheter; no more than 2 eggs are introduced into each tube. Fertilization thus occurs in the fallopian tube as it would during a normal conception. The thought behind the technique is that there may be factors in the fallopian tube which promote fertilization; the procedure also allows for the fertilized ovum to develop into the same sized embryo by the time it reaches the uterine cavity as would be the case in a normal pregnancy. Some researchers believe that the relatively low success rate of IVF results because the fertilized egg is placed directly into the uterus. Because GIFT employs only one basic procedure, it takes less time and is not as expensive as IVF-ET.

IVF-ET and GIFT have unique points of stress for infertile couples. For most, there is the frustration of a waiting list (which can be a year's duration) and the high, sometimes prohibitive cost. Although GIFT is typically less expensive than IVF-ET, it too is a costly procedure and couples frequently have to make hard financial choices to give themselves the chance to bear a biologic child. In that it is almost always the last chance for a couple to have a biologic child, there is intense emotional pressure involved as well as unrealistic expectations for success which, for the most part, consists of the couples feeling that <u>has</u> to be successful. Couples carry into these programs all the frustration and disappointment of previous infertility treatment. Most often, the physician involved in the procedure will be new to the couple which means there will not be the possibility of an established, supportive working relationship. Events which can lead to premature termination of IVF-ET or GIFT treatment cycle include failure of the woman's ovary to produce mature follicles or ovulation prior to laparoscopy. Since the ova must be retrieved just prior to ovulation, this is not an infrequent occurrence. The second phase of the treatment may be the most stressful for the husband as he has to wait out his wife's surgery and must produce a semen sample at a time when his wife may still be in the recovery room. Performance demands at such a time can precipitate impotence. The man may also feel at fault if fertilization fails to occur. The woman may show intense anxiety about the laparoscopy or aspiration, even though she has had previous surgical procedures. Either procedure may also be done with donor sperm or even donor ova; in such cases the same psychological, ethical, legal, and religious questions may arise as with AID.The waiting period following embryo transfer is very emotionally charged. It may be difficult for the couple to accept the blood hormone levels are dropping indicating that the procedure has failed:

After all the novelty of the protocol, the patient may experience the euphoria that accompanies the certainty that her sore breasts and bloated feeling mean pregnancy; more likely, she will face the familiar despair, the onset of menses. Although the despair is not new to her, it carries with it extra bitterness and disbelief (18).

Despite all the stress of these procedures, it is rare for couples to drop out of the program. The treatment program, however, may cause differences between the couple to emerge for which the best recommendation may be to take a time out before pursuing this option.

Surrogate Motherhood:

The use of surrogate when the woman of a couple is unable to conceive or carry a pregnancy to term is one of the most contraversial procedures used for infertility. Nevertheless, there have been more than 500 babies born in this way, and the arrangement continues despite significant ethical and legal concern. The process is complicated only in its legal considerations. Medically, it consists of the surrogate being impregnated with the sperm of the husband of the infertile couple via artifical insemination. Ethically, however, the use of a surrogate is not analogous to AID, but is closer to the considerations involved in the use of donor ova which is occasionally done with IVF-ET and GIFT (16). The additional factor of the pregnancy coming to term in the uterus of the surrogate mother makes the process legally, ethically, and psychologically more complicated. Long term studies of the psychological impact of this process for any of those involved have not been completed. Most instances of the use of surrogates have apparently proceeded without incident. However, the entrepenurial aspect of this particular method of obtaining a partially biological child makes it the potentially most abuseable approach to infertility.

PSYCHOLOGICAL ASPECTS OF INFERTILITY AND THE INFERTILITY SPECIALIST:

A physician specializing in the treatment of infertility may find the emotional responses patients have toward their infertility and its treatment a most difficult part of his or her work. In response, he may reason that management of emotions is not his area of expertise and focus exclusively on the somatic; or he may claim a lack of time and/or knowledge to manage complicated psychological problems. It can no longer be argued that the infertility specialist must confront the psychological aspect of infertility because these tensions have a major etiologic role in infertility. However, there are other reasons for the infertility physician to know about and tend to the psychological component of his patients' medical problems. First of all, the patient's feelings and attitudes towards their infertility and their physician do influence compliance and cooperation with the treatment process. The emotional consequences of infertility and its treatment represent the most difficult aspect of the experience for most patients. Women who undergo infertility treatment say that the psychological suffering is worse than any physical discomfort they endure. Dropping out of treatment is far more likely to be for psychological than for any other reasons. As Gwen Davis says, describing her feeling after her attempt at pregnancy through IVF-ET failed:

"I've gained ten pounds and remain haunted by the idea that I may be suffering a mental breakdown. I believe nothing. I trust nothing. I'm numbed by the pain. Amazed that I'm so fragile. I never thought I could be emotionally crippled by anything. I want to be a mother, plain and simple. What's just as plain and simple, though more difficult to accept, is the fact that I will never be a mother. I can't bring myself to test the IVF clinic's claim that my chances of getting pregnant will improve with each cycle. I can't face again the possibility of failure. It is a matter of self-preservation. It's a matter of freedom. Freedom from want."

Second, the patients' feelings and attitudes toward their illness and their treatment affect their evaluation of the physician's competence. An infertility specialist who can address the psychological aspect of his patient's experience will more likely have their cooperation and respect.

Patients have several common complaints about their experience with infertility specialists. The most frequent is that they have not been provided thorough information (9,12). In fact, the most common complaint from patients about obstetrician-gynecologists in general, is that they do not allow sufficient time for questions (20). There are three other common sorts of complaints from infertility patients (7,12). The first has to do with feeling "worked on" rather than "with." Patients feel that their infertility specialists expect them to follow the treatment plan without question (3). A related complaint is that partners (normally, the husband) are excluded from office visits, difficult procedures and important decision making. A second area of dissatisfaction is the patient's perception that the infertility doctor is not interested in feelings associated with being infertile or with the treatment. Related to this is the patient's perception that infertility specialists are unwilling to inform them of psychological support services. Finally, patients complain that their infertility specialists seem not to do well with failure; patients feel the physicians treating their infertility tend to either delay referring them, prolong treatment beyond what is reasonable, or abandon them when success is not forthcoming. While these complaints are not true of all infertility physicians, they are consistent with what is known about the common personality characteristics of physicians who choose obstetrics and gynecology as a speciality (9).

From this information, several recommendations can be made to the infertility specialist with respect to the psychological needs of their patients. First of all, the goal of the relationship between the infertility specialist and his patient is not pregnancy, rather the goal should be the development of a partnership in which a mutually agreed upon treatment plan can be carried out cooperatively while the psychological well being of the marriage and the individual spouses is protected.

From the beginning to the end of the treatment, infertility should be treated as a problem of the couple. Approaching the problem as a couples problem is a beginning, as in doing so the physician brings the strengths of both spouses into the situation and encourages mutual support. Both partners should be seen together at the initial visit to allow the physician to not only assess physiological problems, but also the emotional state of the couple. During this first interview, it should be possible to assess each partner's attitude toward pregnancy, each other, and the therapy. The physician should realize that this may be the first time that the couple hears each others opinions. Their responses to each other in the interview situation will demonstrate their relationship style. The present state of the couple's marriage and of the individual emotional history of each spouse should be explored. The timing of seeking treatment is of interest; for example, is the attempt at pregnancy a response to some stress in the marriage? Also important is which of the couple is the primary motivator in seeking treatments the level of desire is often not equal. It is a mistake to assume that everyone coming for infertility treatment wants to have a child; the doctor should try to assess the level and nature of the motivation for pregnancy and for raising a child for each spouse. A thorough sexual history including frequency and adequacy of coitus should be taken and discussions of sexual life should be initiated in subsequent visits. Even in this initial interview, the question of what will happen if pregnancy is not achieved should also be broached.

Each member of the couple should also be interviewed separately to allow for other information to emerge. Discrepancies in information or "secrets" that emerge are very revealing of the nature of the couples relationship. It is often convenient to speak with the husband alone while the wife prepares for any physical exam and to the wife alone either before or after the exam.

The capacity to ellicit and tune into psychological information will vary from one infertility specialist to another. Specialists who feel particulary at a loss here should have someone on his or her team who is adept at doing psychological assessements and who can help integrate this information into the treatment plan.

From the initiation of the treatment to its termination, the infertility physician should be accessible to his patients. Ideally, one physician will be responsible for and have sufficient time for all procedures, counseling, and proving information. Time is a major factor in infertility treatment. The waiting period between ovulations "chances" can be excruciating for the patient, as is the waiting to find out if pregnancy has been achieved.

The availability of the physician for questions or reassurance is of immense help to the patient. In contrast, the patient's perception that the physician inaccessibility led to a missed opportunity is a detriment to the doctor-patient relationship. In an infertility waiting room one often hears, "I called him to tell him I felt as if I was going to ovulate but he didn't return my call. Now I have to wait for another month."

The treatment program should be structured to minimize emotional distress. The physician should carefully explain the rationale of the workup and should expect that this will need repeating. The investigation itself should be as comprehensive and as short as possible. The physician must realize that by the time the couple comes for treatment for their infertility, they are already frustrated. In general, couples will do all they can to avoid making emotional demands on the physician because they want to be liked. Typically nothing will come up until there is a crisis. Crises can often be prevented if the physician can help the couple anticipate emotional responses. Patients need acknowledgement from the beginning of treatment that there are common, expectable emotional responses to their situation and to the treatment. Anger is a normal byproduct of infertility investigation and therapy. The physician should be prepared for this and know that his normal reaction will be to withdraw or get angry in return. He can then be in a position to have the "unnatural", learned response of allowing the patient to discharge feelings without getting defensive, appealing to logic, or making counter threats; simply trying to understand will take care of most such situations.

Since 50% of couples will not conceive, the preparation for this possibility should start at the first meeting as part of the overview of treatment. In addition, the infertility specialist should assist his patients in finding and accepting the limits to which they will go to try and achieve pregnancy. In a non-judgmental fashion, he should help them to monitor their level of energy and commitment and to know when to stop. Most infertile couples need to be reassured that they have explored all viable options to be able to let go.

Cancelled appointments, decreased enthusiasm, and questions about "the odds" can serve as clues to the physician and these should be openly confronted.

Professional psychological counseling should be offered during and after the treatment course. In general, the longer infertility treatment continues, the higher percent of patients will express the need for some sort of psychological counseling or therapy. The patient's perception of counseling or psychotherapy will be greatly influenced by the physician's attitude and mode of presentation of the idea. Also, the infertility physician should know about and recommend Resolve, a nationwide support group for infertile couples.

Ideally, the infertility specialist will schedule a termination meeting with patients for whom treatment is unsuccessful. This is to provide them a face to face chance to bring the complex doctor-patient relationship to a close. As it can take up to six months or even more for the couple to do grief work, the responsible physician should have followup contact with the couple one year after the treatment program.

ROLE OF THE PSYCHIATRIST AND OTHER MENTAL HEALTH PROFESSIONALS

The psychiatrist or other mental health professional can be found playing three different roles with respect to infertility programs: as a consultant, as a full infertility team member, or as a therapist to whom patients are referred for psychotherapy.

When a consultant is called in to evaluate the emotional state of the infertile couple, typically the first issue he or she confronts is the couple's concern that this contact indicates that their infertility is "all in their head." This is a concern that can be ameliorated or exacerbated by the way in which the referral is presented to the couple. If the couple senses the referring doctor is motivated by frustration or loss of patience, they will experience the referral as a rejection, a punishment, or as meaning they are "crazy". If the infertility physician can present the referral as motivated by his concern for the level of stress the treatment is causing the couple, the referral will generally be regarded positively. In any case, the consultant should assess the attitude and anxieties with which the couple are approaching his intervention before pursuing the referring question.

Consultants are usually called upon to answer any or all of four questions with regard to infertility patients (3). These questions may or may not be explicitly stated by the referring physician.

1. Is there evidence that the marriage is likely to dissolve in the near future?

2. Is the motivation to become a parent doubtful in either patient?

3. Is there a pre-existing psychological condition that could make either spouse at risk if the procedure were unsuccessful; for example, the precipitation of severe depression by a previous miscarriage.

4. Are there psychological conditions present which would make spouses incapable of assuming parental responsibilities?

The consultant may also be called upon to assess a patient whose treatment poses an ethical dilemma for the infertility specialist; for example, a single woman requestion AID. The answers to these questions must be kept in perspective; as Carol Ackerman Mitchell says, "It is a cruel irony that only the infertile have to look at why they want to be parents" (21).

While the use of consultants is a common model for addressing the psychological component of infertility and its treatment, available research supports the need for an interdisciplinary approach to the management of infertile couples (22). Mental health professionals who are part of an infertility team usually do indepth psychological evaluations of all patients. Given that this is the "routine", the couple usually feels less defensive than they do when a consultation is recommended. The initial evaluation of the couple will cover the type of information recommended the infertility specialist to take in his first interview. In addition, the form and degree of emotional distress the couple are experiencing with respect to their infertility and treatment is carefully assessed. The couple's marital relationship, their relationship with family and friends, and ability to function at work will be looked at. The couples characteristic style of coping with stress, as a couple and as individuals, should be delineated. It is enlightening to ask each spouse for an explanation of the cause of the infertility; responses make it clear that educational level is not directly related to the correct information in this regard. Distorted responses reveal feelings of shame, guilt, denial, or rationalization.

It is a challenge for the evaluator to determine, given the level of distress which can be considered normal or expectable, which responses to the situation are of concern. The following reactions have been suggested to indicate failure to cope in women of infertile couples (9): pervasive doubts about femininity, high levels of anxiety about procedures, entrenched feelings that infertility is a punishment, inability to contemplate not having a biologic child, or having no one to talk to about infertility.

In addition, mental health professionals who are part of an infertility treatment team work toward helping patients to develop realistic expectations and to expect the emotional spectrum of elation, anxiety, and despair that predictably accompanies the treatment regimen. Routine education about the evaluation and treatment procedures is often delegated to this team member. It has been demonstrated that such programs significantly decrease anxiety and provide the couple a feeling of having some control.

For couples who require more intervention, the infertility team psychiatrist, psychologist, or social worker provides counseling and supportive psychotherapy. Brief focus counseling is recommended when any of the following are found in an infertile couple: feelings of isolation, tension, depression, or inferiority related to infertility that interfere with important relationships or other functioning; sexual problems related to attempts to achieve pregnancy; ambivalence about pregnancy (couples must be allowed to explore this ambivalence without the risk that therapy will be withheld); and overwhelming feelings of loss (18). In that people will not follow through for recommendations of counseling if they do not want it, the referrer should carefully assess the couples response to a potential counseling or psychotherapy referral. Counseling is often not needed when the couple has adequate emotional support from family and/or friends, or when the level of stress does not interfere with normal functioning.

A primary sexual dysfunction that antedates the infertility experience is a specific indication for sex therapy rather than psychotherapy. For example, vaginismus is still a cause of infertility; in this case teaching the patient to dialate herself is a more rapid and predictable cure than psychotherapy. Also good results in alleviation of anxiety and frustration associated with infertility can be obtained in groups without the more intensive and expensive forms of psychotherapy.

Psychotherapy with Infertility Patients

Indications that more intensive psychotherapy should be recommended for an infertile individual or couple include: a lack of relief from brief, focused counseling or supportive psychotherapy; and /or the discovery that the emotional or relationship difficulties are long standing and only exacerbated or given focus by the infertility. For example, a woman's chronic low self-esteem may only be given new definition by her infertility.

The psychotherapist who treats an infertile person is challenged to find the optimal perspective. This is one which neither discounts the distress attributable to infertility nor neglects the patient's unique characterological response to the issue. Throughout the therapy, the therapist must assess to what extent the patients' reactions to the situation are primarily normal and expectable and thus need to be validated and dealt with supportively; and to what extent the reactions contain a component of the patients' pre-existing psychological problems, and need to be understood and interpreted to allow for psychological growth.

Frequently, the task of such treatment is helping the patient identify his or her feelings about infertility. As previously mentioned, the feeling of loss is often central. Putting the nature of the loss into words is in itself therapeutic and can be the first step in mourning a biologic child or otherwise coping with the situation. Getting patients to end their pursuit of infertility therapy and accept childlessness or adoption may even be the goal of the psychotherapy. Infertile couples often have an unrealistic view of a life without children. The therapist can help them to develop another perspective, reminding them that they will not always feel as miserable about not being parents as they do at the moment. Once a decision is made and they are no longer in limbo, they can go on to find new meaning and direction to what seems like a permanent void in their lives. When the nature of the loss is primarily narcissistic, or that is of self-esteem, the psychotherapeutic work may consist more of a redefinition of the self. Concepts of sexuality, self-image, and self-esteem have to be disconnected from childbearing, while remaining complete. People with self-esteem problems seem particularly vulnerable to guilty or shameful thoughts about infertility, requiring the therapist to help them understand these feelings and find a healthier perspective.

The psychotherapist may also be useful in helping with feelings about a child obtained through adoption or through a successful treatment. Realistically, adoption now often involves accepting a child from another culture or ethnic background, or an older or disabled child. Couples can be helped by being encouraged to focus on parenthood instead of pregnancy, and on the unique challenges of developing a good adoptive bond with such a child. Couples who are successful in having a child through infertility treatment may also have problems. Because of the extremes they went through to have a child, their need to be perfect parents or their expectation that they not have ambivalence may cause emotional conflict and require psychotherapy.

ETHICS OF REPRODUCTIVE INTERVENTION

Difficult ethical issues have followed in the wake of excitement over new reproductive techniques. Dennis Doherty (23) succinctly stages the ethical dilemma: "Something is not moral simply because it is possible: because something can be done does not mean that it may or should." Public attention was drawn most intensely to the ethical issues of infertility treatment by the custody dispute for Baby M between her biologic father and her biologic mother who contracted as surrogate. The question raised by surrogate use of who are the baby's real parents when either sperm or egg that do not belong to the infertile couple are used to induce pregnancy is only one example of many complicated ethical questions in the field. Other ethical questions include: Are unmarried women and men entitled to avail themselves of this technology? Does a child have the right to know of its method of birth? Who do frozen embryos belong to? Does the embryo have rights? To date, there has been inadequate public discussion in the United States of appropriate legal policies, ethical guidelines, and medical practices of infertility treatment. Unfortunately, the interest and well-being of the baby-to-be-made seem to be the last addressed if they are addressed at all. The question of whether scientific intervention enhance or debase the meaning of parenthood as we understand it will for better or worse be answered case by case in the courts and in legislative bodies. Physicians involved in infertility treatment must daily confront their own feelings, and hopefully will take it upon themselves to be a part of the development of legal guidelines.

CONCLUSION

The recent and ongoing technological innovations in the field of infertility are impressive. However, the challenge of providing infertile couples with an evaluation and treatment program that optimally meets their psychological needs is in no way diminished by these advances. While emotional factors are not longer considered a primary etiology of infertility, the psychological impact of infertility and its treatment remains a major factor in the field.

REFERENCES

1. Seibel, M.; Taymor, M.: Emotional aspects of infertility. Fertility and Sterility, 37: 137-145, 1982.

2. Sarrell, P.; DeCherney A.: Psychotherapeutic interventions for treatment of couples with secondary infertility. Fertility and Sterility, 43: 897-900, 1985.

3. Fagan P.; Schmidt C. et al: Sexual functioning and psychological evaluation of invitro fertilization couples. Fertility and Sterility, 46: 668-672, 1986.

4. Freeman, E.; Boxer, A. et al: Psychological evaluation and support in a program of in vitro fertilization and embryo transfer. Fertility and Sterility, 43: 48-53, 1985.

5. Bensley L.: Counseling the Infertile Couple. Medica: Women Practicing Medicine, pp 1-2, 1986.

6. Hammond M.; Talbert L.: Infertility: A Practical Guide for the Physician. Medical Economics Books, Oradell, N.J. 1985.

7. Menning, B.E.: The emotional needs of infertile couples. Fertility and Sterility, 34: 313-319, 1980.

8. Mazor, M.: Barren couples. Psychology Today, pp 101-112, May 1979.

9. Martinez D; Henry, L.; Kobos J. Infertility treatment: Doctors and patients. Presented January 23, 1987 at "Evaluation and Management of the Infertile Couple" Conference, San Antonio, Texas.

10. Given J., Jones G. et al: A comparison of personality characteristics between in vitro fertilization patients and other infertile patients. J of In Vitro Fertilization and Embryo Transfer, 2: 49-54, 1985.

11. Abarbanel A.; Bach G.: Group psychotherapy for the infertile couple. Internatl. J. of Fertility, 4: 151-160, 1959.

12. Mahlstedt, P.: The Psychological component of infertility. Fertility and Sterility, 43: 335-346, 1985.

13. Wabrek A.; Reddick D. "Psychosocial issues in donor insemination" in Ramon-Garcia C., Mastroianni L. et al (eds) Current Therapy of Infertility, B.C. Decker, Inc. Ontario, 293-298, 1984-85.

14. Richardson, J: The role of a psychiatric consultant to an artificial insemination by donor program. Psychiatric Annals. 17:101-105, 1987.

15. Aiman, J.: "Artificial Insemination" in Aiman, J. ed. Infertility: Diagnosis and Management, Springer-Verlae, NY, 277-287, 1984.

16. Brozan, N.: Babies from donated eggs: growing use stirs questions. New York Times, January 18, 1988.

17. Kremer, J; Frijling, B.W., et al: Psychosocial aspects of parenthood by artificial insemination donor. Lancet, 1(8377):p 628, March 17, 1984.

18. Greenfeld, D.; Maguire, C. et al: The role of the social worker in the in vitro fertilization program. Social Work in Health Care. 10: 71-79, 1984.

19. Davis, G.: The private pain of infertility. The New York Times Magazine, p 106, December 6, 1987.

20. Fooner, A.: Can you talk to your doctor? American Baby, p 8ff, November 1986.

21. Mitchell, C.A.: "Adoption counseling" in Ramon-Garcia, C. Mastroianni, et al (eds) Current Therapy of Infertility, B.C. Decker, Inc., Ontario, pp 272-276, 1984-85.

22. Leader, A.; Taylor, P. et al: Infertility: Clinical and psychological aspects. Psychiatric Annals 14:461-467, 1984.

23. Doherty, D.: "Ethics of reproductive intervention" in Aiman, J. (ed), Infertility: Diagnosis and Management, Springer-Verlae, NY, pp 337-344, 1984.

SEXUAL DYSFUNCTION: PSYCHOSOMATIC PERSPECTIVES

KENNETH J. REAMY, M.D., M.P.H.

Associate Professor, OB-GYN
Behavioral Medicine and Psychiatry
West Virginia University
School of Medicine

CONTENTS:

SEXUAL DYSFUNCTION: PSYCHOSOMATIC PERSPECTIVES

Kenneth Judson Reamy, M.D., M.P.H.

"We must, then, no more ask whether the soul and the body are one, than whether the wax and the figure impressed on it are one, or generally inquire whether the material and that of which it is the material are one."

Galen (1)

Sex is psychosomatic. Kaplan (2), in articulating a psychosomatic concept of sexual dysfunction, discusses the vulnerability of the "complex sequence of hormonal and physiologic events" to fear, anger, and depression. Adverse stress can interfere with sexual arousal and can inhibit desire by the depression of circulating androgen through its effect on the hypothalamic pituitary axis. In addition, sexual responses such as erection or orgasm, can be thwarted by learned inhibition from negative contingencies such as associated anxiety, sexual guilt, or threat of injury. The psychosomatic concept views the person as a "biological organism, a self-aware person, and a social being" (3). And sexual dysfunction is seen as the consequence of impaired dynamic interaction of biologic, psychologic, and social factors (4,5,6).

SEXUAL RESPONSE AND FUNCTION

Masters and Johnson (7), in their monumental research work, "Human Sexual Response," detail the anatomic and physiologic parameters following psychophysiological stimulation. They have divided the sexual response cycle into the four phases of excitement, plateau (heightened excitement), orgasm, and resolution. Physiologic responses consist of incremental vasocongestion and myotonia, culminating in orgasm. Extragenital preorgasmic responses include tachycardia, tachypnea, an increase in blood pressure, a skin flush arising in the epigastrium, nipple erection and breast swelling. Genital congestive features of the male during the excitement phase include penile tumescence and scrotal thickening and during the plateau phase penile rigidity, testicular swelling and perineal apposition, and bulbourethral (Cowpers) gland secretion, which lubricates the penile meatus.

In the female during excitement vaginal lubrication (a transudate from the circumvaginal venous plexus) and vulvar swelling (clitoris and labia) occur. During plateau, the clitoris retracts under the clitoral hood or prepuce from its normal pudendal overhang position and the major vestibular gland (Bartholin's) secretion is produced, which provides introital lubrication. Additionally, vasocogestion and edema of the perivaginal tissue and vestibular bulbs form the orgasmic platform which, teleologically, has a grasping effect and abets the mounting response. There is maximal expansion of the distal vagina or "vaginal barrel" and elevation of the uterine body and cervix.

The male orgasm or ejaculation consists of the two stages: 1) emission, characterized by contractions of the prostate, seminal vesicles, and vasa deferentia and collection of semen in the prostatic urethra and 2) expulsion or true ejaculation at which time seminal propulsion through the penile urethra is effected be contraction of the bulbospongeosus, ischiocavernosus, and pubococcygeus muscles as well as the sphincter urethrae. The emission phase is accompanied by a feeling of "ejaculatory inevitability" of two to three seconds prior to ejaculation. After ejaculation, there is a finite "refractory period" of time in men which is age related (3 minutes to 24 hours and beyond) in which further ejaculation cannot occur.

Female orgasm is characterized by the sequential enhancement of "intense clitoral-pelvic awareness," a "suffusion of warmth" from the pelvic region, and finally "pelvic throbbing" as involuntary pelvic contractions (7). Masters and Johnson (7) state that physiologically, an orgasm is an orgasm irrespective of the sexual stimulus and that the clitoris is the receptor and transmitter of erotic sensation. During coitus clitoral stimulation is indirect and often minimal (compared to direct digital or orolabial stimulation) and is provided by the "labial-preputial mechanism" in which traction on the labia minora during coital thrusting moves the clitoral hood, thus providing stimulation to the erogenous receptor and transmitter, the clitoris. Women do not have a refractory period and have a multiorgasmic potential as long as plateau levels of sexual tension are maintained.

Helen Singer Kaplan (2) in her highly acclaimed "The New Sex

Therapy" introduces some useful conceptual viewpoints. She conceives of sexual response as being a biphasic response consisting of arousal (Subsuming the excitement and plateau phases of Masters and Johnson) and orgasm. Arousal is essentially a parasympathetic response and anxiety the final common pathway of sexual dysfunction. Cetecholamine release has a parasympatholytic effect on vasodilatation, be it penile erection or vaginal lubrication.

Kaplan (2) considers orgasm to be a reflex, and like the patellar reflex having a neurophysiologic threshold related to the degree of central inhibition. Krantz (8) has distinguished anatomic differences, i.e., varying clitoral and vulvar distribution of Pacinian corpuscles among human females, through the dissection of a number of cadavers.

Freud (9), of course, had believed that an important maturational task of females was to "transfer" the erogenous site from the clitoris to the vagina, that a coital orgasm was superior to one derived from digital stimulation, and that a woman incapable of having a "vaginal orgasm" was psychosexually immature, hence frigid. Although this theory was challenged by Kinsey (10) and seemingly repudiated by Masters and Johnson (7), other workers and numerous individual women argue that orgasms associated with coital thrusting are often experienced as quite different from those triggered by direct clitoral stimulation (11,12). Master and Johnson (7) reported that clitorally induced orgasms were the strongest on objective measure, although many

women report these to be much less pleasurable than a weaker
orgasmic response on coition. Singer (12) suggests that the
perceived orgasmic differences may be more than "psychological"
and describes distinct vulval, uterine, and blended orgasms.
Recent publicity on the "Grafenberg spot," a purported major
erogenous zone on the anterior vaginal wall (and female homologue
of the prostate) distinct from the clitoris and on "female
ejaculation" (estimated to occur in perhaps 10% of women in the
United States according to Perry and Whipple) has sparked heated
controversy (13,14,15). Weisberg (15), after patient examination
and extensive review has written, "My personal evaluation of the
G spot ejaculation issue is one of interested skepticism. I have
felt the G spot. I have witnessed the expulsion of fluid, and I
have read letters of thousands of people.......I am confused by
the conflicting data and the unproven hypotheses, and I am
fascinated by the possibility of a new discovery of something
that has always been there" (15).

NEUROLOGIC AND ENDOCRINOLOGIC ASPECTS OF SEX

The lower centers for the sexual reflexes and responses are
located in the spinal cord or brain stem. Higher centers of the
human, found in the midbrain, limbic cortex, and subcortical
nuclei exercise hierarchical control. Hence, learned experience,
memories, thoughts, and emotions can profoundly influence and
condition the neural discharge of the lower motor neuron (2).

The neuroanatomy and neurophysiology of penile erection and
ejaculation are remarkably complex. Knowledge is incomplete and

concepts are controversial. Current understanding is derived primarily from animal studies, patients with spinal cord injuries, and patients who have had operative transection and resection of pelvic nerves. Data on analogous female lubrication-swelling and orgasm have been largely extrapolated from findings on male sexual response (16).

Penile erection is initiated by psychic and physical stimulation. Erection (and by inference vaginal lubrication and vulvar swelling) appears to be primarily a parasympathetic phenomenon (2,17). Erection has been arbitrarily and simplistically divided into "reflexogenic" and "psychogenic" erections (16,17,18). As conceptualized, in response to tactile stimuli, afferent impulses from the sensory branches of the dorsal nerve of the penis, supplying the glands and penile skin, are carried in the pudendal nerve to a reflex center in the sacral cord. Efferent impulses originate from parasympathetic fibers in sacral cord roots S2, S3, and S4 and pass via the nervi erigentes (pelvic nerve) to the penis (16,17). In response to suprasegmental stimuli from cerebral sex centers, impulses traverse the brain stem to the thoracolumbar spinal cord. Efferent impulses originate in the thoracolumber cord and travel via sympathetic pathways in the hypogastric nerve to genital structures (16,17). These autonomic nerves from the thoracolumbar cord have been found to contain cholinergic (vasodilator) as well as adrenergic (vasoconstrictor) fibers (17). They are believed to act synergistically with the nervi erigentes from the sacral cord to mediate erections. Numerous clinical reports have indicated that even radical sympathectomy will not predictably impair erection but will alter emission and ejaculation (17). Recent work by Zue and co-workers (19), involving electrostimulation of dogs and dissection of human cadavers, has confirmed the presence of the spinal nuclei for control of erection in S2, S3, and S4 and localized the thoracolumbar segments to T10, T11, T12, L1, and L2. Penile erection is atropine resistant and it has been hypothesized the VIP (vasoactive intestinal polypeptide), widely distributed throughout the female genital and male genitourinary tracts, and not acetylcholine, may be the neurotransmitter mediating the relaxation of vascular and cavernous smooth muscle (20).

The hemodynamic contributions of increased arterial flow, arteriovenous shunting, and decreased venous outflow in the production and maintenance of penile erection are controversial (21) as is the existence of functioning (constricting) vascular polsters (22). These muscular polsters or Ebner's pads have been believed, since the turn of the century, to function in the distribution of penile blood flow to the cavernous spaces (corpora cavernosa and corpus spongiosum) during erection and detumescence. They have likewise been described in women (16). Benson and co-workers (22), in a recent histologic study of penile vasculature, determined that "polsters" appear to represent myoepithelial proliferation secondary to intimal damage.

Emission, the collection of semen in the proximal urethra, is mediated by sympathetic nerve fibers from T11 to L2 of the spinal cord via the hypogastric plexus supplying the prostate, seminal vesicles and vasa deferentia. Expulsion or "true ejaculation" is additionally mediated by somatic spinal nerves (pudendal) from S2 to S4 sacral cord segments (16,17). The neurological basis of female orgasm has not been established but has been considered similar to the male and sympathetic (2,16).

Ejaculation, independent of erection, can be produced by stimulating regions of the brain stem, midbrain, and limbic cortex (23). A separate erection center, as well as ejaculatory center, has been located in monkeys (23).

Sexuality is dominated by the "pleasure principle" rather than by pain avoidance and neuroanatomic and neurophysiologic investigations have revealed a close association between psychosexual centers and pleasure centers and pleasure centers of the brain (2), an importance for species survival. Close central anatomic relationships have also been found between sexual response and olfaction. Although the presence of odoriferous and sexually stimulating pheromones has been established in a wide variety of animal species including mammals, its presence and role in human sexual attraction have not been established (2,16). Although chemically similar substances have been identified in vaginal secretions, these are not believed to comprise a "sex-attractant pheromone system" (24). Male reaction to vaginal odors, according to Levin (16), has been characterized by one sexologist as "affectionate distaste." Clearly odors and aromas can serve as impediments and enhancers of sexual attraction.

Releasing hormones, produced in the hypothalamus, regulate the release of pituitary hormones which, in turn, mediate the production and secretion of hormones from target organs, including sex steroids from the ovaries and testes (25). These steroid hormones, including testosterone, play a role in effecting sexual differentiation of the brain during fetal life, initiating puberty, and regulating adult sexual behavior (22). Testosterone appears to be an essential libidinal hormone in women as well as men (2,24,26). Androgens are important for erection and ejaculation as well (27). In addition to the maintenance of sexual drive or appetite, testosterone also enhances energy and aggressive behavior (2). Estrogen, in spite of its importance in receptivity, proceptivity, and attractiveness in animals (28), does not have a direct effect on sexual desire in humans (2). Estrogens are necessary for optimal sexual function of the vagina. Synthetic progestins such as medroxyprogesterone can suppress sexual desire (27). Gonadotrophin-releasing hormone, a polypeptide produced by the hypothalamus, appears to increase sexual desire, even in the absence of testosterone (2) and evokes mating behavior in animals of both sexes (25). Research suggests inconclusively that dopamine and serotonin have important functions in the neurotransmission of sexual stimuli to the sex centers of the brain; dopamine is stimulatory and serotonin inhibitory (2).

ILLNESS AND SEXUALITY

Any disease accompanied by pain, malaise, lassitude, or nausea or associated with anxiety, fear, guilt, or depression has the strong potential for diminishing sexual desire and impairing function and gratification. "Among the determinants of sexual impairment are the psychological stress induced by the illness, previous past experiences, nature of current relationships, and the possible effects of metabolic imbalance, abnormalities of peripheral nerve conduction, and pituitary gonadal function" (29).

There are a number of good references detailing the effects of illness on sexuality (30,31). Only a very brief review is possible. Coronary artery disease, especially myocardial infarction, is associated with fear of sudden death, dyspnea, angina and palpitations. Thirty to 50 percent of men report a decrease in sexual desire and coital frequency several years later (30). Maximal heart rate from many activities of daily living is actually greater than that sustained in coitus. Less than one percent of sudden deaths is related to coitus. Frequently coitus can be resumed following M.I. before 8-12 weeks, as exercise tolerance increases (31). Supine and lateral coital positions as well as oral and manual stimulation can be utilized with less work expenditure.

The association of sexual dysfunction and hypertension is usually due to the effects of antihypertensive drugs. Untreated hypertension can result in hypertensive heart disease with a decreased cardiac output. Rises in blood pressure during cardiac activity can be marked. Certain patients with hypertension can be effectively treated by diuretics, hydralazine, and beta antiadrenergic drugs such as propanalol, which do not usually cause inhibition of desire, excitement, and orgasm (31).

Over 50 percent of diabetic men experience erectile dysfunction because of autonomic neuropathy aggravated by performance anxiety. Neuropathy can be metabolic as well as vascular. Good diabetic control and sexual counseling may resolve much of the sexual concerns and dysfunction. Orgasmic dysfunction may occasionally obtain and is often associated with a neurogenic bladder (29). A decrease in vaginal lubrication and sexual desire have been reported in women (32).

Sexual dysfunction is seen in a large proportion of men and women with renal failure. Reduction of testosterone levels is associated with hypoactive sexual desire and impotence and may respond dramatically to zinc supplementation in the dialysate (31).

Various debilitating diseases can produce sexually inhibiting organic and psychosocial deficits; these include arthritis, genitourinary diseases, hypothyroidism, hypopituitarism, Addison's disease, cirrhosis, hepatitis, chronic respiratory disease, and cancer and the effects of surgery and radiation treatment (30,31).

DRUGS AND SEXUALITY

Many pharmacologic agents have been reported to have adverse effects on sexual functioning. Antihypertensive drugs probably interfere with sexuality more than any other prescribed drug (33). Thiazide diuretics are frequently associated with impotence. Centrally acting sympatholytics such as methyldopa (Aldomet) and clonidine (Catapres) can frequently cause impotence. Ejaculatory failure has been reported with these drugs less frequently. Peripheral sympatholytics such as guanethidine (Ismelin) can produce both of these sexual dysfunctions. Alpha-adrenergic blockers such as phenoxybenzamine (Dibenzyline) often retard ejaculation. Beta-adrenergic blockers such as propanolol (Inderal) can cause decreased sexual desire and impotence. Reserpine (Serpasil) and others can cause depression and loss of desire which can lead to impotence. The arteriolar dilator hydralazine (Apresoline) is not believed to cause sexual dysfunction (33).

Psychoactive drugs have been associated with sexual dysfunction (34) which, of course, is seen frequently in untreated depression and schizophrenia as well (35). The tricyclic anti-depressants have been implicated in erectile dysfunction including imipramine (Tofranil), protriptyline (Vivactil), desipramine, and amitriptyline (Elavil) (34). Most of these represent small case report studies. Monoamine oxidase inhibitors have also been implicated in impotence. Phenelzine (Nardil), mebanazine, and tranylcypromine (Parnate) have been reported. Lithium is a psychoactive drug that causes impotence in a minority of patients. Among the neuroleptic drugs chlorpromazine (Thorazine) has not been found to cause impotence but thioridazine (Mellaril) has been associated with impotence and priapism (and commonly with ejaculatory inhibition). Fluphenazine (Prolixin) has caused frequent impotence. Minor tranquilizers in normal dosage should not impede erection.

Many psychiatric drugs also impair ejaculation (34). According to a small number of case reports, both tricyclic antidepressants and MAO inhibitors can either delay or prevent ejaculation and inhibit female orgasm (36). Most of the major tranquilizers, except for chlorpromazine, used for over five years will inhibit ejaculation. Thioridazine surpasses the other psychoactive drugs multifold in reported retarded ejaculation. Retrogade ejaculation has not been conclusively established according to Seagraves (34). Female orgasmic dysfunction is associated as well (36). Cimetidine (Tagamet), a histamine-H2-receptor antagonist, has antiandrogenic activity, can cause hyperprolactinemia, and inhibits sexual desire in men and women, and can cause impotence (33).

Libidinal or aphrodisiacal effects have been reported from L-Dopa and nomifensine (Merital) and spontaneous orgasm has been reported with chlomipramine (Anafranil) (37).

There is a great deal of folklore surrounding licit and illicit recreational drugs. Alcohol decreases inhibitions but is frequently associated with erectile dysfunction. Autonomic neuropathy is associated with chronic alcoholism (38). Marijuana is believed by users to increase libido and heightens awareness.

High doses are associated with decreased desire and impotence associated with decreased testosterone (38). Cocaine has a great street reputation as an enhancer of libido and performance. Habitual use of cocaine and opiate use are both associated with inhibited sexual desire, excitement and ejaculation (33,38). Sedatives have not usually been heralded as aphrodisiacs but the introduction into this country of methaqualone was followed by illicit use and false claims concerning its mystical sexual properties (39). Sedatives depress the central nervous system and can diminish desire and performance (33,39). Amphetamines in acute doses are reported to enhance libido and orgasm (40). Chronic sustained use is associated with a diminution of libido and sexual functioning (39,40). Amylnitrite has been a remarkably popular sex drug especially among homosexual men (39). Intensified sexual arousal and especially orgasm has been reported on ingesting a "popper" just prior to orgasm (39,40). Severe transient headache is frequent and hypotension, tachycardia, and diminished cardiac output are hazardous to people with known or unsuspected cardiac disease (39).

SEXUALITY IN PREGNANCY AND THE PUERPERIUM

The effects of pregnancy on sexuality have been reviewed in detail elsewhere (41,42,43). Perkins believes pregnancy itself to be the most important or overriding variable influencing gestational sexuality (43). Although there are clearly individual variations, in general there is a decrease in sexual desire, coital frequency, sexual enjoyment, and orgasmic attainment as pregnancy progresses, the mid-trimester, which in some respects most closely resembles the pre-pregnant state (44), may be associated with an increase in sexual desire and satisfaction approaching or surpassing pre-pregnancy levels (7,41). Dyspareunia, as well as apareunia, increases as pregnancy progresses (44). There is a consensus that coitus and orgasm do not precipitate obstetric or perinatal complications and need not be prohibited in normal pregnancies (42). Several cases of fatal air embolism following vaginal insufflation associated with cunnilingus have been reported (42).

An extensive review of postpartum sexuality including sexual aspects of lactation has been recently written (45). A temporary decrease in sexual desire is frequent. Superficial dyspareunia is frequent among breast feeding mothers because of hypoestrinism secondary to hyperprolactinemia and resultant vaginal atrophy. A medio lateral episiotomy is associated frequently with poor healing and dyspareunia. A midline episiotomy usually heals within three weeks permitting coital resumption. A vertical scar from a Cesarean delivery is not only cosmetically inferior to a low transverse Pfannenstiel ("Bikini") scar but may occasionally result in painful orgasmic spasms.

SEXUALITY AND AGING

Peak desire and responsiveness for men is 16-17 years of age with a steady gradual diminution thereafter (46). Peak desire and responsiveness for women is the late thirties to the early forties with a gradual diminution, although there is greater individual variation among women (10). There are, also, a substantial number of women who experience a decrement of these sexual variables at the menopause, which is related to sociocultural mores (sexuality is equated with youth and beauty), prior sexual dissatisfaction, and the absence of an interested and interesting sexual partner. Other women, freed from concerns of contraception and caretaking, and building on positive reinforcement of satisfying sexual interaction, experience a surge of interest and responsiveness. Sexual activity persists well into old age provided the individuals are in relatively good health and, (a variable especially important for women) that there is the availability of a loved and socially-sanctioned partner (2,24).

The aging process is associated with less intense and slower to develop vasocongestion and myotonia during sexual arousal (7). Atrophy of skin, subcutaneous tissue, and elastic tissue are associated with skin wrinkling and sagging. Ovarian failure associated with the menopause precipitates vaginal atrophy, decreased and slower vaginal lubrication (47), dyspareunia, vaginitis, and vaginismus. Hot flashes and progressive osteoporosis are frequently encountered. These symptoms respond well (as do painful orgasmic contractions of the uterus at orgasm) to hormonal replacement therapy (7,47). Premarin 0.625 mg the first through the twenty-fifth of each month and Provera 10 mg, day 15 through 25 (the progestin negates the risk factor of exogenous estrogen for endometrial carcinoma) is a popular and effective regimen. Women maintain their multiorgasmic potential.

Men from their twenties onward experience a gradual decrease in sexual desire, ejaculatory demand, spontaneity of erections, and in middle years a diminution of penile turgidity, a loss of the feeling of ejaculatory inevitability, decreased force and volume of the ejaculate (accompanied by less intense sensation), prolongation of the refractory period, and a gradual decrease in the frequency of coital ejaculation.

Since men do not menstruate, it is inane to speak of a male menopause. There is a gradual decrease in spermatogenesis from the forties on (although persistence of sperm production in the eighties); after age 50 there is a gradual decrease in the bioactive free testosterone as the concentration of sex binding globulin increases (24).

PSYCHOSOCIAL INFLUENCES ON SEXUALITY

Masters and Johnson believe that the fear of inadequacy is the main deterrent to sexual functioning and that "sociocultural deprivation and ignorance, rather than psychiatric or medical illness" (48) is etiogenic. A performance demand generates performance anxiety. Anxiety is seen, psychophysiologically, as the "final common pathway" of sexual dysfunction (2). Ignorance of stimulus requirements, more common in women, who generally have had less autoerotic experience than men, and ignorance of such aspects as the sexual effects of aging are sexual deterrents. Evidence indicates that sexual dysfunctions and dissatisfactions are multicausal or multifactorial and are believed to result from remote (unconscious conflict) and immediate (performance anxiety) causes (2). Sexual conflicts may include sexual guilt, fear, and disgust as well as sexual identity conflicts. There are numerous potential intrapsychic sources of sexual anxiety (49). Various potent irrational ideas include conscience - sex is sinful, anticipated loss of control, aggression and fear of injury, secret revelation - disclosure of hidden desires and fantasies. A psychodynamic perspective attributes most sexual problems to unresolved Oedipal conflicts and the inappropriate son-mother and daughter-father transferences into the marital dyad. Hypothetical developmental influences that may affect sexuality and produce sexual dysfunction are premature separation, parental rejection, excessive intimacy, and sexual trauma.

Interpersonal or relationship influences that are believed to be causes of sexual dissatisfaction and dysfunction include partner rejection, destructive transferences, lack of trust, power struggles, contractual violations, poor communication, and sexual sabotage within the dyad, e.g., creating pressure and tension, using poor timing, poor grooming, fitness, and hygiene, and frustrating the partner's sexual wishes (2). In addition to intrapsychic and relationship factors, sociocultural factors that influence one's sexual value system and sexual expression are culture, race and ethnicity, class, subculture, religion, and world view.

THE SEXUAL DYSFUNCTIONS

Masters and Johnson (48) have estimated that sexual dysfunctions occur in approximately 50 percent of American couples. Frank and associates (50) found a similar incidence among 100 normal couples and their questionnaire did not include dyspareunia. The Diagnostic and Statistical Manual of Mental Disorders of the American Psychiatric Association (DSM-III-R) includes the currently defined dysfunctions (Table 1) (51). Certain neurotic traits are often associated with specific dysfunctions - histrionic traits in women with inhibited excitement and inhibited orgasm and compulsive traits in men with inhibited desire and inhibited excitement (52). Although the literature is contradictory, Derogatis and associates (53) found, in addition to disproportionate levels of psychological distress, defined psychiatric illness (apart from psychosexual dysfunction) in about one third of the men and one half of the women, out of 325 sexually dysfunctional patients.

EVALUATION OF SEXUAL DYSFUNCTION: A BIOPSYCHOSOCIAL APPROACH

Kaplan (54) indicated that to optimally assess an apparent sexual disorder the following eight questions should be answered:

1. Does the patient actually have a sexual disorder?

2. What is the disorder?

3. Differential diagnosis: Is the symptom primarily organic or psychogenic?

4. Is the problem secondary to some other psychiatric illness?

5. What are the immediate psychologic causes?

6. Are there deeper psychologic causes and if so what are they?

7. How severe are the psychologic factors?

8. What are the relationship aspects?

Most individuals and couples have sexual questions and concerns from time to time that do not merit the label of "dysfunction" but must not be minimized or discounted. Concerns often center around such things as forbidden fantasies, sexual behaviors, and expected changes of sexual variables in pregnancy, menopause, and aging. Patients frequently wish to know whether their thoughts, feelings, or behavior or their husbands requests and behavior are "normal" and seek informed support or reassurance (6,55). Sometimes, schizophrenics present with bizarre sexual complaints (54,56) and patients with incipient depression with lack of desire (40,54).

In order to arrive at the correct diagnosis it is essential to know which of the three phases of sexual response is involved - desire, excitement, or orgasm. Where in the sexual response cycle does the symptom occur? Is there another sexual dysfunction present? Which came first? As a rule, the situational nature of the complaint establishes psychogenicity and rules out illness or drug effects (54).

Psychological assessment includes the assessment of proximate and earlier (and typically deeper) psychological factors that may have precipitated or aggravated the symptom. Determination of the presence of another psychiatric disorder is essential and the workup should include a psychiatric history and a mental status evaluation. Historically the "standard psychological test battery" for the evaluation of sexual disorders has included the Wechsler Adult Intelligence Scale, the Minnesota Multiphasic Personality Inventory, the Bender Gestalt Test to screen for organicity, and the Thematic Apperception and Rorschach Tests. Little of the data have predictive value concerning sexual functioning (57). The MMPI has been the most useful and provides levels and patterns of psychological functioning. Most recently the Derogatis Sexual Functioning Inventory (DSFI) (57) has shown promise in detailing the patient's current sexual functioning or "sexual status" (54) and has demonstrated reliability. Measures or "substantive domains" are sexual information, experience, drive, sexual attitudes, psychological symptoms, affects, gender role definition, sexual fantasies, body image, and sexual satisfaction (57). Kaplan believes "the sexual status examination," i.e., a detailed description and analysis of the couple's current sexual interaction to be the single most important diagnostic technique available (54).

The single patient with sexual dysfunction can be problematic because most of the structured treatment is conjoint. Patients with anorgasmia, many with vaginismus, those with dyspareunia, and I believe many with rapid ejaculation, however, can be seen singly. Those with other dysfunctions are often suitable for group therapy or "sexually oriented individual psychotherapy" (54).

A recent, general physical exam is recommended for all patients. Women with sexual dysfunctions, including primary anorgasmia, should be seen by a gynecologist with expertise in psychosomatic and sexual medicine for a diagnostic evaluation and an educational pelvic exam, which is often an important intervention because of its permission giving, desensitization and reassurance (58). Men with sexual dysfunction should be evaluated by a urologist with expertise in andrology and sexual medicine to rule out organic disease. General screening tests include a complete blood count, a urinalysis, an automated chemical profile, and a chest x-ray (59).

THE SEXUAL DYSFUNCTIONS

INHIBITED SEXUAL DESIRE

Hypoactive Sexual Desire Disorder and 302.79 Sexual Aversion Disorder (51).

Doctor, "I'm just not interested in sex." Kaplan, citing the independent experiences of Dr. Harold Lief and herself, believes low, hypoactive, or impaired sexual desire to be "probably the most prevalent of all the sexual dysfunctions" (40). The literature is contradictory as to whether low desire is more common among men or women (51,60,61). Sexual desire is defined as the frequency and intensity with which a person desires to participate in sexual activity. Sexual desire varies within life cycles and among individuals. Circulating testosterone maintains sexual desire. When a patient's sex drive is constitutionally low, or when he has a subnormal testosterone level, or is depressed, or on drugs such as narcotics, high doses of sedatives, alcohol, central acting antihypertensive drugs, or one of many offending psychotropic drugs, sexual desire is impaired because it is not generated. In _inhibited_ sexual desire, libido is actively but unconsciously suppressed because of psychological conflict (40). Sexual desire is a much more subjective measure than orgasm or painful coitus. Impaired sexual desire usually becomes evident when there is disparate desire within a dyad. It may, of course, be primary (lifelong) or secondary (acquired) and global or situational. Diagnostic parameters include frequency of coitus, coital initiation, fantasies, sexual dreams, and masturbation.

McCarthy (62) believes the "mold of performance - failure-avoidance" to be "a main cause of ISD in males." LoPiccolo (63), in a current review of male dysfunctions, cites three main categories of proposed causal factors: hormonal factors (decreased testosterone, increased estrogen, increased prolactin, decreased gonadotropin releasing hormone), family of origin explanations, and relationship dynamic theories. He indicates the low prevalence of hormonal abnormalities among men with impaired sexual desire and the poor correlation between hormonal levels and sex drive. Family of origin explanations, largely unsupported by empirical data, include Oedipal conflicts and a poor relationship between the parents. Relationship dynamic theories stress the adaptive value of low desire for the man of unconsciously maintaining "equilibrium" as a passive-aggressive means of using power and control or as a way of maintaining distance and preventing intimacy.

Although specific psychosocial barriers and psychodynamics are not unique to the individual dysfunctions, anger in the context of marital discord is especially prevalent with ISD of either partner. Other interpersonal factors that have been suggested as etiologic include loss of attractiveness, boring marital and sexual routines, infidelity, and situational distress (64).

The medical evaluation of impaired sexual desire, in addition to a history and physical examination and routine laboratory tests should include a two hour post-prandial blood sugar and plasma testosterone on men. An LH and FSH should be obtained to clarify a subnormal testosterone value and hyperprolactinemia should be assessed by a visual field study and a coronal CAT Scan (60).

Diabetes and defects of the hypothalamic-pituitary axis need to be ruled out as well as other medical illnesses and the effects of drugs (30,31,33). It is essential to rule out depression which is frequently associated with low libido. Loss of desire may precede or accompany loss of sleep and appetite (40).

MALE ERECTION DISORDER (51)

Doctor, "I've lost my manhood!" Men live by the myth of phallic primacy. Zilbergeld, in an excellent book for professionals and laity alike (65), speaks of the male fantasy model of sex: instant erection, two feet long, hard as steel, and ready to go all night. Masculine self-esteem demands sexual potency, prowess, and performance. "Impotence" with its broad implications, including a basic characterological deficit, reflects its catastrophic, humiliating, and often times histrionic expression.

Studies have shown that erectile dysfunction or impotence is present in 0.1 percent of men under 20, 1-4 percent of 35 year olds and in 75 percent of men by age 80 (46,52). More than 50 percent of men treated for sexual dysfunction have impotence as their presenting concern (52). Probably at least 50 percent of all men have sporadic, transient episodes of impotence which is not considered abnormal (2). Much less prevalent is primary erectile dysfunction, whereby a man has never been able to attain or maintain an erection firm enough to complete coitus (66).

Levine recommends that 4 basic questions be asked during history-taking to help distinguish a psychogenic etiology from a primarily organic one (67).

1. What is the problem? Is it the inability to obtain an erection, the inability to maintain an erection, the inability to maintain an erection during intercourse, or some combination of these factors?

2. How firm does the penis become? Is it soft or slightly firm with the erection not self-supporting, is there decreased firmness but enough to permit coitus, or is it fully turgid?

3. Is the impairment constant or intermittent? Under what circumstances is the pattern not present: with other partners, with masturbation, with sleep, upon awakening, during the day, when engaging in other erotic activity?

4. What life events were occurring at the onset of the problem?

Impotence is the most likely of all the sexual dysfunctions to have an organic cause (54). Organicity is particularly common after age 40 because of the increased prevalence of diabetes, arteriosclerosis, and medication side-effects. However, Kaplan believes that only a small percentage of impotent patients require a complete urological workup. Like, Levine (67), she suggests that a skillful anamnesis by a clinician knowledgeable in sexual medicine can rule out organic factors in the large majority of cases "by establishing that the difficulty fluctuates with the patient's emotional state" (48).

In 1970, Masters and Johnson indicated that 95 percent of erectile failure was psychogenic (48). More recent studies suggest that 30 to 50 percent of impotence has an organic basis (68,69). Segraves and co-workers (70) discovered, however, that frequency data was dependent on the "medical care system entry point." In their study, an organic etiology was found in 26 percent of the urology referrals but in only 4 percent of the patients referred for sex therapy (70). In a number of discrepant studies, one is unable to discern what distinguishing criteria were used to establish organicity. In many cases, organic and psychogenic causes cannot be differentiated. There is currently no test or diagnostic paradigm that is unequivocally discriminating (63,69). Conceptually, researchers have erred in attempting to dichotomize patients into mutually exclusive psychogenic or organic subsets. In many cases, both organic and psychogenic factors are etiogenic in erectile failure (63).

Kaplan (2), in stressing a psychosomatic concept, hypothesizes that men with erectile dysfunction have a constitutional organ vulnerability (the vasocongestive genital system) to emotional stress. And the "final common pathway" appears to be performance anxiety, reflecting a fear of failure, irrespective of predisposing psychodynamic factors.

Patients who present an organic or ambiguous pattern of erectile dysfunction, demand careful medical evaluation. Illness, drugs, surgery, and traumatic effects must be considered. One needs to consider vascular, neurologic and endocrinologic causes.

On physical examination, the patient's affect, and especially clinical signs of depression should be assessed (this can, of course, be antecedent or subsequent to impotence). The presence or absence of gynecomastia, suggesting hypogonadism, is noted. Palpation of the abdomen and auscultation for bruit over the aorta and iliac arteries should be performed. The external genitalia are examined for inflammation, penile plaques suggestive of Peyronie's disease, and testicular atrophy or swelling. The prostate and seminal vesicles (if palpable) are examined. Normal rectal sphincter tone suggests an intact bulbocavernosus reflex and neurologic integrity. Saddle sensation is tested for light touch and pinprick. Sensation, including vibratory sensation at the malleoli, strength, and reflexes of the lower extremities and femoral and pedal pulses should be checked. Trophic skin changes such as hair loss as well as absent pulses suggest peripheral vascular disease or neuropathy (69,71).

Laboratory studies include a routine CBC, standard automated chemical profile, and urinalysis. Abnormal liver function studies may reflect alcoholic cirrhosis. Over 50 percent of diabetic men are impotent with psychogenic as well as organic causal factors. Plasma testosterone is normally within the wide range of 300-1200 ng/ml, reflecting diurnal variation and intermittent release. Melman (72) estimates that hormonal abnormalities account for only 1-2 percent of impotence, although three published studies between 1980 and 1984 revealed disorders of the hypothalamic-pituitary axis (decreased testosterone with or without decreased or increased FSH and LH and with or without hyperprolactinemia) in between 15 and 30 percent of impotent patients (73,74,75). LoPiccolo (63) believes a more representative range to be between 5 and 10 percent. Low testosterone levels have been related to low libido and the lack of early morning erections (74). In the absence of clinically evident hypogonadism or low testosterone, a more complete hormonal investigation was not found to be cost effective in one study (75) but plasma or serum prolactin may be recommended (54,69) to rule out the occasional prolactinoma of the pituitary.

There has been a recent proliferation of various physiologic tests to help elucidate organic deficits, subtle as well as major, in the individual patient with impotence (63). Current procedures used to evaluate vascular causes include penile blood pressure, penile blood velocity, and penile blood volume assessments via Doppler ultrasonography and penile plethysmography. The pelvic steal test must be considered in the assessment of Doppler findings, i.e., Doppler testing after exercising the thighs and buttocks. The external iliac steal syndrome occurs when blood is diverted from the pudendal artery to the gluteal muscles, which in some individuals become ischemic during coital thrusting, effecting penile detumescence (72). Corpus cavernography and arteriography are selective invasive procedures performed on an individual basis. Although a direct cause and effect relationship has not been established between impotence and subtle neurologic deficits (69), electromyographic testing of bulbocavernosus reflex latency times is utilized in some centers.

Nocturnal penile tumescene monitoring (NPT) has been heralded as a non-invasive diagnostic technique that was capable of clearly differentiating organic from psychogenic impotence (68). It has been widely publicized and increasingly used in medical centers and "do it yourself, take home" modification consisting of a ring of perforated gummed stamps or a plastic snap gauge, have proliferated. An 80-85 percent efficiency (the percent of all results that are true results whether positive or negative) has been described for hospital based NPT but several authorities do not believe the procedure to have been adequately validated (63,69). The effects of profound stress or depression may decrease NPT specificity so that an abnormal record is less valuable than a normal sleep record in differentiating psychogenicity from organogenicity (54). A new diagnostic test using the intracorporeal injection of papaverine is purportedly the best screening test for diagnostic differentiation, obviating the need for preliminary NPT testing (76).

FEMALE SEXUAL AROUSAL DISORDERS

Like erection, genital vasocongestion in the female is mediated through cerebral sex centers, but in spite of central inhibition, psychogenic dysfunction appears to be infrequent (54). Female genital vasocongestion is reported to be substantially more resistant to the effects of illness and drugs than male (24), perhaps since it does not require the complex hydraulic system of erection (54). Nonetheless, drugs and illness can produce analogous effects involving the desire, excitement and orgasm phases of the sexual response cycle. Additionally, inhibited female excitement may be under-reported because the female anatomic and physiologic concomitants of sexual excitement are less obvious and less essential for coital connection. Even under normal conditions, lubrication decreases as plateau levels of sexual excitement are reached, especially following prolonged stimulation (24). Also vaginal lubrication is an internal phenomenon and women with adequate lubricity may be unaware of vulvar wetness. A frequent discrepancy between affective arousal and genital vasocongestion has been recently documented by vaginal photoplethysmography (77).

McGuire and Wagner have reported inhibited sexual excitement as a frequent pattern among women who were sexually molested as children and seek sexual therapy. Their clinical profile included little sexual desire, aversion to touching and caressing of their body and their partner's body, and restricted foreplay, but the presence of coital orgasms. Treatment was sought either because husbands desired more physical and emotional contact, the women were feeling guilty over their feelings of revulsion, or the husbands in the absence of emotional or manual stimulation, were losing their capacity for erections (78).

Impaired vaginal lubrication is a frequent consequence of estrogen deficiency and is experienced in the menopause, in the puerperium especially with lactation (45), and with hyperprolactinemia and anovulation. Whatever the etiology, inhibited sexual excitement is characterized by decreased lubricity and vaginal accomodation (44) (vaginal tenting and uterine elevation) and dyspareunia, vaginitis, and vaginismus are frequent sequellae. Secondarily, inhibition of desire and orgasm may occur (54).

INHIBITED FEMALE ORGASM (51)

The orgasmic threshold varies among women along a continuum (2,54). This theoretically could be related to constitutional factors, e.g., number and concentration of vulvar nerve endings (8), relationship and proximity of clitoris to introitus, or experiential, e.g., developmental influences, amount of inhibition, amount of stimulation. A representative continuum was portrayed by Lief (79) who showed 10 percent of women with total orgasmic inhibition, 20 percent able to climax by (self) masturbation only, 40 percent by clitoral stimulation from partner, 20 percent coitally orgasmic (some of whom need "clitoral assistance" - e.g., associated digital stimulation), and 10 percent highly responsive (multiple orgasms during coitus). Levine and Rosenthal, in describing women with primary orgasmic phase dysfunction, state that they "perceive the intensity of arousal as a threat to their psychic integrity rather than as opportunity for pleasure" (80). Although some anorgasmic women have inhibited sexual excitement, many get highly aroused but "stuck" due to psychological inhibition, e.g., intimacy fears, dependency fears, fears of loss of control. The most prevalent immediate mechanism is obsessive self-observation during sexual relations (54) or "spectatoring" (48) with the result that a natural response or reflex is not allowed to occur.

The overwhelming majority of cases of inhibited female orgasm are psychogenic although three alleged physical causes have been proposed but not substantiated (54). These are weak pubococcygeus muscles, clitoral adhesions, and inadequate attention to the G spot (13,14,15). Kaplan (54) suggests that less than half of women complaining of orgasmic problems are totally anorgasmic. In these patients, an organic source should be ruled out to include medication effects, e.g., antihypertensives and antidepressants, absence of the clitoris - congenital or from infibulation ("female circumcision," a misnomer), or true phimosis. Brindley and Gillan (81) report the frequent absence of the bulbocavernosus reflex with primary anorgasmia and hypothesize a structural defect of the spinal cord. Secondary anorgasmia, often consequent to relationship failure, can be also due to neurologic diseases including multiple sclerosis, diabetes, spinal cord tumors, and degenerative diseases (54). Inhibited female orgasm is seen frequently in late pregnancy (42,43), secondary to dyspareunia, and in women embarrassed by urinary stress incontinence (14).

INHIBITED MALE ORGASM (51)

The inability to ejaculate and experience orgasm despite the presence of erection has been known as retarded ejaculation, ejaculatory incompetence, ejaculatory inhibition, and, at one time, the conceptually unsound "impotencia ejaculandi" or ejaculatory impotence (82,83). It is, clinically, the least frequently encountered male dysfunction, and probably the least prevalent among the population (2,48,82). It can be primary, i.e., always present or secondary, i.e., acquired. In its severest form, and least prevalent, even nocturnal emissions are inhibited; more commonly is the situation in which there is a selective incapacity for intravaginal ejaculation. The mildest form is characterized by inordinately prolonged periods of coital thrusting prior to ejaculation (48,82). The dysfunction can be continuous or intermittent. Desire and excitement are usually not inhibited (54). However, some men who contend with their difficulty or inability to ejaculate with increasing performance demands may develop impotence secondarily (48).

Although Kaplan (54) indicates that inhibited male orgasm or "retarded ejaculation" is analogous to inhibited female orgasm, certain phenomenological differences are apparent. Orgasm is a cerebral event or cortical sensory experience and is not synonymous with ejaculation (84,85). Seminal emission, (antegrade) ejaculation, and orgasm are separate entities, although they are normally associated (84,85). However, orgasm can occur without ejaculation - in pre-adolescent males, in the aged, and in certain disease states (54,85). Additionally, ejaculation can occur without erection and can occur without the pleasurable feelings of orgasm (2,48,85).

Nonejaculatory intercourse can be subdivided into "anejaculation", retrograde ejaculation, nonemission, and "aspermia" (85). This classification is based on etiology and pathogenesis, sexual history including duration of sexual intercourse, orgasmic experience, and presence of nocturnal emissions, and urologic assessment including the presence or absence of spermatozoa and fructose in a post-ejaculatory urine sample (85).

Proposed psychological determinants include castration anxiety (the "vagina dentata"), intimacy fears, hostility, sexual guilt and inhibition, and relationship deterioration (48,54,82). "Spectatoring" (48), i.e., vigilant observation or compulsive monitoring with its attendant anxiety can clearly exacerbate retarded ejaculation (86) and is believed to be the most common immediate psychological barrier (54). Patients with this syndrome have been described as "....super-rational, emotionally controlled (and) overly critical..." (86). Men with retarded ejaculation, like those with impotence, may suffer from a deficiency of physical and emotional stimulation. Like women with inhibited orgasm, some male individuals seem to have high orgasmic thresholds and may not get sufficient enough stimulation (as they do with masturbation) to effect release (86).

Although organic causes of ejaculatory impairment have been considered rare (54), a number of them have been recently publicized (63). Most patients with this syndrome below the age of 50 can ejaculate on masturbation, establishing psychogenicity. Kaplan indicates that aging, with the prolongation of the refractory period, alpha adrenergic drugs, e.g., clonidine (Catapres), and thioridazine (Mellaril) are virtually the only organic factors to selectively impair male orgasm (54). Brindley and Gillan (81), believe that some men and women with primary anorgasmia may have subtle structural cord defects as reflected in an absent bulbocavernosus reflex (81) and, hence, recommend neurologic testing. According to LoPiccolo, ejaculatory impairment may be the first symptom of multiple sclerosis and may be one effect of the "post-concussion syndrome" (63). The inability to ejaculate can be associated with spinal trauma, syringomyelia, and Parkinsonism (82). Ejaculation (antegrade) depends on the synchronous deposition of the vasal contents into the prostatic urethra and the closure of the internal urethral sphincter to prevent retrograde ejaculation. These physiologic processes, i.e., seminal emission and bladder neck closure, are mediated by the sympathetic nervous system. Prostate surgery and Y-V plasty of the bladder neck can result in retrograde ejaculation because of a patulous bladder neck postoperatively (84). This may be associated with thioridazine and other drugs (54) and occasionally with diabetes as well (84). Anejaculatory orgasm must be distinguished from retrograde ejaculation and includes "aspermia" associated with hypogonadism and nonemission, associated with alpha adrenergic blockers, sympathectomy, and retroperitoneal lymph node dissection and other abdomino-pelvic surgery with resultant damage to the sympathetic nerves supplying the genital viscera (84,88). Vasectomy is the most frequent cause of anejaculatory orgasm (54).

Additional inhibitors of ejaculation include fatigue, short interval from prior ejaculation, and chronic alcoholism (85). Genitourinary tuberculosis can obstruct the vasa deferentia and ejaculatory ducts and impair ejaculation (86).

PREMATURE EJACULATION (51)

Premature ejaculation is considered to be the most frequent

male dysfunction and the most readily cured (48,82).   Kinsey   et al reported that 75 percent of men ejaculated within 2 minutes of intromission (46).   They believed "rapid ejaculation" to be normative and a product of   natural   selection   (46).   Premature ejaculators frequently have strong desire and   potency   but   have not acquired voluntary control, perhaps because of a low orgasmic threshold   or   the   diminished   awareness   of   the   premonitory sensations of orgasm (54,82).   In some cases there is a suggestion of response conditioning because of adolescent   fears of interruption and discovery (48,54,82).

The large majority of cases, especially primary prematurity, have psychogenic causes. Primary premature ejaculation can be associated with spina bifida. Secondary prematurity necessitates a urologic or neurologic evaluation (48). Spinal cord tumors and multiple sclerosis should be ruled out with persistent symptoms. Premature ejaculation can also be   secondary   to   erectile dysfunction. A man may be conditioned to ejaculate rapidly before losing his "tenuous" erection (54).

FUNCTIONAL DYSPAREUNIA (51)

Organic causes of male dyspareunia include   various genitourinary inflamations and infections,   i.e.,   phimosis, balanitis, balanoposthitis, herpes genitalis,   scabies,   and urethritis due to gonococcus, chlamydia, and chemical irritants and allergens, as well as chordee and traumatic abrasions (88). Sexual pain may occur during erection and ejaculation as well.

Psychological factors in sexual pain, including dyspareunia of men and women, include conversion or hysterical pain, chronic pain associated with depression (depression - pain syndrome), chronic pain with latent schizophrenia, "hypochondriacal preoccupations and obsessive over reactions to normal physical sensations," and pain from local trauma associated with sadomasochism or rape (54).

Dyspareunia is the most frequent female dysfunction other than orgasmic dysfunction according to reported clinic series (89). Women with dyspareunia need to be assessed by a gynecologist by vaginal speculum and "bimanual" examinations of the vagina and rectum and selective laparoscopy and pelvic sonography. Representative organic causes include vulvitis, vaginitis, pelvic inflammatory disease, pelvic cancer, endometriosis, scars from mediolateral episiotomy and posterior colporraphy, broad ligament varicosities and pelvic congestion (44,45,48,89). Thirty to 40 percent of women referred to sex therapy clinics with dyspareunia have an organic cause (52,89).

FUNCTIONAL VAGINISMUS (51)

Vaginismus, the spastic contraction of the vaginal outlet, is precipitated by perceived attempts at vaginal penetration and prevents or markedly impedes coitus (48). The diagnosis is suggested by the history of an unconsummated marriage or apareunia or severe and persistent superficial dyspareunia (58). Many women report difficulty or inability to tolerate pelvic examinations and to insert tampons. Vaginismus has been reported as the least prevalent female sexual dysfunction and the most incapacitating (89). There are suggestions, however, that it is more common than the literature has suggested (58,90). It can be primary or secondary and absolute or situational.

Vaginismus is a classic example of a psychosomatic disorder (48), with a specific penetration phobia and somatically expressed vaginospasm. The traditional psychoanalytic formulation of vaginismus is that of a conversion reaction representing an unconscious hostile desire to castrate the male (91). Current consensus, however, is that vaginismus is a (involuntary) conditioned reflex to the threat of vaginal penetration (2,48). It has been compared to the blink reflex when corneal contact is anticipated (91).

Most vaginismus has a psychogenic etiology. Proposed causes include sexual trauma, traumatic pelvic examinations, strict religious orthodoxy, ignorance and misconceptions concerning sexuality and childbirth, homosexual orientation, and impotence of the male partner (2,48,91). In these cases, anxiety causes vaginospasm which in turn causes pain. A minority of vaginismus cases are consequent to painful coitus from organic disease, e.g., vulvovaginitis, endometriosis, pelvic inflammatory disease, cystitis. In these situations, pain causes anxiety which in turn causes vaginospasm (58).

THE TREATMENT OF SEXUAL DYSFUNCTION

Masters and Johnson, in their 1970 book, "Human Sexual Inadequacy," proclaimed that most sexual problems are not the result of deep-seated sexual problems, but rather are derived from sexual ignorance and sociocultural deprivation (48). Further, they emphasized that the interpersonal relationship is the appropriate therapeutic focus rather than the identified patient, and that short-term psychoanalytic or dynamic approach, can be highly successful in resolving sexual problems.

Other short-term techniques of sex therapy for individuals, couples, and groups, all of which can be designated as directive and behavioral, including those by Wolpe and Lazarus and LoPiccolo and Lobitz, were published within a few years of the Masters and Johnson work (93). The goal of treatment in general is that of the (direct) removal of symptoms rather than the (dynamic) attainment of insight. Behavioral modification is founded on learning theory, where dysfunctions are seen as consequences of disturbed learning, conditioning, or habit (94). The behavioral approach emphasizes "skill training in effective sexual behavior, reducing anxiety about performance, and increasing communication between partners" (93).

Marital discord accounts for a substantial proportion of sexual problems. If a patient is married or has an ongoing sexual relationship, it is useful to see her with her husband or sexual partner at some point in order to observe their communication. Seeing the sexual partner individually is helpful in obtaining a different "viewpoint." It is mandatory that information obtained at individual sessions not be shared with the other partner without expressed consent.

Masters and Johnson's (sex therapy) program, focusing on

short-term, directive, action-oriented therapy, produced outcome statistics that, for the first time, offered the promise of a rapid, highly effective treatment "for sexual dysfunction" (95). The Masters and Johnson approach consists of a group of problem - centered procedures that address the immediate etiologic factors of sexual dysfunction including performance anxiety, obsessive monitoring or "spectatoring," a lack of sexual information, and communication deficits (48,96). Three main components of the "new sex therapy" (48,96,97) are:

1. Educational counseling to eliminate sexual myths and misconceptions

2. Facilitation of open verbal communication of sexual and non-sexual issues, and

3. A graded series of home tasks designed to enhance communication, eradicate performance demands, and mitigate sexual anxiety.

Many of the departures from traditional dynamic therapy are obvious - the direct, rapid problem or symptom-oriented approach, conjoint (couple) therapy, the dual-sex team approach, the contention that sexual dysfunction is not necessarily a product of deep-seated psychopathology. Masters and Johnson see couples, outside their home environments for an intensive two week course of therapy, with "home assignments" performed in hotel rooms, isolated from many of the diverting and fatiguing stresses of everyday living. Cotherapy is believed to minimize transference, being designed to facilitate identification and communication within the patient dyad rather than emotional dependency on the therapist. It also has a built in provision of peer review.

There have been many modifications of the Masters and Johnson approach. Most frequent changes have been weekly or biweekly one hour sessions, between 3 and 20 (often 10-14), the use of one therapist rather than a dual-sex team, individual therapy and group therapy.

Helen Kaplan and others stress the importance of a dynamic understanding of the patient especially when difficulty develops with a specific behavioral exercise (2). Avoidance or resistance might be manifested by a refusal to do the exercise, preoccupation, or boredom. Although behavioral approaches are generally used first to deal with avoidance and resistance - repeating the assignment, modifying the task, or bypassing, interpretation may be useful, especially if cognitive restructuring or "reframing" is ineffectual.

Lobitz and LoPiccolo have utilized sexual self awareness tasks and masturbation training for women with primary orgasmic dysfunction (98). Lazarus and Wolpe have utilized Jacobsonian muscle relaxation and systematic desensitization to decondition or extinguish anxiety (97). Adjunctive anti-depressant therapy has been useful when depression is a major contributor to inhibited sexual desire or impotence (2). Tranquilizers have generally been ineffectual. Many therapists have eclectic approaches, merging old techniques and paradigms with new but relying on a behavioral core.

THE TREATMENT OF THE MAJOR PSYCHOSEXUAL DYSFUNCTIONS

SEXUAL DESIRE DISORDERS

Most sex therapists believe that inhibited sexual desire is more difficult to treat and has a poorer prognosis than the other sexual dysfunctions (24,40). Kaplan believes etiogenic sexual anxieties to be "more tenacious and profound" (40). The impression also exists that it is difficult to facilitate or enhance the motivation of a client with ISD to change sexual behavior (60). (I think of this difficulty as a similar problem to teaching a child to learn to like liver.) Often the ISD patient is coerced to seek treatment with the threat of infidelity or divorce (60).

The other desire phase disorder, sexual aversion or aversion to sex, is believed by Schover and LoPiccolo to be on the end of the continuum of sexual avoidance behavior, whereas Kaplan believes sexual aversion to be a sexual phobia (40,51,60). Schwartz, in presenting etiologic and treatment concepts of the Masters and Johnson institute for the treatment of ISD, stresses the heavier emphasis on integrating marital therapy techniques (98). Their social skills package includes information exchange, assertiveness training, active listening, negotiation and creative problem solving, conflict resolution, socializing and courtship, play, time management and maintenance of changes, and levels of intimacy (98).

PSYCHOSEXUAL THERAPY FOR ISD   (24,40,60,62,98)

1.   Identification of inhibitions blocking sexual desire if

possible.

2. Educate couple that sexual pleasure and gratification are not contingent upon initial sexual interest.

3. Educate couple that sexual activity need not culminate in penile vaginal intercourse. "Sexplay" rather than foreplay, a means to an end, has intrinsic value.

4. Social skills package to enhance communication and eliminate destructive patterns.

5. Sensate Focus (S.F.1) at least 3 times during the week.

6. S.F.2 (genital sensate)

7. Exploring fantasies to increase desire and reveal psychological blocks.

8. Vaginal (penile) containment and slow, non-demand thrusting.

9. Focus on the emotional climate before sexual relations. Do not attempt sexual activity unless each individual feels calm and receptive.

SEXUAL AROUSAL DISORDERS

Impotence of the male is the most likely of all the sexual dysfunctions to have an organic cause (54). Rigid control of diabetes, bromocriptine for hyperprolactinemia, antidepressants for depression, testosterone for hypogonadism, and intracavernous injection of papaverine/phentolamine for cases of neurogenic and vasculogenic erectile dysfunction have been used (54,99). Selective surgery such as operative penile revascularization for large vessel arteriosclerosis and ligation and cauterization for abnormal drainage of the corporal bodies is indicated in a small proportion of men with organic impotence and offers curative potential (72,99). Many urologists will implant a penile prosthesis, after "psychiatric clearance" in some cases, if any organic deficits are diagnosed. It is, however, apparent that many cases of partial organic impairment can be treated successfully by sex therapy (63). Although the use of the penile prosthesis, first reported in 1952, achieves the goal of allowing intromission and coitus in the majority of reported cases, the frequency of post operative complications is appreciable, whatever degree of preoperative tumescence occurred may be arrested, and long term satisfaction and sexual adjustment is reportedly poor in some cases (63,100). In spite of the expressed reservations concerning penile prostheses, individuals with marked organic impairment, irreversible by other treatment methods, whose coital connection is perceived as a necessary ingredient of sexual expression, may be good candidates for prosthetic implantation (24,100).

PSYCHOSEXUAL THERAPY FOR ERECTILE DYSFUNCTION (40,48)

1. Coital prohibition

2. No man can will an erection. Eliminate performance demands with their attendant anxiety and spectatoring.

3. S.F.1

4. S.F.2. Non-demand, reassuring genital stimulation may proceed to erection but not to orgasm, cessation until detumescence, return to play to achieve resurgence of

erection, thus assuring man of his ability for erection.

5. Female partner stimulates man's penis when astride and inserts penis in introitus if erect, slowly and without demand, thrusts a few times and separates.

6. Prolonged vaginal containment.

7. Coitus to orgasm in female superior position.

8. Coitus to orgasm in male superior position.

FEMALE SEXUAL AROUSAL DISORDER

The treatment objective of this relatively uncommon dysfunction is to inhibit anxiety that interferes with genital vasocongestion including vaginal lubrication.

PSYCHOSEXUAL THERAPY FOR INHIBITED FEMALE EXCITEMENT (40,48)

1. S.F.1

2. S.F.2

3. Slow, teasing stimulation of the breasts, nipples, and external genitalia with interruption prior to orgasm and resumption.

4. Intromission after the woman is well-lubricated.

5. Vaginal containment in female superior position.

6. Coitus.

INHIBITED FEMALE ORGASM

Sensual and sexual self-awareness tasks including masturbation appear to be an effective treatment vehicle especially in women with primary anorgasmia. (6,10,101) Secondary and situational orgasmic dysfunction (absence of coital orgasm) show better improvement and symptom resolution when sexual and nonsexual communication techniques are stressed. (48,102)

THE PSYCHOSEXUAL THERAPY OF PRIMARY INHIBITED FEMALE ORGASM (6,101)

1. The sin of Onan was coitus interruptus and not masturbation.

2. Know thyself intellectualy, emotionally, sensually and sexually.

3. Educational pelvic exam with positive genital imagery and Kegel pubococcygeal exercises to increase cognitive awareness of vaginal sensation.

4. Sensual baths.

5. "Mirror work" - viewing her nude body in a noncritical appreciative sense.

6. Tactile self-exploration.

7. Clitoral stimulation but "don't have an orgasm." This principle of paradoxical intention can be singularly successful in mitigating performance anxiety, diminishing inhibition, and allowing orgasm to occur.

8. If orgasm does not occur explore various orgasmic "triggers," act out an orgasm, directed stimulation with lubrication (it may take 20 minutes).

9. Vibrator stimulation if all else fails.

PSYCHOSEXUAL THERAPY OF SITUATIONAL INHIBITED FEMALE ORGASM (48)

1. S.F.1

2. S.F.2

3. With man seated at head of bed in slightly reclining position and woman seated with back to him between his thighs, he accesses her body with caresses. This position provides security for woman (back-protected phenomenon and dissipates self-consciousness or obsessive monitoring.

4. Instruction to man in stimulative technique avoiding direct or rough stimulation to clitoris, use vaginal lubrication to clitoral area. Do not force responsivity and accommodate her desires, requests, and nonverbal cues.

5. If orgasm does not occur during next session have woman masturbate to orgasm in same position.

6. Vaginal containment when highly excited.

7. Coitus in female superior condition when woman ready, prolonged nondemanding coitus.

8. Additional digital stimulation to clitoral area can be provided with coitus if desired.

INHIBITED MALE ORGASM

This is an uncommon dysfunction. The man should provide himself with emotional, partner, physical, and fantasy stimulation and avoid spectatoring.

PSYCHOSEXUAL THERAPY OF INHIBITED MALE ORGASM (Ejaculatory Incompetence)

1. Woman provides penile stimulation to penis and asks for direction to maximize and optimize stimulation, a water-soluble lubricant is used.

2. Continue manual stimulation until ejaculation occurs and

wife becomes associated in man's mind with ejaculatory release.

3. Vibrator stimulation can be used if #2 is ineffectual.

4. Effect intromission as orgasm is imminent and inevitable and woman provides active thrusting.

5. If #4 is unsuccessful repeat manual stimulation.

PREMATURE EJACULATION

Many treatment methods have been devised for the treatment of rapid or premature ejaculation to increase one's "staying power." An early focus was on means not only to delay orgasm but to diminish arousal. Methods have included topical anesthetic ointment, and non-sexual, anxiety-producing, distracting, or aversive fantasies. Semans in 1956, giving credit to Hirsch, published a new approach, the pause or stop-start technique (extravaginal stimulation of the penis until sensations premonitory to orgasm are experienced and cessation of stimulation until sensations have disappeared and cycles are repeated), the Masters and Johnson coronal squeeze technique, the intracoital basal or bulbar squeeze, and the intra (or extra) coital testicular tug (48,103). ("And if all else fails, slam it in the refrigerator door.") Another treatment suggestion is simply to increase ejaculatory frequency which helps appreciably in some cases. It is uncertain why the pause and squeeze techniques are effective; it may be a reflection of "crowding the threshold" and extinguishing the response by gradually increasing the intensity of the stimulus but remaining below the threshold for eliciting the response (63). An alternative explanation for the Semans' and Masters and Johnson's success at delaying ejaculation is that a patient is trained at monitoring his arousal level and increases his self-awareness and ejaculatory control (2,63).

PSYCHOSEXUAL THERAPY OF PREMATURE EJACULATION (40,48)

1. Unequivocal assurance that premature ejaculation can be reversed.

2. Manual stimulation of penis by woman until he approaches climax at which time he tells her to stop. On diminution of sensations he tells her to resume stimulation. Cycles are repeated thrice until ejaculation is allowed to occur.

3. The stop-start technique series is repeated using a water-soluble lubricant.

4. Non-demand slow coitus with woman astride. The man does not thrust. He ejaculates on the third cycle of stimulation.

5. Repeat after attaining control with male thrusting.

6. Repeat coital cycle in male superior position.

FUNCTIONAL DYSPAREUNIA

A situational pattern suggests psychogenicity. Gynecologic (Urologic for males) evaluation to rule out organic disease is necessary. Functional female dyspareunia can be frequently treated like vaginismus (89).

FUNCTIONAL VAGINISMUS

The diagnosis of vaginismus is confirmed at the pelvic

examination. In vivo systematic desensitization eliminates the phobic avoidance of vaginal penetration and deconditions progressively its somatic expression, i.e., the acquired vaginospasm (58). Systematic desensitization is a method or process whereby anxiety-response habits are eradicated by the gradual and progressive exposure of the patient to a hierarchy of perceived threats beginning with the least anxiety producing (104). The treatment emphasis in on active patient participation rather than on passive accommodation or acquiescence.

THE PSYCHOSEXUAL THERAPY OF VAGINISMUS (58)

1. Formation of a therapeutic alliance with the patient during the first session. Coital prohibition.

2. Educational pelvic exam, during the second session, the extent of which is controlled by the patient's comfort. Vaginospasm observed by patient with help of female assistant in positioning mirror.

3. Prescription of Kegel contraction _and_ relaxation exercises to increase cognitive awareness of vaginal tension.

4. Follow up pelvic examinations - one finger, medium Pedersen speculum, 2 fingers, medium Graves speculum.

5. Digital self dilatation, progressive, with lubricant.

6. Partner dilatation.

7. Vaginal containment.

8. Coitus in female superior position.

9. Selective adjuncts:

a.   conjoint counseling - especially important with non-consummation or apareunia.

b.   sensate focus.

c.   verbal communication tasks.

d.   progressive muscle relaxation

e.   in vitro desensitization (evocative imagery)

f.   sexual self-awareness tasks

g.   adjunctive bibliotherapy

OUTCOME OF THE NEW SEX THERAPY

Historically, the psychoanalytic treatment of sexual dysfunction, in spite of its great depth, cost and length of treatment, has been singularly unsuccessful (105). Many, if not most, women with orgasmic dysfunction and men with premature ejaculation and erectile problems, remained dysfunctional after months, if not years, of therapy (105). Ignorance of sexual physiology and the failure to consider the role of the sexual partner in the sexual distress were two variables that were lacking. In the late 50's and 60's, prior to the landmark publication of Masters and Johnson's "Human Sexual Inadequacy," a variety of short term behavioral approaches emerged from Wolpe, Hastings, and Ellis that stressed the reduction of sexual anxiety, the changing of negative and irrational sexual beliefs, and couple communication. These short term direct approaches with a behavioral core effected reported cure rates of 60-80% (105).

Masters and Johnson reported, in 1970, an overall success

rate of 80 percent, upon treating 510 married couples (56% of whom had "unilateral dysfunction"), 54 single men, and 3 single women (68). Their success rates (with the number of cases in parentheses) were: primary impotence (32)=60%, secondary impotence (213)=74%, premature ejaculation (186)=98%, ejaculatory incompetence (17)=82%, vaginismus (29)=100%, primary orgasmic dysfunction (193)=83%, situational orgasmic dysfunction (149)=77%, total male (448)=83%, and total female (342)=81%. This successfully treated group had essentially no relapses with an 80% success rate at the end of 5 years (48).

Recent papers have critically reviewed the treatments of psychogenic impotence, premature ejaculation, orgasmic dysfunction, and inhibited sexual desire (63,97,102,106,107,109). There was no controlled research supporting the effectiveness of "depth" or psychoanalytic treatment of male sexual dysfunction (106). The use of Masters and Johnson's "extensive retraining program" or a modification by therapists including Kaplan, LoPiccolo, and McCarthy achieved a 60-90% success rate with impotence and almost 100% success rate for premature ejaculation (106). Cooper, who treated a lower middle class sample of 41, most of whom came in because of pressure from their wife, was the only one to report poor success rates - 40% for impotence and only 10% (including the Seman's "stop-start" technique) for premature ejaculation (106). Various methods of systematic desensitization have been effective in treating vaginismus, functional dyspareunia, orgasmic dysfunction, and sexual aversion

(102,107). Retraining programs such as the Masters and Johnson method have been successful in treating orgasmic dysfunction. Muscle reeducation (Kegel's) exercises have shown some success in the treatment of vaginismus and orgasmic dysfunction. Hall successfully treated 16 out of 24 women with vaginismus, a 67% success rate; Kegel reported attainment of coital orgasm for 78 out of 123 women, a 63% success rate (107).

Kaplan reports a success rate similar to Masters and Johnson but offers no empiric data. Although utilizing a similar behavioral approach, she stresses the use of the dynamic attainment of insight when psychological resistances are encountered. Chapman, utilizing couple reeducation ad coital prohibition, had an 80 percent success rate in the treatment of 74 married couples with sexual dysfunction including orgasmic dysfunction and vaginismus. Friedman reported successfully treating 70 out of 100 vaginismus patients with vaginal dilatation and supportive psychotherpay (107). Reamy has reported a 93 percent success rate in treating vaginismus patients using in vivo desensitization (58).

Research has indicated that, in spite of some theoretical advantages of cotherapy (dual-sex team) over a single sex therapist, it is neither more successful nor cost-beneficial (108,109). Daily therapy has been found to be no more effective than the more commonly used weekly session (95). Group treatment seems to be effective for (female) orgasmic dysfunction and erectile dysfunction (110).

On the basis of the studies of the directive sex therapies, many authors have indicated great successes and low recurrence rates (97). LoPiccolo, while indicating that the most significant components of the behavioral "packages" have not been identified, has emphasized seven integral commonalities (105). These are; (1) mutual responsibility within the relationship, (2) information, education, and permission, (3) attitude change, (4) anxiety reduction, (5) communication and feedback, (6) intervention in destructive sex roles, life-styles, and family-interaction, and (7) the prescription of changes in sexual behavior (105).

In spite of the apparent successes of the new sex therapy, research methodology and outcome data have not been without criticism or challenge. Critics have claimed that follow-up by Masters and Johnson, for instance, had been accomplished with on "45 percent of their original sample" and that their follow-up ratings were based on unstructured interviews (102,106,107). Criticism of much of the research data of the numerous studies has been that treatment procedures have been confounded, groups have varied in the presence of psychopathology and other subject variables, some studies have combined various dysfunctions, patient self reports have been relied upon, diagnostic categories have varied, criteria for e.g., inhibited sexual desire diagnosis remain highly subjective, and outcome measures have not been standardized (63,97,102,107,109). Suggestions for improvement of research methodology include standardized interview methods, more careful specification of therapy techniques, assessment of psychosocial as well as sexual functioning, clearly designated diagnostic and outcome criteria, use of control groups, the consideration of alternatives to the DSM-III to improve standardization, prognostication, and comparison, e.g., a multi-axial problem-oriented system, and methodical in-person follow-up (63,111).

SEX AND DEPRESSION

Depression is a frequent cause of decreased sexual interest (105) and individuals with incipient depression may present with lack of desire (40,54). The depressed person "typically loses much of his appetite for food, fun, and sex" (105). Although sexual dysfunction related to ignorance and sociocultural deprivation may be decreasing, sexual dysfunction associated with depression seems to be increasing (105). Research has indicated that "one out of five patients who comes to a clinic for the treatment of sexual and marital problems is moderately to severely depressed" (106).

Depression reduces interest and energy which impairs sexual function. A vicious cycle is maintained as sexual dysfunction aggravates the depression. As depression intensifies, a loss of sexual responsivity (inhibited sexual excitement) and orgasm may follow. Sexual aversion may develop in addition to erectile and orgasmic dysfunction (106).

A loss of sexual interest is reported to occur in between 50 and 100% of cases of severe depression (64). Although less severe depression may be associated with an increase in activity including sexual activity, ostensibly an ego-enhancing device (64), decreased activity and interest are often present with milder depression that may be unrecognized or unacknowledged (105).

In a random sample of 500 psychiatric outpatients Woodruff, Clayton, and Guze found that 42% of 43 men and 33% of 115 women with a diagnosis of primary depression had a decrease in sexual desire following the onset of the depressive episode (107). Impotence occurred in 19 percent of the men. Of the 247 patients without depression, only 12 percent of the men and 21% of the women had a decreased libido. Beck has reported similar findings (106).

According to the conventional wisdom, depression is a primary cause of impotency (106). Recent empirical research at the University of Pennsylvania, however, concluded that only 18 percent of men with secondary impotence were depressed (108). Additionally, 83% of the depressed patients had impaired sexual desire.

A sudden or definite change in a person's sexual interest or activity should alter the clinician to the presence of a depressive syndrome. The recognition and successful treatment of the depressive symptoms may facilitate the return to the patient's premorbid level of sexual functioning, although sex therapy may be necessary with firmly established sexual dysfunction. The pharmacologic treatment of depression can produce autonomic side effects that can further impair sexual function (34-38). The individual and idiosyncratic nature of drug and dose response must be carefully considered to obviate iatrogenic impairment.

CONCLUSIONS

1. The evaluation of a patient with a sexual dysfunction should include medical as well as psychological approaches.

2. Some sexual dysfunctions could be secondary to physical illness, psychological conflicts, or drugs (licit or illicit) use or abuse.

3. Primary sexual dysfunction may reflect organic causes, psychological conflicts, or more commonly, a combination of both.

4. The treatment of psychosexual disorders should include the patient and his/her partner most of the time, although some exceptions are possible to this rule and some specific sexual dysfunctions could be approached individually.

5. Any psychopharmacological treatment for concomitant psychiatric illness should consider the side effects of psychotropic drugs in the genital organs.

TABLE I

NOSOLOGY OF SEXUAL DYSFUNCTION

(Code Numbers from DSM-III-R, 1987)

<u>Sexual Desire Disorders</u>

Hypoactive Sexual Desire Disorders--302.71

Sexual Aversion Disorder--302.79

<u>Sexual Arousal Disorders</u>

Female Sexual Arousal Disorders--302.72

Male Erection Disorder--302.72

<u>Orgasm Disorders</u>

Inhibited Female Orgasm--302.73

Inhibited Male Orgasm--302.74

Premature Ejaculation--302.75

<u>Sexual Pain Disorders</u>

Dyspareunia--302.76

Vaginismus--306.51

REFERENCES

1. Siegel, R.E.: Galen on Psychology, Psychopathology, and Function and Diseases of the Nervous System, Basel, S. Karger, 1973.

2. Kaplan, H.S.: The New Sex Therapy. Active Treatment of Sexual Dysfunctions. New York, Brunner/Mazel, 1974.

3. Lipowski, Z.J.: Psychosomatic medicine in the 70's: An overview. Am J Psychiatry, 134:234, 1977.

4. Engel, G.L.: The need for a medical model: A challenge for biomedicine. Science 196:129-136, 1977.

5. Heinrich, R.L.: Behavioral medicine: Approaches and applications. Psychiatr Clin North Am, 1:323, 1978.

6. Reamy, K.J.: Sexual counseling for the non-therapist. Clin Obstet Gynecol, 27:781-789, 1984.

7. Master, W.H., Johnson, V.E.: Human Sexual Response. Boston, Little, Brown, 1966.

8. Krantz, K.E.: Anatomy of the urethra and anterior vaginal wall. Transactions of the American Association of Obstetricians and Gynecologists and Abdominal Surgeons. 61:31-59, 1950.

9. Freud, S.: Three Essays on the Theory of Sexuality. New York, Basic Books, 1962.

10. Kinsey, A.C., Pomeroy, W.B., Martin, C.E.: Sexual Behavior in the Human Female. Philadelphia, WB Saunders, 1953, p. 584.

11. Fox, C.A., Fox B.: Blood pressure and respiratory patterns

during human coitus. J Reprod Fertil 19:405-415, 1969.

12. Singer, I.: The Goals of Human Sexuality. New York, W.W. Norton, 1973.

13. Perry, J.D., Whipple, B.: The varieties of female orgasm and female ejaculation. Siecus Rep 15-16, May-July, 1981.

14. Ladas, A.K., Whipple, B., Perry, J.D.: The G spot and other recent discoveries about human sexuality. New York, Holt, Rinehart, and Winston, 1982.

15. Weisberg, M.: Physiology of female sexual function. Clin Obstet Gynecol 27:697-705, 1984.

16. Levin, R.J.: The physiology of sexual function in women. Clin Obstet Gynaecol 7:213-252, 1980.

17. Weiss, H.D.: The physiology of human penile erection. Ann Intern Med 76:793-799, 1972.

18. Bors, E., Comarr, A.E.: Neurological disturbances of sexual function with special reference to 529 patients with spinal cord injury. Urol Surv 10:191-222, 1960.

19. Lue, T.F., Zeineh, S.J., Schmidt, R.A., et al: Neuroanatomy of penile erection: Its relevance to iatrogenic impotence. J Urol 131:273-280, 1984.

20. Benson, G.S.: Penile erection: In search of a neurotransmitter. World J Urol 1:209-213, 1983.

21. Lue, T.F., Zeineh, S.J., Shmidt, R.A., et al: Physiology of penile erection. World J Urol 1:194-196, 1983.

22. Benson, G.S., McConnell, J.A., Schmidt, W.A.: Penile polsters: Functional structures or arteriosclerotic changes.

J Urol 125:800-803, 1981.

23. MacLean, P.: New finding relevant to the evolution of psychosexual functions of the brain. J Nerv and Ment Dis 135:289-301, 1962.

24. Kolodny, R.C., Masters, W.H., Johnson, V.E.: Textbook of Sexual Medicine. Boston, Little, Brown, 1979.

25. Speroff, L., Glass, R.H., Kase, N.G.: Clinical Gynecologic Endocrinology and Infertility. Baltimore, Williams and Wilkins, 1978.

26. Sherwin, B.B., Gelfand, M.M., Brender, W.: Androgen enhances sexual motivation in females: A prospective, crossover study of sex steroid administration in the surgical menopause. Psychosom Med 47:339-351, 1985.

27. Bancroft, J: Endocrinology of sexual function. Clin Obstet Gynaecol 7:253-281, 1980.

28. Beach, F.A.: A review of physiological and psychological studies of sexual behavior in mammals. Physiol Rev 27:240, 1947.

29. Schiavi, R.C., Schreiner-Engel: Physiologic aspects of sexual function and dysfunction. Psychiatr Clin North Am 3:88, 1980.

30. Myerscough, P.R.: Sexual function in illness. Clin Obstet Gynaecol 7:387-400, 1980.

31. Levay, A.N., Sharpe, L., Kagle, A.: Effects of Physical illness on sexual Functioning. Human Sexuality, AMA, 1982.

32. Schreiner-Engel, P., Schiavi, R.C., Vietorisz, D., et al:

Diabetes and female sexuality: A comparative of study of women in relationships. J Sex Marital Ther 11:165-175, 1985.

33. Med Lett Drugs and Ther. Drugs that cause sexual dysfunction. 25 (issue 641):73-76, 1983.

34. Seagraves, R.T.: Male sexual dysfunction and psychoactive drug use. Postgrad Med 71:227-233, 1982.

35. Mitchell, J., Popkin, M.: The pathophysiology of sexual dysfunction associated with antipsychotic drug therapy in males. Arch Sex Behav 12:173-183, 1983.

36. Shen, W.W., Sata, L.S.: Inhibited female orgasm resulting from psychotropic drugs. J Reprod Med 28:497-499, 1983.

37. Seagraves, R.T.: Drug effects on female sexuality. Paper presented at the annual meeting of Society for Sex Therapy and Research (SSTAR), Philadelphia, 1986.

38. Reproductive Toxicology, a medical letter 4(1):1-4, 1985.

39. Hollister, L.E.: Drugs and sexual behavior in man. Life Sci 17:661-668, 1985.

40. Kaplan, H.S.: Disorders of Sexual Desire. New York, Simon and Schuster, 1979.

41. Reamy, K., White, S., Daniel W.C., et al: Sexuality and pregnancy: A prospective study. J Reprod Med 27:321-327, 1982.

42. White, S.E., Reamy, K.: Sexuality and pregnancy: A review. Arch Sex Behav 11:429-444, 1982.

43. Perkins, R.P.: Sexuality during pregnancy. Clin Obstet Gynecol 27:706-716, 1982.

44. Reamy, K.J., White, S.E.: dyspareunia in pregnancy. J Psychosom Obstet Gynaecol 4:263-270, 1985.

45. Reamy, K.J., White, S.E.: Sexuality in the puerperium: A review. Arch Sex Behav, in publication, 1986.

46. Kinsey, A.C., Pomeroy, W.B., Martin C.E.: Sexual Behavior in the Human Male. Philadelphia, WB Saunders, 1948.

47. Semmens, J.P., Semmens, E.C.: Sexual function and the menopause. Clin Obstet Gynecol 27:717-123, 1984.

48. Masters, W.H., Johnson, V.E.: Human Sexual Inadequacy. Boston, Little, Brown, 1970.

49. Levine, S.B.: Marital sexual dysfunction: Introductory concepts. Ann Intern Med 84:448-453, 1976.

50. Frank, E., Anderson, C., Rubinstein, D.: Frequency of sexual dysfunction in "normal" couples. New Eng J Med 299:111-115, 1978.

51. American Psychiatric Association Diagnostic and Statistical Manual of Mental Disorders, DSM-III-R, 1987.

52. Sadock, V.A.: Psychosexual dysfunctions and treatment in Comprehensive Textbook of Psychiatry. Edited by Kaplan HI, Sadock BJ, Baltimore, Williams and Wilkins, 1985.

53. Derogatis, L.R., Meyer, J.K., King, K.M.: Psychopathology in individuals with sexual dysfunction. Am J Psychiatry 138:757-763, 1981.

54. Kaplan, H.S.: The Evaluation of Sexual Disorders. New York, Brunner/Mazel, 1983.

55. Annon, J.S.: The Behavioral Treatment of Sexual Problems:

Brief Therapy. New York, Harper and Row, 1976.

56. Donlon, P.T.: Sexual symptoms of incipient schizophrenic psychoses. Med Asp Hum Sex 10:69-70, 1976.

57. Derogatis, L.R.: Psychological assessment of sexual functioning. Psychiatr Cl North Am 3:113-130, 1980.

58. Reamy, K.: The treatment of vaginismus by the gynecologist: an electic approach. Obstet Gynecol 59:58-62, 1982.

59. Horwith, M., Imperato-McGinley, J.: The medical evaluation of disorders of sexual desire in males and females in The Evaluation of Sexual Disorders. Edited by Kaplan HA, New York, Brunner/Mazel, 1983.

60. Schover, L.R., LoPiccolo, J.: Treatment effectiveness for functions of sexual desire. J Sex Marital Ther 8:179-197, 1982.

61. Levine, S.B.: an essay on the nature of sexual desire. J Sex Marital Ther 10:83-96, 1984.

62. McCarthy, B.W.: Strategies and Techniques for the treatment of inhibited sexual desire. J Sex Marital Ther 10:97-104, 1984.

63. LoPiccolo, J.: Diagnosis and treatment of male sexual dysfunction. J Sex Marital Ther 11:215-232, 1985.

64. Munjack, D.J.: The recognition and management of desire phase sexual dysfunction in Gynecology and Obstetrics. Edited by Sciarra JJ, Philadelphia, Harper and Row, 1983.

65. Zilbergeld, B.: Male Sexuality. Boston, Little, Brown, 1978.

66. Kedia, K.R.: Vascular disorders and male erectile

dysfunction. Urol Cl North Am 8:153-168, 1981.

67. Levine, S.B.: Marital sexual dysfunction, erectile dysfunction. Ann Intern Med 85:342-350, 1976.

68. Karacan, I.: Nocturnal penile detumescence as a biological marker in assessing erectile dysfunctions. Psychosom Med 23:349-360, 1982.

69. Van Arsdalen, K.N., Wein, A.J.: A critical review of diagnostic tests used in the evaluation of the impotent male. W J Urol 1:218-226, 1983.

70. Segraves, R.T., Schoenberg, H.W., Zarins, C.K., et al: Characteristics of erectile dysfunction as a function of medical care system entry point. Psychosom Med 43:227-234, 1981.

71. Montague, D.K.: Clinical evaluation of impotence. Urol Clin North Am 8:103-118, 1981.

72. Melman, A., Leiter, E.: The urologic evaluation of impotence in The Evaluation of Sexual Disorders. Edited by Kaplan HS, New York, Brunner/Mazel, 1983.

73. Spark, R.F., White, R.A., Connolly, P.B.: Impotence is not always psychogenic. JAMA 243:750-755, 1980.

74. Segraves, R.T., Schoenberg, H.W., Ivanoff, J.: Serum testosterone and prolactin levels in erectile dysfunction. J Sex Marital Ther 9:19-26, 1983.

75. Nickel, J.C., Morales, A., Condra, M.: Endocrine dysfunction in impotence: incidence, significance, and cost-effective screening. J Urol 132:40-43, 1984.

76. Abber, J.C., Lue, T.F., Orvis, B.R., et al: Diagnostic tests for impotence: a comparison of papaverine injection with the penile-brachial index and nocturnal penile tumescence monitoring: J Urol 135:923-925, 1986.

77. Shreiner-Engel, P., Schiavi, R.C., Smith, H.: Female sexual arousal: relation between cognitive and genital assessments. J Sex Marital Ther 7:257-267, 1981.

78. McGuire, L.S., Wagner, N.N.: Sexual dysfunction in women who were molested as children: one response pattern and suggestions for treatment. J Sex Marital Ther 4:11-15, 1978.

79. Lief, H.I.: Controversies over female orgasm. Med Asp Hum Sex 11:136-138, 1977.

80. Levine, S.B., Rosenthal, M.: Marital sexual dysfunction: female dysfunctions. Ann Intern Med 86:588-597, 1977.

81. Brindley, G.S., Gillan, P.: Men and women who do not have orgasms. Brit J Psychiatr 140:351-356, 1982.

82. Levine, S.B.: Marital sexual dysfunction: ejaculation disturbances. Ann Intern Med 84:575,579, 1976.

83. Munjack, D.J., Kanno, P.H.: Retarded ejaculation: a review. Arch Sex Behav 8:139-150, 1979.

84. Lipschultz, L.I., McConnell, J., Benson, G.S.: Current concepts of the mechanisms of ejaculation: normal and abnormal states. J Reprod Med 26:499-507, 1981.

85. El-Bayoumi, M., El-Mokaddem, H., El-Sherbini, O., et al: Experience with the classification, diagnosis, and therapy of non-ejaculatory intercourse. Fert and Steril 39:76-79,

1983.

86. Shull, G.R., Sprenkle, D.H.: Retarded ejaculation: reconceptualization and implications for treatment. J Sex Marital Ther 6:234-246, 1980.

87. Dow, M.G.: Retarded ejaculation as a function of non-aversive conditioning and discrimination: a hypothesis. J Sex Marital Ther 7:49-53, 1981.

88. Reckler, J.M.: The urologic evaluation of male dyspareunia in The Evaluation of Sexual Disorders. Edited by Kaplan HS, New York, Brunner/Mazel, 1983.

89. Fordney, D.S.: Dyspareunia and vaginismus. Clin Obstet Gynecol 21:205-221, 1978.

90. Lamont, J.A.: Vaginismus. Am J Obstet Gynecol 131:632, 1978.

91. Kroger, W.S., Freed, S.C.: Psychosomatic Gynecology. Hollywood, Wilshire Book Co., 1962.

92. Tolstoy, L., in Wahl, C.W.: Sexual Problems: Diagnosis and Treatment in Medical Practice. New York, Free press, 1967, p. 22.

93. LoPiccolo, J., Miller, V.H.: A program for enhancing the sexual relationship of normal couples, Counsel Psychol 5: 203, 1975.

94. Meyer, J.K.: The treatment of sexual disorders. Med Clin North Am 61:811, 1977.

95. Heiman, J.R., LoPiccolo, J.: clinical outcome of sex therapy. Arch Gen Psychiatry 40:443-449, 1983.

96. Masters, W.H., Johnson, V.E.: Principles of the new sex therapy. Am J Psychiatry 133:548-554, 1976.

97. Wright, W., Perreault, R., Mathieu, M.: The treatment of sexual dysfunction. Arch Gen Psychiatry 34:881-890, 1977.

98. Schwartz, M.: Inhibited sexual desire. Paper presented at annual conference of the Society of Sex Therapy and Research (SSTAR), Phila., March, 1986.

99. Sotile, W.: The penile prosthesis: a review. J Sex Marital Ther 5:90-102, 1979.

100. Sotile, W.: The penile prosthesis: a review. J Sex Marital Ther 5:90-102, 1979.

101. LoPiccolo, J., Lobitz, W.: The role of masturbation in the treatment of orgasmic dysfunction. Arch Sex Behav 2:163-171, 1972.

102. Kilmann, P.R.: The treatment of primary and secondary orgasmic dysfunction: a methodological review of the literature since 1970: J Sex Marital Ther 4:155-176, 1978.

103. Semans, J.H.: Premature ejaculation: a new approach. South Med Jour 49:353-358, 1956.

104. Wolpe, J.: Quantitative relationships in the systematic desensitization of phobias. Am J Psychiatry 119:205, 1963.

105. Mead, B.T.: Depression and sex. Sex Behav Aug: 75-79, 1971.

106. Beck, H.I.: Sex and depression. Med Asp Hum Sex 20:38-53, 1986.

107. Woodruff, R.A., Jr., Guze, S.B., Clayton, P.J.: Personal communication cited in Baker M, Discussion of Mead BT:

Depression and sex. Sex Behav Aug: 77, 1971.

108. Shrom, S.H., Lief, H.I., Wein, A.J.: Clinical profile of experience with 130 consecutive cases of impotent men. Urol XIII: 511-515, 1979.

PSYCHIATRIC ASPECTS OF OBSTETRICS AND GYNECOLOGY

Leslie Hartley Gise, M.D.

Associate Clinical Professor
Department of Psychiatry
The Mount Sinai School of Medicine
New York, N.Y.

CONTENTS:

PSYCHIATRIC ASPECTS OF OBSTETRICS AND GYNECOLOGY

Leslie Hartley Gise, M.D.

INTRODUCTION

The field of obstetrics and gynecology provides many opportunities to study the psychobiology of women. Postpartum depression poses an important challenge regarding the detection of common and treatable psychiatric illness among obstetrical patients. Pseudocyesis, vomiting during pregnancy, and chronic pelvic pain are all classic examples of mind-body interaction. In addition, these clinical syndromes impose a significant strain on the doctor-patient relationship and demand a biopsychosocial approach. Many of these patients are unwilling to accept psychiatric referral, at least initially, forcing the obstetrician/gynecologist into a primary care/counselling role. Pseudocyesis remains a mysterious and fascinating dilemma which often defies rational management. Both postpartum depression and vomiting during pregnancy illustrate the spectrum from "normal" changes to pathological phenomena. Considering what is currently known about these clinical syndromes will hopefully pave the way for future research to clarify the mechanisms and complex interactions between multiple causes of these problems in mind-body interaction.

POSTPARTUM DEPRESSION

Postpartum psychological reactions have been described since the fourth century BC (1). Yet information on childbirth-related psychiatric disorders remains inadequate (2). It is known that clinical depression in predisposed individuals can be precipitated by stress, and the postpartum period - a critical time of identity reformation and role transition for the new parent - can certainly exert such a stress (3,4). But the usefulness of existing reports is limited by several factors:

1. Poor understanding of the psychological correlates of hormonal changes.

2. Lack of uniformity in the definition of the postpartum period (ranging from 2 days to 2 years after delivery).

3. Variation in the definition of psychological characteristics (ranging from the "blues" to major affective disorder, including psychotic depression).

4. Different methods of measurement (e.g., self-report, interviews, objective measures).

5. Variation in populations studied (e.g., race, culture, socioeconomic status, normal vs. women with pathologic diagnoses).

6. Variation in the definition of postpartum depression (e.g., occurring in adoptive mothers, husbands, grandparents) (5).

The birth of an infant is usually joyous for the family. It is particularly upsetting when a new mother feels in turmoil, is depressed, or even thinks of harming her infant. Furthermore, postpartum emotional disturbance jeopardizes the mother-child relationship, disrupts the entire family, and has been associated with future psychiatric problems (6). It can create problems in the doctor-patient relationship, is a demanding clinical situation which requires a biopsychosocial approach, and presents an example of how the obstetrician may be faced with the task of detecting mental disorders in his/her role as a primary care physician (7).

THE SIGNIFICANCE OF POSTPARTUM DEPRESSION

Postpartum depression is an especially significant clinical entity for several reasons.

1. Postpartum depression is common. From 10 to 20% of women suffer a major depressive episode within three months after childbirth.

2. Postpartum depression is largely undetected.

3. Postpartum depression is a treatable psychiatric disorder.

4. Postpartum depression has attracted considerable attention in recent years despite the lack of major research findings or technological developments. The women's movement may have contributed as well as an increased concern for the emotional hazards of childbirth as the obstetric risks decline and obstetric units are increasingly dominated by high technology (11). In addition, the possibility of harm to the newborn baby is always a concern.

5. Because more women, particularly married women, are active in the work force, the effects of postpartum depression have obvious **economic** consequences (8-10).

6. Postpartum depression presents an opportunity for primary prevention and has important preventive mental health implications for the whole family including the effects on young children.

7. Postpartum depression presents an opportunity and a challenge

for **research** to better understand the nature of these disorders and offers a **paradigm** to understand the psychological and somatic aspects of a much wider range of psychiatric disorders (11).

The Detection of Postpartum Depression

Recent data have clearly documented the prevalence of depression in the community with regards to age and sex (12). Depression is more common in women than in men, and the reproductive years (ages 25-45) are the time in a woman's life cycle when she is at greatest risk for the development of a depressive syndrome (13). Previously it had been assumed that the prevalence of depression increased with age and that the risk of depression in women was greatest at menopause.

The failure to detect and treat mental disorders, including major depressive syndromes in medical and surgical patients is well documented (14 -16). Fifteen percent of Americans suffer from some form of mental disorder (17), only 21% of these people go to psychiatrists or other mental health specialists, and 54% are seen exclusively by their primary care physician or by other health professionals (18). Up to 50% of patients with physical complaints who visit primary care physicians have some emotional or cognitive disorder (19). These disturbances are largely undetected and even when detected, they are generally poorly treated (20-22). Furthermore, medical psychiatrists have concentrated their attention primarily on general medical patients and relatively little on obstetrical and gynecologic patients, despite the fact that obstetrics and gynecology is a primary care specialty and that most women of childbearing age consult no other physician than an obstetrician/gynecologist. In view of these facts, it is not surprising that psychiatrists are only very rarely involved with the treatment of postpartum depression (23).

Numerous studies have reported that 10-15% of mothers become depressed within six weeks following childbirth (24-25). These studies have largely used structured interviews which are both time-consuming and impractical for use in a postpartum clinic. Therefore, a self-report questionnaire which could identify major depression associated with pregnancy would be of great importance. Currently available self-report questionnaires have been reported to have limitations for the detection of postpartum depression (23). The Edinburgh Postnatal Depression Scale (EPDS) has been developed for this purpose and shown to be valid and reliable in the United Kingdom (26). Because cultural factors and attitudes towards postpartum depression differ in the United States, this scale should be retested for validity and reliability prior to advocating its widespread use in the United States.

Etiology

Because of the profound hormonal changes of pregnancy, many researchers have postulated a biological basis for postpartum depressive disorders (27-29). But to date, no consistent link between hormone levels and mood has been demonstrated (30). Biological studies have largely looked at women with postpartum blues as opposed to women with postpartum depression, so that they are not generalizable to the more clinically relevant disorder. To address the problem of the biological basis of postpartum depression, future research should utilize neuroendocrine research strategies currently used in studies of affective disorders (31). At present the status of biological theories of postpartum depression is equivocal.

While the specific cause of postpartum emotional disorders remains unknown, the debate about whether they are essentially the same as psychopathology occurring at other times or whether they are specific and distinct disorders continues. The majority of postpartum psychoses (about 2/3) seem to have a course of illness similar to that of nonpuerperal psychopathology (32). More follow-up studies are needed to better categorize women with exclusively puerperal decompensation, as they seem to be nosologically independent from other psychoses. The lack of family history of psychiatric disorder and the lack of nonpuerperal recurrence suggest that this group represents a separate clinical entity. Frank found that depressed women who had had pregnancy-related episodes had an earlier age of onset of illness, a more severely depressed baseline, less emotional stability, longer REM sleep time, and more REM activity than depressed women who had not had pregnancy-related episodes (33). Future studies need to consider three specific groups of women: those who become depressed during pregnancy, those with affective episodes only postpartum, and those with both puerperal and non-puerperal episodes.

Because hormonal shifts are so marked during and after pregnancy, postpartum psychiatric disorders have been assumed to have a specific hormonal etiology, but controlled evidence of a causal relationship is lacking and hormonal differences between postpartum women with and without these disorders has not been demonstrated (34). Why some women develop these syndromes and others do not is unknown. Endocrine, biochemical, neurophysiological, genetic, psychological, social, cultural, and sleep-related causes have been proposed but not confirmed (35-40)(3). Hormonal changes may be precipitating causes of postpartum mood disorders in women with an underlying predisposition, perhaps combined with the stress of the postpartum state. There are probably a variety of causes which interact to determine the form and timing of the episode. It is important that both psychological and neuroendocrine factors be studied. Childbirth is currently understood to function as a nonspecific stress and thus postpartum psychiatric disorders are classified with other psychopathology and not as separate diagnostic entities. Data which support this position include: 1) similar family histories among women who are depressed postpartum and those depressed at other times, 2) similar clinical syndromes and outcomes between postpartum psychiatric disorders and those in nonparturient women, and 3) the occurrence of similar syndromes without the hormonal changes of pregnancy as after adoption, in fathers, and in grandparents (41).

The role of cultural factors is not clear. Some have felt that postpartum depression in the United States represents a culture-bound phenomenon, yet postpartum depression has been described in other cultures in essentially similar form

(42-43)(38).

THE THREE KINDS OF POSTPARTUM DEPRESSIONS

Three types of postpartum reactions can be distinguished: **Postpartum blues,** the most common and the mildest, are a transient mood disturbance or a precursor of postpartum depression, characterized by tearfulness, feelings of dysphoria, and emotional lability (44);

Postpartum depression which is similar to an untreated or outpatient, clinical or major depression (45); and

Psychotic depression with delusions, similar to a non-puerperal psychotic depression.

The failure to clearly distinguish the three types confuses much of the literature on postpartum depression, especially that prior to DSMIII in 1980.

Postpartum Blues

Definition

Postpartum blues are fleeting, mild, benign, and common, and are often called "maternity blues" or "baby blues". Since they occur in up to 80% of women during the first postpartum week, they may be regarded as normal. They are transient situational disturbances or adjustment disorders which typically occur after delivery within the first few days or weeks, but may occur within three months. They may last from a few minutes to a several days, but if a consistently depressed mood persists for two weeks or more, what started out as a mild postpartum emotional disorder may have progressed into a major depression.

Etiology

Because "baby blues" are so common, they have been assumed to have a biological rather than a psychological cause, although as yet none has been clearly demonstrated.

Maternity blues have been described as a reflection of our culture in which women may not get a great deal of support after childbirth. But baby blues have been described in similar form in other cultures, such as at least two in East Africa (38)(43).

Clinical Characteristics

Typical symptoms of the blues include tearfulness, fatigue, apathy, irritability, somatic complaints, headache, sleep disturbances, excessive dreaming, nightmares, lability of mood, crying, and hostile thoughts or feelings toward the baby or other children (46). Women typically weep without apparent cause and may feel that they are falling apart. Postpartum blues have been reported in women who lack marital support and are having difficulties with their babies, but they are also seen in women without obvious psychosocial morbidity (47). Sleep deprivation may contribute to the emotional distress of new parents as the sleep-wake cycle and feeding habits of the infant become regulated during the early weeks and months. Depressed mood has been reported to peak on the 5th day postpartum independent of breastfeeding or number of days in the hospital (48). Although postpartum blues have not been associated with psychopathology, they have been found to be associated with pessimism in late pregnancy, severe premenstrual tension, unplanned pregnancy, and marked ambivalence toward the pregnancy as reflected by consideration given to elective termination in early pregnancy (49,50).

Psychodynamics

Unrealistically high expectations for the rewards of new motherhood and insecurity about her ability as a mother, may result in feelings of failure and lowered self-esteem. Depressive feelings after delivery may also be related to the loss of the pregnant state, women may feel depleted and unable to tolerate even minor burdens or stresses.

Treatment

The obstetrician should acknowledge how frustrating the care of an infant can be, and the new mother should be encouraged to set aside time for her own enjoyment. Psychiatric consultation should be recommended for women who seem overly anxious or who are preoccupied with thoughts of harming their babies, since mild disturbances may escalate into more serious disorders, a psychiatric consultation can help determine whether or not hostile thoughts towards the baby are within the range of normal maternal ambivalence.

MAJOR DEPRESSION

Clinical Characteristics

The risk of postpartum depression begins in the early days following childbirth, but many major depressive symptoms do not emerge until several weeks postpartum. This means that the traditional 6 week postpartum visit is an excellent time to screen women for depression. Unfortunately many postpartum depressions never come to medical attention although they may last for several weeks up to a year or more (11). This may be one of the reasons they have been studied so little. Postpartum depression has been defined as occurring up to one year following childbirth.

Typical prodromal symptoms include irritability, crying, and insomnia which is characterized by a woman being unable to sleep even when the baby is sleeping. Obviously sleep is disturbed by the baby crying. To make a diagnosis of a major depressive episode by DSM-III-R criteria, depressed mood or anhedonia must be present for at least two weeks. In addition three or four of the following symptoms must also be present: change in weight, sleep, psychomotor agitation or retardation, fatigue, feelings of worthlessness or excessive guilt, diminished concentration or indecisiveness, and recurrent thoughts of death or suicidal ideation (51). Other symptoms include feelings of inadequacy and difficulty coping, guilt over not loving the baby enough, and severe anxiety over the baby's health or feeding. In most respects, however, postpartum depressions are typical depressive illnesses (11). Just as with other depressions, the symptoms may not be obvious unless specific inquiry is made. For example, anxiety and depression may be manifested by somatic symptoms. The recurrence rate for postpartum depression is 20-30%, but a past history of postpartum depression is not a contraindication for future pregnancy (52).

Differential Diagnosis

Medical causes of psychopathology must be ruled out before the diagnosis of postpartum depression can be made. Thyroid dysfunction, toxic metabolic problems after hard labor, psychiatric side effects of medical drugs such as bromocriptine (a prolactin inhibitor to suppress lactation in postpartum women) or scopolamine or barbiturates, vitamin deficiency, neurological disorder, or exacerbation of chronic illness such as lupus must be ruled out (53,54).

Psychodynamics

In addition to the neurochemical basis of major depression, characteristic psychodynamic features are often present. Hostility toward the infant may stem from reactivated unconscious oedipal or sibling rivalry conflicts. An inadequate or hostile relationship with her own mother may result in a lack of an adequate role model with resultant identity confusion and a rejection of the mothering role. In this context, the infant's cries are experienced ambivalently both as a desperate call for help and as an angry rejection of the mother. Furthermore, a woman may be intolerant of the infant's demands because of her own unfulfilled dependency needs. Ego weakness may make her unable to accept the newborn's absolute dependency. Childrearing may conflict with career interests. And advice from friends and relatives may add more confusion.

Risk Factors

Psychological risk factors have been described including a past psychiatric history (especially of major affective disorder), a family history of mental illness or alcoholism, and a difficult adaptation during pregnancy (55,56,2,57,58). Dissatisfaction with the marital relationship has been found to be a risk factor for postpartum depression just as it is a risk factor for depression occurring at other times (59,13). O'Hara found depression during pregnancy to predict depression postpartum (60). Saks also found psychological and psychosocial variables to predict postpartum depression (61). But it is not always easy to predict which women are vulnerable to postpartum depression, and women without apparent risk factors can be affected.

Treatment

The treatment of a postpartum depression usually consists of antidepressant medication and psychotherapy. A woman who is depressed after having a baby should receive extra support and particularly relief from childcare responsibilities. Contact with other mothers with new babies in either informal or organized settings can be especially supportive. In addition, the woman's wishes or fears regarding harming the baby must be assessed and monitored. Aside from these considerations, the treatment of postpartum depression is similar to the treatment of major depressive disorders occurring at other times. Although hormonal treatment for postpartum depression has been proposed, there have been no controlled or long-term studies of it (62).

The concentration of tricyclic antidepressants in breast milk has been found to be similar to that in blood and no adverse effects on infants have been demonstrated, but infants' metabolism is immature and long-term effects of even small amounts of drugs are unknown (63). For this reason, any woman taking medication is best advised not to breastfeed her infant.

POSTPARTUM PSYCHOSIS

Classification

Whereas postpartum depression is more commonly seen as similar to major depressions occurring at other times, postpartum psychosis is often viewed as a separate psychiatric disorder. This issue is discussed in the section on etiology above.

Clinical Characteristics

The incidence of postpartum psychosis is generally said to be between 1 to 2 per 1000 live births (1,46,64,65,66). This rate is low enough that the disorder is seen infrequently by an obstetrician, although it is familiar to psychiatrists. These are severe illnesses which usually require psychiatric hospitalization. Some have found that they are more common in primiparae (11). McNeil has suggested that early and late onset psychoses may differ in demographic and psychiatric characteristics (67). The early onset group (within the first 3 weeks) was found to be primiparous, younger, with affective disorders, while the late onset group tended to be older, multiparous, nonmarried, of lower social class, with schizophrenic-like disorders.

A typical course consists of the onset of depression during the first three weeks after childbirth and lasting three months or more. Prodromal symptoms of irritability, crying, and insomnia are common. A flamboyant manic picture may occur soon after delivery and may have a good prognosis (68-71). A dramatic presentation may include excitement, restlessness, pressured speech, and grandiosity. Rapid fluctuations to a euthymic or depressed state may occur and a delirious-like state is also described with clouding of consciousness, confusion, disorientation, irritability, restlessness, and visual hallucination (68,2). Often delusional material will incorporate elements of the childbearing experience, for example, the belief that there were snakes in her abdomen, that the baby was exchanged, lost, kidnapped, or killed, or not born by natural means.

Treatment

The treatment of a postpartum depression characterized by psychosis, suicidal, or homicidal ideation may be carried out on an inpatient, outpatient, or partial hospitalization basis (72). Because of potential destructive acts towards herself or the baby, adequate monitoring of symptoms and supervision is a priority. Inpatient units where the mother and baby, and perhaps even the father, can be hospitalized may provide the best setting to facilitate bonding and to reinforce the woman's ability to function as a mother, but such units are costly and are not generally available in the United States (73,74).

Antidepressants with or without neuroleptics are used as they are in the treatment of nonpuerperal depressions. Even when somatic treatment is required, psychotherapy can foster compliance as well as help the woman understand the psychological issues (psychodynamics), increase her self-knowledge, and help her to recognize danger signals in the future.

Immediate contraception should be provided for women at risk, as unstable moods may make them prone to unprotected

809

intercourse.

When medication fails or if there is pressure of time (e.g., when there is fear of harm to the mother or baby, or risk of impairing mother-child bonding), electroconvulsive therapy has been used with good results (75,76). From extensive clinical experience, Gabriel reports no problems with dislodged clots or pulmonary emboli either during pregnancy or during the first 4 weeks postpartum (77).

DEPRESSION DURING PREGNANCY

Recent data have challenged previous reports of reduced psychopathology during pregnancy and increased risk of psychiatric syndromes occurring only postpartum. Particularly regarding depression, prospective studies have found rates of depression **during** pregnancy comparable to those **after** pregnancy (78-80,60,67). Furthermore, prenatal depression has been found to be a predictor of depression postpartum (78-80,60). In addition, Bridge found that first trimester anxiety and hostility, as well as first trimester depression, correlated with postpartum depression. It seems that women with a past psychiatric history are at risk for psychiatric disturbance both during as well as after pregnancy. Controlled, prospective studies using clear diagnostic criteria and large sample sizes are needed to clarify the risks of recurrent major affective disorders at each stage of the childbearing process (81).

Although lithium and diazepam (Valium) are the only two psychotropic drugs clearly linked to birth defects, an attempt should be made to withdraw women from medication either prior to their becoming pregnant or when the pregnancy is discovered. Nevertheless, if, during the course of the pregnancy, it becomes evident that medication is required, it can usually be reinstituted safely after the first trimester. Although exacerbations may occur during pregnancy, with close monitoring, many patients will remain in remission during pregnancy and will not need psychotropic medication.

The management of a pregnant bipolar patient may be difficult. First, bipolar patients are at risk of recurrence both during and after pregnancy. Second, lithium is teratogenic and relatively contraindicated especially during the first trimester. Third, women with major affective disorders may be concerned about the genetic transmission of these disorders adding guilt and even more anxiety to the pregnancy. Although lithium is teratogenic, tertogenicity is very low, so that most women who take lithium during pregnancy bear normal infants. In addition, bipolar women may remain in remission off lithium during pregnancy although they may relapse postpartum (82). In any event, lithium levels should be monitored weekly during pregnancy since the clearance of lithium may increase during pregnancy and drop to prepregnancy levels at delivery (83). The dose should be halved the week before the expected date of confinement, and omitted during labor. Salt restriction and the administration of diuretics can induce lithium retention and toxicity, and dialysis is indicated if the patient is severely toxic, or if renal failure occurs (84). Infants born of lithium-treated mothers may show poor sucking, hypotonia, tachypnea, tachycardia, and thyroid abnormalities (85,86).

A Past History of Depression

A past psychiatric history seems to be a risk factor for the development of postpartum psychiatric disorders. A past history of a depressive episode increases the risk of depression in the puerperium. A past history of depression has also been associated with depression during pregnancy (80). In contrast to past psychiatric history which is a risk factor for postpartum psychiatric illness, age and parity have not been consistently related as risk factors for postpartum depression (10).

Effect on Children

One reason postpartum depression is so important is because of its prominent preventive mental health aspect. Although earlier reports failed to document negative effects on children whose mothers suffered from postpartum depression, recent reports have shown intellectual deficits in children whose mothers suffered depression during the first year of the child's life (87). Preliminary data suggests that postpartum depression does indeed have an adverse effect on both the infant and the mother-infant relationship (88-92,3).

Postpartum Psychiatric Hospitalization

Although previous reports have suggested that there is an increased risk of psychiatric hospitalization for women postpartum, a recent study reviewing published international research indicates that the post-pregnancy-related risk of admission to a psychiatric hospital is about the same as compared with the three-month admission rate to psychiatric hospitals for all women of similar age (93). Thus it is not yet clear whether or not the postpartum period is associated with an increased risk of psychiatric hospitalization for women.

Recurrence and Outcome

If a woman has had a postpartum psychiatric disorder, she may be reluctant to become pregnant again. The recurrence rate is about 30% and a history of postpartum psychiatric disorder is not regarded as a reason to dissuade a woman from becoming pregnant or carrying a pregnancy to term. Davidson reported a follow-up of postpartum psychiatric illness and found 70% to have major affective disorders (52% unipolar and 18% bipolar) (94). the overall prognosis was good. The risk of developing another postpartum illness varied from 1 in 3 to 1 in 5 pregnancies. Five percent ultimately committed suicide in this series.

Neonaticide

Neonaticide is the correct term to describe mothers who kill their babies shortly after delivery, as opposed to infanticide, or the killing of older children. Neonaticide is a postpartum phenomena, whereas infanticide is more closely related to the problem of child abuse and not specifically tied to the postpartum period.

Neonaticide has received scant attention in the psychiatric literature, but has been related to unwanted pregnancies, other psychological problems, and sociological factors such as poverty, adolescence, and deprivation (95). A variety of psychodynamic explanations have been offered such as blurred distinction between mother and baby during pregnancy and postpartum when the baby may come to represent the bad part of the self and become the victim of displaced suicidal drives (41). Another explanation is that the fear of abandonment may be denied during pregnancy, but becomes overwhelming after delivery when these women become acutely disorganized and murder their infants (96).

In a follow up study of postpartum psychiatric disorders, Davidson reported the probable incidence of infanticide to be 4% (94). The rates of infanticide are higher in schizophrenic women than in depressed women, and some women who kill their babies are not found to have diagnosable mental disorders.

<u>Prevention</u>

The potential adverse effects of postpartum depression on the mother and her baby pose an important problem in preventive mental health. With multifactorial causation, reducing any of the contributing factors may lessen the likelihood of a major depression postpartum.

Any woman who appears excessively anxious or who is having difficulty with her baby during pregnancy, in the hospital, or at the first postpartum visit should be considered for a psychiatric consultation. Often providing information, discussion, and reassurance may be all that is needed. Simple inquiry about mood, worries, eating, sleeping, and how things are going in general will detect most postpartum mood disorders. Maternal anxiety and depression result in emotional deprivation for the new baby so it is important to try and prevent these reactions (97).

Childbirth education classes are a good place to educate

women about the risk factors for the development of postpartum depression and this can facilitate early referral. This approach does not seem to "put ideas into their heads", but rather to reduce postpartum emotional disorders (98).

Conclusion

Postpartum depression covers a spectrum from mild early emotional setbacks to profound disruption requiring psychiatric hospitalization. These disorders are common, largely undetected, and generally treatable as well as having important implications for the mother-child relationship and for maternal adaptation. The causes of postpartum depressions are yet to be clarified, and present a challenge to both the obstetrician and the psychiatrist for research and treatment.

PSEUDOCYESIS

Definition

Pseudocyesis is a fascinating but mysterious condition. It is a very rare psychiatric syndrome marked by the conviction of a nonpregnant woman that she is pregnant. Signs and symptoms of pregnancy typically appear. Pseudocyesis has also been described in men and in animals (99,100).

History

Pseudocyesis has been called the oldest known psychosomatic condition (101). Hippocrates gave the first and classic description - "women who imagine they are pregnant" - in 300 B.C. In 1823, Good introduced the term pseudocyesis, which was derived from the Greek pseudes, (false), and kyesis, (pregnancy) (102). Other cases include Mary Tudor, Queen of England and daughter of

Henry VIII, a famous case of recurrent pseudocyesis in the 16th century; Joanna Southcott, a 19th century prophetess and religious leader who believed herself pregnant with the second messiah at the age of 64; and Breuer's patient "Anna O", discussed by Freud, developing pseudocyesis while under treatment (103).

Incidence

Pseudocyesis is rare and the incidence seems to be decreasing (104). Reasons may be lack of reporting, increasing patient sophistication, or social change whereby women can fulfill themselves in roles other than motherhood, diminishing the psychological need to be pregnant (103).

Five hundred and forty-six cases have been reported in the English language medical literature since the 18th century (104a). One 79-year-old mother of 10 had symptoms lasting 7 years. Recurrence is rare, but one woman developed the condition every 9 months from the time of her marriage to death. Pseudocyesis has been described in all races, all nations, and all strata of society from British royalty to Chinese coolies to American plantation slaves to German hausfraus to African Zulus to Tennessee mountain people.

Clinical Course

Pseudocyesis typically occurs in older women who have an emotional need for childbearing or affection from a child or spouse, or who may have infertility (105). It may occur months or even years after sterilization surgery, before menarche, or after menopause - and males are not immune (106-109,99).

Subjects are most typically aged 20-39, married, often for the second time, and 41% had previously given birth, so that they were not totally naive in matters of reproduction. Evans described a "simulated pregnancy" in a male analysand who enacted a pregnancy on the analytic couch and in everyday life over a period of about 10 days (110). Aronson reported a delusion of pregnancy in a male patient which ceased when the diagnosis of a papillary carcinoma of the kidney was made (111).

Signs and symptoms of pregnancy actually develop in pseudocyesis and many able clinicians have been fooled. A dramatic case has been reported illustrating extent of the mind's influence over the body. This woman had toxemia with hypertension, albuminuria, and edema (112).

The following signs and symptoms, listed in order of frequency, may occur, sometimes in exaggerated form:

1. Menstrual disturbance (amenorrhea or hypomenorrhea);

2. Abdominal enlargement (sometimes to term size, but with an inverted umbilicus in contrast to the flattened or everted umbilicus of pregnancy);

3. Breast changes similar to those of pregnancy (sometimes with colostrum);

4. Fetal movements reported by the patient (often earlier than in a real pregnancy);

5. Softening of the cervix with signs of congestion (although careful examination usually reveals a normal-sized uterus);

6. Nausea and vomiting; and

7. Weight gain (often greater than in normal pregnancy);

8.   Labor pains (these can be severe, last for days and usually occur at the due date) (103,104,107,113).

Murray has summarized the mechanical factors responsible for abdominal distention and a 1889 obstetrical journal reports intestines distended with gas found on caesarean section for pseudocyesis (103,113). d'Orban has described an association with child stealing (114).

Diagnosis

The diagnosis of pseudocyesis may be made during the course of prenatal care or it may present as an unproductive episode or "labor". By presenting obstetrical symptoms in the absence of an obstetrical diagnosis, pseudocyesis strains the doctor-patient relationship.

When obesity or lack of patient cooperation hamper physical examination, the diagnosis of pseudocyesis may be made by sonography (115). Pseudocyesis should be distinguished from:

1.   **Delusional pregnancy.** This is when the patient is psychotic with other signs of psychotic illness as well as delusions of pregnancy.

2.   **Simulated pregnancy.** This is when a woman professes to be pregnant knowing she is not. A woman with pseudocyesis believes she is pregnant, whereas a woman with simulated pregnancy knows that she is not.

    a.   **Factitious Illness or Munchausen's Syndrome.** This is a case of simulated pregnancy when a woman professes she is pregnant knowing she is not, but she does not know why she is doing it. The reasons for professing pregnancy are unconscious.

b. **Malingering.** This is where a woman is professing pregnancy for an obvious, conscious, specific reason (116).

3. **Pseudopregnancy.** This is caused by a hormone-secreting tumor creating changes suggestive of pregnancy such as dysgerminomas or other feminizing ovarian tumors (117).

Etiology

There are currently three hypotheses regarding the etiology of pseudocyesis. First is the classic psychosomatic hypothesis that fantasies of pregnancy initiate alterations in physiology just as sexual fantasies result in elevations of gonadotropins (118,119). The second is the somatopsychic hypothesis that minor bodily changes initiate the false belief in pregnancy (120). The third is a psychophysiologic hypothesis that major depressive disorder, with its concomitant alterations in brain biogenic amines, may be an important initiating event in pseudocyesis, as biogenic amines are involved in the regulation of gonadotropin-releasing hormone (GnRH), which in turn controls follicle-stimulating hormone (FSH) and luteinizing hormone (LH) (121). Starkman et al conducted the first investigation combining psychiatric characterization and radioimmunoassay techniques of measuring pulsatile gonadotropin secretion and concluded that there is no one common endocrine profile of patients with pseudocyesis (122).

Psychological Factors

Despite the above, pseudocyesis has generally been regarded

as psychogenic according to the first hypothesis. Many underlying unconscious purposes have been suggested, such as:

to resolve conflicts over childbearing and sexual functioning;

to effect self-punishment;

to please a husband;

to have an heir;

to force marriage;

to prove youthfulness;

to compete with mother;

to resolve incestuous conflicts; or

to resolve conflicts over threatened object loss or over physical illness

The symptom frequently is over-determined and has many meanings (108).

Support for the somatopsychic hypothesis comes from the idea that minimal bodily changes or subtle physical symptoms which occur from the side effects of psychotropic medication may interact with the wish to be pregnant and result in pseudocyesis (110,123). Anticholinergic side effects of both antidepressant and antipsychotic medications include ileus and intestinal dilatation, and weight gain also occurs. Furthermore, elevated serum prolactin and lactation are side effects of antipsychotic medication. The somatopsychic formulation is supported by Aronson's case of abdominal malignancy and Cramer's case of pseudocyesis in a woman with antipsychotic-induced lactation (111,123).

PSYCHIATRIC DIAGNOSES

Pseudocyesis has been conceptualized as a **conversion disorder** in a suggestible woman with a **histrionic personality**, possibly with infertility and yearning for a baby (107). But it appears in women without conversion disorder or personality defects.

Pseudocyesis has also been conceptualized as an **affective equivalent** (124). If this is true, hormonal changes should be mediated through the neuroendocrine mechanisms of major affective disorder, but endocrine changes are not consistently found. If pseudocyesis is an affective equivalent, antidepressant medication should help (108).

Actually pseudocyesis has been associated with a wide variety of psychiatric disorders from mild anxiety states to very severe disturbances. Pseudocyesis may reflect adaptive mourning activity, a defense against psychotic decompensation, or the subjective interpretation of physiological changes.

Endocrine Factors

Endocrine functioning in psuedocyesis is not well understood. But appears to be of central hypothalamic-pituitary origin similar to polycystic ovarian disease (125). Observations by Forsbach et al indicate that the amenorrhea of pseudocyesis is associated neither with a persistent corpus luteum nor with chronic hyperprolactinemia (126). Elevated gonadotropins have been reported, but in general changes in estrogen or progesterone levels have not been observed. Starkman et al, however, found elevated testosterone and estradiol levels, abnormal growth hormone secretory patterns, but normal prolactin levels and concluded that there was no consistent linkage between psychiatric and neuroendocrine abnormalities in pseudocyesis (122). Tulandi reported a derangement in hypothalamic-pituitary function suggestive of an underlying impairment in dopaminergic function (127). Devane et al report a hormone pattern most consistent with polycystic ovarian disease (128). In any event, hormone levels fall immediately, as does abdominal distension, when the patient gives up her belief (129).

Treatment

Curiously, telling the patient that she is not pregnant does not seem to work. In the past, patients were allowed to "go into labor", "deliver", and then told that the "baby" "died" (107). This dishonesty is not compatible with today's awareness of the need for open doctor-patient communication.

Traditionally, the patient is confronted and an attempt is made to persuade her that she is not pregnant. Alternatively, no interventions are made and the condition is allowed to run its course. Weddington et al point out the role of the pseudofather in helping the woman accept the diagnosis (130).

The obstetrician should share the negative results of the pregnancy test with the patient to try and help her begin to understand that she may not be pregnant. The physician's attitude should be one of empathy with the patient's paradoxical dilemma of a visible "pregnancy" and a negative pregnancy test. The obstetrician should encourage the patient to seek psychiatric consultation, while at the same time scheduling regular follow-up visits to reassure her that she is not being abandoned.

Sonography may help with diagnosis and with helping the patient to accept it. But Starkman emphasizes the importance of exploring the patient's fears and fantasies before the ultrasound examination (e.g., she may be afraid of cancer), as well as eliciting any observations from the patient during the ultrasound procedure which she could use to bolster her fantasy (e.g., that she saw a baby's hand) (131).

Some patients may not be willing to accept psychiatric help initially. But if the obstetrician follows the patient, develops more of a trusting relationship with her, and as the patient gets nearer to "term", she may eventually be willing to accept psychiatric help. Psychotherapy is generally believed to be the most effective measure, and patients who continue to be unable to accept psychiatric help are at increased risk of psychotic decompensation.

Conclusion

Pseudocyesis is a striking example of the mind's influence over the body, specifically the role of the central nervous system in the control of ovarian function. Unanswered questions about pseudocyesis include: how often it does to "term", how often it recurs, what the prognosis is for further psychiatric disorder, and why it is on the decline (107). Hopefully further study of pseudocyesis will help elucidate mind-body interactions.

VOMITING DURING PREGNANCY

Introduction

Vomiting during pregnancy has been described in the earliest medical writings, about 2000 B.C. (132). Formerly the difference between "morning sickness" and hyperemesis gravidarum was thought to be only a matter of degree, but today they are generally viewed as qualitatively distinct. Actually four types of vomiting during pregnancy must be distinguished:

1. vomiting due to nonpregnancy causes,

2. third trimester vomiting,

3. "morning sickness", and

4. hyperemesis gravidarum.

The literature, however, often fails to clearly define "morning sickness", or mild-to-moderate vomiting during the first trimester, as opposed to hyperemesis gravidarum, the "pernicious vomiting of pregnancy", which persists into the second trimester, may seriously affect nutritional state or weight, and is associated with hospitalization. The term hyperemesis gravidarum is often used to refer to the mild vomiting of early pregnancy or used in a general sense to include both the mild, early vomiting and the severe, later, true hyperemesis.

Vomiting Due To Nonpregnancy Causes

The first task in the diagnosis of vomiting during pregnancy is to rule out vomiting due to nonpregnancy causes. Vomiting in pregnancy may be due to any cause which affects nonpregnant women, such as infectious (e.g., urinary tract infections), gastrointestinal disturbances (e.g., appendicitis, intestinal obstruction), drug reactions, brain tumors, and endocrinologic disorders (e.g., thyrotoxicosis) (133). Vomiting is an often forgotten manifestation of hyperthyroidism. The incidence of thyrotoxicosis during pregnancy is about two per thousand (134). Given the ease of laboratory confirmation, excellent therapy, and the seriousness of delay in diagnosis, thyrotoxicosis should be considered in patients with vomiting during pregnancy. Transient elevations of thyroid function tests have also been reported in patients with severe hyperemesis, but no way to distinguish this from true thyrotoxicosis is apparent (135).

Third Trimester Vomiting

Third trimester vomiting is frequently linked with liver disease and preeclampsia, and hospitalization should always be considered (97).

"MORNING SICKNESS"

Definition

"Morning sickness" is mild-to-moderate vomiting during the first trimester. It is so common as to be considered normal, does not seriously affect nutritional state or weight, and seems to have **little psychological significance.** Early nausea and vomiting are considered among the earliest diagnostic symptoms of pregnancy and affect about 50% of pregnant women, peaking at the 8th to 12th week, and generally disappearing by the 12th and 16th week (136,137). These early symptoms are distinguished from the severe vomiting of hyperemesis which may persist after the first trimester.

Etiology

The hypothesis that elevated estrogen levels early in pregnancy are responsible for vomiting in pregnancy is supported by recent findings of higher serum estradiol levels and higher sex hormone binding-globulin binding capacity (SHBG-BC) in patients with vomiting as opposed to those without vomiting during pregnancy (138). SHBG-BC levels would be expected to accompany an elevated level of estradiol, because estradiol is the stimulus for synthesis of SHBG (139). An extremely rapid rise in estradiol in early pregnancy is likely to be a cause of vomiting, especially if SHBG production accelerates with some delay after the rise in estradiol.

Maternal risk factors for vomiting during pregnancy which were found in this study and which also support the estrogen hypothesis include nulliparity, high body weight, and non-cigarette smoking status during pregnancy (138). Higher circulating and urinary estrogen levels have been reported in nulliparous women as compared with parous women and higher first-trimester estrogen levels have been reported in primigravidas as compared with multigravidas (140). Cigarette smokers have lower levels of endogenous estrogens than do non-smokers, so the protective effect of cigarette smoking may also have an estrogen basis (141). Furthermore, women who vomit during pregnancy have been found to be less likely to smoke and this effect has been found to be preexisting and not a response to either the pregnancy or to the vomiting (142,143).

Pregnancy outcome factors which may be related to elevated estrogen levels include fewer spontaneous abortions, fewer stillbirths, and an increase in central nervous system and related skeletal malformations in the offspring of women who vomit during pregnancy. The occurrence of congenital dysplasia of the hip and undescended testicles in the offspring of women who vomit during pregnancy support the hypothesis that vomiting during pregnancy is related to higher estrogen levels (144). The estrogen hypothesis is also supported by the fact that exogenously administered estrogens often produce nausea and vomiting.

Early pregnancy vomiting has also been ascribed to the high and rising human chorionic gonadotropin levels of the first trimester (145,146), but other investigators have been unable to relate human chorionic gonadotropin levels to vomiting (138,147). Support for HCG in the etiology of vomiting comes from the association of Down's syndrome in offspring of women who vomit during pregnancy. Since many Down's embryos and fetuses are aborted spontaneously, those with the best functioning placenta with the highest hormone production might have an advantage and survive to birth. This could cause the association of high HCG producers, vomiting, and Down's syndrome (144). Vomiting during pregnancy has also been associated with raised pregnancy-specific beta-1-glycoprotein (SP-1) concentrations by Kauppila et al (146).

Elevated thyroid function tests had been reported in women with vomiting during pregnancy, but subsequent study suggests normal function of the thyroid gland and of the pituitary-thyroid axis in women who vomit during pregnancy with an enhanced peripheral conversion of T4 to reverse T3 which is most probably related to dietary factors, especially carbohydrate deficit (148).

Vomiting is a nonspecific symptom often of multifactorial origin. In contrast, motion sickness is considered entirely reflexogenic on the basis of a disturbance of central reflexogenic mechanisms. Since the rates of motion sickness in the non-pregnant condition do not differ between women who vomit during pregnancy and those who do not, a central reflex mechanism is considered unlikely for vomiting during pregnancy (149).

Early psychoanalytic investigation regarded the lack of nausea as a possible sign of denial of pregnancy, indicating conflicts about the feminine role (150). Subsequently Uddenberg found women with moderate first trimester nausea to have fewer adjustment difficulties during and after pregnancy than either the symptomless or the severe hyperemesis groups (151).

Sociocultural factors have been implicated by the lower incidence among native American, native African, Eskimo, and Asian populations with the exception of industrialized Japan. Also, symptoms are more common in urban than in rural populations (152).

Clinical Characteristics

Vomiting during pregnancy has generally been reported to be more common in primigravidas (153), but one study reported it to be more common in multigravidas (149). Younger age has been found to be a maternal risk factor for the development of vomiting during pregnancy (138). Morning sickness has also been reported to be more common in those with short intergestational intervals, and to be associated with significantly higher diastolic blood pressure in late pregnancy (149).

Delivery outcome was studied by Kallen in 3068 pregnancies with vomiting during pregnancy in the Swedish Medical Birth Registry from 1973-1981. Vomiting during pregnancy was found to be associated with low maternal age, first parity, the infant being a girl, twinning, shorter gestational length, lower birthweight, and congenital malformations. The congenital malformations may possibly due to antiemetic medication use and included undescended testicles, hip dysplasia, and Down's syndrome (144).

Treatment

Morning sickness may require no treatment or may respond to education (e.g., informing the woman that it almost always clears spontaneously by the 12th week of gestation), placebos (including prenatal vitamins which produced as 75% cure rate in one study) (152), and emotional support and/or reassurance, (e.g., informing the woman that it is a normal reaction in pregnancy).

Antinausea medication is usually effective in severe cases. Although antiemetics have not been proven teratogenic, the thalidomide tragedy has produced an understandable reluctance to use medication during pregnancy, especially during the first trimester. If there is an increased incidence of birth defects after vomiting, they could be due to hormonal factors such as increased estrogen levels as well as to antiemetic medication. Commonly used antiemetics include antihistamines such as meclizine (Bonine) and cyclizine (Marezine), and phenothiazines such as prochlorperazine (Compazine).

Lone et al reported successful outpatient treatment of

vomiting with behavioral techniques in 4 patients who refused medication (154).

HYPEREMESIS GRAVIDARUM

Introduction

Hyperemesis gravidarum, the "pernicious vomiting of pregnancy", is a classic illustration of mind-body interaction and requires a biopsychosocial approach (152,155). It strains the doctor-patient relationship in 3 ways. First, after treating a hyperemetic patient, the obstetrician may fear that other patients with mild symptoms may develop the same problem. Second, the doctor must decide whether to give medication to a pregnant woman. And third, vomiting during pregnancy has traditionally been associated with the idea of rejection of the child which is understandably disturbing to the doctor. Before intravenous therapy was adopted, ketosis, neurologic disturbances, and death would often occur. Hyperemesis has a relatively low incidence and occurs in 1 per 1000 births in the United States and 0.5 to 10 per 1000 births cross-culturally (153).

Definition

Hyperemesis gravidarum is a much more severe type of vomiting than "morning sickness", persists into the second trimester, may assume life threatening proportions with weight loss, dehydration, electrolyte imbalance, even disturbed protein metabolism, and is associated with psychological problems in many cases (152). It is often defined as vomiting during pregnancy severe enough to require hospitalization with associated features including weight loss greater than 5% body weight, ketosis, and acetonuria.

Psychological Factors

Although psychological factors have been associated with hyperemesis for almost a century (154), the tendency to presume psychogenic causes for unexplained physical symptoms should be avoided. Most illnesses are neither psychogenic nor organically caused, but rather are the result of a number of causes each of which may either predispose, precipitate, or sustain the symptoms (155a).

Early psychoanalytic studies posited the rejection of feminity, oral impregnation fantasies, or an overly close relationship between the patient and her mother, among other predisposing factors (7,156). The latter concept is supported by the fact that women frequently return to their mothers' homes when they start to vomit, or their mothers come to stay with them. However, the widely held but oversimplified view that vomiting is a symbolic rejection of the pregnancy, an unconscious attempt to reject the child (a throwing up and out of the unborn child), or an oral attempt at abortion, has occasionally resulted in punitive, rejecting treatment of such patients (157-159). In the past, denial of visitors, keeping the shades drawn, isolating the patient, etc. were part of this punitive approach for which there is no rationale.

Up to 80% of cases of hyperemesis gravidarum have been associated with psychological factors (153,160) and today, hyperemesis gravidarum is conceptualized as a stress reaction to difficult circumstances, not as a symbolic rejection of the pregnancy. The hyperemetic woman is often overburdened by social and psychological difficulties, and vomiting may be understood as a physiological response to extremely high levels of stress. She appears to need to protect herself from being overwhelmed and "to need a hole to crawl into, one in which (she) could protect (her) unborn child" (161). When her coping skills and social supports are limited, hyperemesis becomes a maladaptive coping behavior which results in relief from stressful home environments and in care from her physicians and family.

The concept of ambivalence is useful in understanding the relationship between hyperemesis and the woman's attitude toward childbirth in her particular circumstance. Vomiting does not seem to be the result of rejection of pregnancy, but rather of an ambivalent attitude expressing in wartime (156), and below-average intelligence (160).

Psychiatric Diagnoses

Hyperemesis gravidarum has been associated with a variety of psychiatric syndromes such as Histrionic Personality Disorder, Borderline Personality Disorder, and Somatization Disorder (51,152).

Biological Factors

Endocrine, metabolic, and immunologic causes of hyperemesis gravidarum have been postulated but not confirmed (7).

Wernicke's encephalopathy has been reported and should be considered and anticipated in women with hyperemesis gravidarum particularly if parenteral fluids are employed. Typically symptoms include delirium, ophthalmoplegia, nystagmus, and ataxia which responded to parenteral thiamine within a few days, but delirium may be absent (165). Although horizontal nystagmus improved dramatically within hours, vertical nystagmus may persis for several months. The Wernicke-Korsakoff syndrome has a high mortality and morbidity rate and may be precipitated by the use of intravenous fluids containing glucose by rapidly depleting the remaining thiamine body stores and may be aggravated by deficiency of magnesium and associated with other deficiency disorders.

Treatment

Hospitalization can represent much needed "time out" from the external stressful world. In fact, most women stop vomiting with the separation from their home environment by hospitalization and supportive care (152). Intravenous fluid replacement is usually necessary and sometimes antiemetics are required as well. The obstetrician is best advised to adopt a supportive attitude and to encourage the patient to talk about her troubles by using open ended questions such as, "How are things going?", "What's on your mind?". Psychotherapy, mainly supportive, has been reported successful in conjuction with hospitalization. Many patients are resistant to psychotherapeutic intervention, but others may benefit from treatment of underlying psychiatric disorders or reduction of interpersonal conflicts. Behavioral approaches including hypnosis and behavior modification have also been used. Placebos have been used as well but it is important to remember that their success does not imply a nonorganic cause, since they are effective in 1/3 or "normal" people even for "real" postoperative pain. Placebos also interfere with the doctor-patient relationship, so a homeopathic dose of a benign medication may be a better choice than a true placebo. Firmness may be called for at times, but a punitive approach, used in the past, is not indicated.

Patients with hyperemesis gravidarum should be referred for psychiatric consultation to determine the nature of the psychological stress which may be contributing to their symptoms and to document any concurrent psychopathology. They should also be referred for social work service evaluation to identify stressful conditions such as lack of financial and social support and inadequate housing (152).

CHRONIC PELVIC PAIN

Background

The modern literature on pain centers on organic lesions and peripheral pathways, relatively little concern is shown for the central nervous system. But pain is a subjective phenomena, and cannot be measured directly. Furthermore, the perception of pain requires psychological processing by the central nervous system. In addition, the central nervous system has a powerful effect on the perception of pain. Soldiers wounded in battle often report that they felt no pain. Religious mystics can walk on burning coals without experiencing pain. Just as the central nervous system can suppress the experience of pain, so it has been hypothesized that the central nervous system may augment or amplify bodily sensations which may be experienced as pain (166,167).

Chronic pelvic pain is a common gynecologic problem in young, adult women. The symptoms are often not specific; the clinical examination is often negative; and further investigation, such as laparoscopy, often fails to reveal pelvic pathology. Psychological problems are frequently present, yet the patient may refuse psychiatric referral. The patient expects the doctor to propose and discuss the cause of the pain and then to cure or decrease the pain.

ANATOMY AND PHYSIOLOGY OF GYNECOLOGIC PAIN

Whereas the perineum, vulva, lower part of the vagina, uterus, fallopian tubes, and ovaries are well innervated and sensitive to painful stimuli, the upper vagina is less sensitive. Clamping or dilating the cervix is painful for most women, possibly due to a great density of nerve terminals at the level of the internal os. The body of the uterus also has a variety of nerve endings which respond to painful stimuli and which are activated by dilation or contraction of the uterus or inflammatory processes. Painful stimuli generate impulses which are transmitted by A-delta- and C-fibers in somatic and visceral nerves. Somatic pain fibers supply the skin, muscles, bones, joints, and parietal peritoneum while visceral pain fibers supply the cervix, uterus, and adnexa. Painful stimuli to the cervix, uterus, and adnexa are transmitted through afferent fibers in sympathetic nerves which enter the spinal cord at T10, 11, 12, and L1. These fibers enter the uterine, cervical, pelvic, and superior hypogastric plexuses, the hypogastric nerve, and the lumbar and lower thoracic chain (168,169).

THE MEANING OF PAIN - PSYCHODYNAMIC FACTORS

Pain is involved in the development of interpersonal relationships. A baby has hunger pains and the mother feeds it. A child falls and feels pain and runs to the mother to "kiss it and make it all better". So from an early age, the child learns to associate pain with human relationships, especially with that of the mother. Pain and punishment are associated from an early age. Since pain is associated with being bad, pain itself may provoke guilt feelings. For children who are neglected by their parents, getting punished may be the only attention the child gets. Since pain and punishment are preferable to utter rejection and abandonment, this pattern may persist into adult life. To the small child, pain is associated with power since the adult can hurt the child and thereby control him or her. As the child gets bigger, the child can hurt those who are smaller and learns to control aggression by hurting himself or herself when experiencing pain instead of hurting someone else (166).

There are a variety of psychodynamic formulations and Castelnuovo-Tedesco concluded that no specific psychodynamics were typical of chronic plevic pain (170). Engel postulated the following psychodynamics for the "pain-prone" patient. As a result of distant relationships in childhood, these patients had no role models, and are subsequently unable to form close relationships. Since pain was a familiar experience for them, they learned to form relationships through pain. As children, parental rejection must have engendered anger which had to be suppressed to avoid complete rejection by their parents. Guilt would be associated with this anger and when such a person feels the forbidden feeling of anger in the future, she could develop pain as a way of coping (171). If the parent made the child feel guilty about sexual feelings, sexual arousal could also provoke pain (166). Some women develop pain when things are going well for them. They have a need to suffer because of their anger and the resulting guilt.

Another precipitant for pain is loss. Through the pain of mourning, the pain of the lost person, or the pain in the relationship, the lost person can be kept alive, and the pain of grief can be diminished. When threatening feelings are about to overwhelm a person, and decompensation is imminent, they can be warded off by the development of symptoms such as pain.

Gidro-Frank concluded that although the psychopathology varied, the primary difficulty in women with chronic pelvic pain was in establishing and maintaining a sense of feminine identity (172). Walker supports Gidro's hypothesis that conflicts about sexuality and intimacy are repressed until the initiation of regular sexual activity and that chronic pelvic pain serves to help these women avoid sexual activity and intimacy and the severe anxieties and painful memories associated with it (173). Furthermore, secondary gain may arise through sexual dysfunction, dyspareunia, and avoidance of sexual activity.

METHODOLOGIC PROBLEMS IN STUDIES

Our understanding of the problem of chronic pelvic pain is

hampered by methodological flaws in studies done to date (174).
Problems include:

1. The Diagnosis of Psychopathology - structured interviews and operational criteria have generally not been used.

2. The Diagnosis of Chronic Pelvic Pain - criteria of 0 to 6 months duration have been used as well as criteria of consistent pain in one location as opposed to variable and changing symptoms.

3. The Diagnosis of Physical Findings - there have not been valid measures of the degree and nature of organic pathology, i.e., findings on laparascopy. The American Fertility Society Classification fof Endometriosis has been used by Walker (173).

4. Appropriate Control Groups have not been used.

5. Casual Relationships have been assumed between gynecologic pathology and pain symptoms.

6. Samples have been biased by samples containing women with psychopathology.

7. Sample size has been small.

Clinical Characteristics

Castelnuovo-Tedesco reported on a group of women with chronic pelvic pain of 5 months duration and compared them to women with pelvic pathology without pain. He found high levels of psychopathology, mainly mixed character disorders with difficulty in forming relationships, which fits with Engel's formulation. The women described the pain as variable in both quality and location. When questioned further, they were unable to clarify the location of the pain. Pain was described as lower abdominal, suprapubic, pelvic, lumbosacral, with radiation down the thighs, and as both sharp and dull. Depressive symptoms such as fatigue, and sleep and appetite disturbances were common as were headache, musculoskeletal pain, low back pain, and obesity. Anxiety symptoms were also present and included anxiety attacks, hyperventilation, shortness of breath, dizziness, and dissociative phenomena. These findings were consistent across socioeconomic groups (170). Magni reported that women without pelvic pathology were more likely to report continuous as opposed to episodic pain (174).

Patients with chronic pelvic pain have been described as young (age 20-40), with symptoms starting during or after the first pregnancy (166). They have been found to be immature and dependent with anxiety, depression, and suicidal ideation. Their past histories are often characterized by turbulent childhoods, parental loss, violence, threat of injury, sexual abuse, marital problems in the parents, and multiple losses and abandonment. Sexual and marital problems, infertility, abortions, and negative attitudes toward pregnancy and child care have been described. Interpersonal relations have been characterized as fleeting, casual, and superficial. On examination these women were found to be detached and bland with affective poverty. Many seemed depressed but denied it. Psychological tests confirmed the presence of schizoid tendencies and significant difficulties in relating to others. Psychological tests also showed hypochondriasis and hysteria indicating the use of somatization, repression, and denial as compared with women with pelvic pathology without pain who were more likely to be overtly depressed (170).

A number of authors have noted that symptoms arise in the context of depression and may be precipitated by stressful life events, especially during and after the first pregnancy (166,172,174,175).

Effect on the Physician

Since pain is unpleasant and the physician sees himself or herself in the role of helper and reliever of this distress, it is frustrating if the patient does not respond and become free of pain. Patients with chronic pelvic pain may be seeking a human relationship through pain. They have pain because they cannot face their problems and may therefore refuse a referral to a psychiatrist.

ETIOLOGY

The Relationship Between Chronic Pelvic Pain and Psychopathology

A word of caution must be given about the concommitant findings of gynecologic and psychologic pathology. Finding pathology, either gyncologic or psychologic, does not prove that either is a significant causative agent in the production of pain symptomatology. Pelvic pathology on laparoscopy and/or significant psychopathology are not infrequently found in women without pain. The finding of a gynecologic disorder does not prove that this physical pathology is the cause of the patient's pain. Similarly, finding psychopathology does not prove that this is a cause of chronic pain either, since psychopathology may be a result of the pain syndrome and also because psychopathology has been found in control groups of gynecology patients without pain. Likewise, pelvic pathology on laparoscopy has been demonstrated in women without chronic pelvic pain.

Physical and psychogenic findings may be present separately or they may be concommitant findings. If a causal relationship is postulated, it can be either a psychosomatic one (i.e., the psychological factors cause the physical findings) or a somatopsychic one (i.e., the physical symptoms secondarily cause the psychologic symptoms). In reality, the causal mechanisms are probably more complicated. There are likely a multitude of both physical and psychological causes which may be predisposing causes, precipitating causes which trigger symptoms, and/or sustaining causes which aggravate the symptoms and make them worse once they are already there (155).

The Psychosomatic Hypothesis

Castelnuovo-Tedesco and others support the psychosomatic hypothesis, viewing the psychopathology as primary, and the pain as a resultant symptom, a product of the psychological conflict and the need to form a relationship through pain. Levitan hypothesizes that the central nervous system affects pelvic blood flow and thereby produces pain (176). For this reason he recommends psychologic treatment prior to laparoscopy.

The Somatopsychic Hypothesis

Renaer studied women with chronic pelvic pain with and without pelvic pathology on laparoscopy. The duration of the pain was unspecified. He found evidence of similar psychopathology on psychological test scores of pain patients regardless of the presence of pelvic pathology (169). He concluded that the psychological findings were secondary to the pain rather than their cause, that is, somatopsychic as opposed to psychosomatic. On the basis of psychological tests, Renaer found anxiety, depression, somatization, social withdrawal, lower ego strength, and marital problems in chronic pelvic pain patients. One problem in this study was that patients without pelvic pathology on laparoscopy were more likely to refuse to participate and may have had more psychopathology. The finding of equivalent psychopathology in pain patients regardless of physical findings has been found with other pain syndromes as well (177). The longer patients have chronic back pain, the more likely they are to have psychopathology. A prospective study of psychopathology, prior to the onset of the pain, is needed to confirm whether or not psychopathology predisposes pain to become chronic. Another problem with the Renaer study is that control gynecologic patients without pain differed from the norms on which the psychological tests were standardized. Psychopathology in the gynecologic control group patients without pain is another problem. It seems that going to the doctor is stressful, so that the selection of control groups is critical.

PHYSICAL FACTORS

Duncan introduced a consideration of psychological factors in patients with chronic pelvic pain into the gynecologic literature in 1952 with a study documenting increased vaginal blood flow with anxiety in women with chronic pelvic pain (175). Taylor then proposed predisposing and precipitating causes, namely pelvic vascular congestion (a vascular disorder of the pelvic autonomic nervous system) in the presence of stress in psychiatrically predisposed individuals (178). However Gidro-Frank found only 3% of these patients to have pelvic congestion and Castelnuovo-Tedesco found 3% (170,172). Lundberg reported no pelvic congestion in a series of 95 patients with chronic pelvic pain, 37 with negative laparoscopies (179). More recently Beard has demonstrated pelvic varicosities on pelvic venography in women with chronic pelvic pain and negative laparoscopy (180). He hypothesized that abdominal pressure over the "ovarian point" occludes the ovarian vein causing back pressure on the hilum of the ovary and resultant pain.

Levitan reported an 81% incidence of irregular menses and a 30% incidence of pelvic tenderness on pelvic examination in his series of women with pain for 6 months (176).

Pelvic Pathology on Laparoscopy

Gynecologic pathology in women with chronic pelvic pain includes ovarian cysts, adhesions, endometriosis, uterine fibroids, pelvic inflammatory disease, uterine retroversion, uterine prolapse, cystocele, rectocele, and urethrocele.

Rates of pelvic pathology on laparoscopy in women with chronic pelvic pain have varied widely depending on patient selection and sampling and on the definition of chronic pelvic pain. In patients with pain for 6 months, Levitan found an 8% incidence of pelvic pathology (176). In patients with pain for 6 months in the same location, Kresch found an 83% incidence of pelvic pathology (181). In a series of patients where duration and location were not specified, the rates of organic pelvic pathology in patients with chronic pelvic pain ranged from 8% to 74% (173,173,182-186).

In Kresch's series, 29% of the pain-free control group had positive findings of pelvic pathology on laparoscopy. Adhesions (38%) and endometriosis (32%) were the most common. Patients who did not initially complain of pain, but were subsequently diagnosed with endometriosis on laparoscopy, stated that they did in fact have pain but that they did not seek medical help for it. Kresch feels that chronic pelvic pain is usually a symptom of pelvic pathology and recommends laparoscopy for women who have pain in the same location for a minimum of six months. But most women with chronic pelvic pain have vague symptoms, so Kresch may be selecting a biased sample with clear symptoms and pain in one location.

PSYCHOLOGICAL FACTORS

In a classic paper in 1970, Castelnuovo-Tedesco introduced chronic pelvic pain into the psychiatric literature. Using the criterion of a duration of 5 months of chronic pelvic pain, he found high levels of psychopathology, mainly mixed character disorders with difficulty forming relationships, in women with chronic pelvic pain as compared with women with pelvic pathology without pain.

Although the gynecologic literature indicates that psychological factors should be studied only in women without organic pathology, Castelnuovo-Tedesco advocates psychological study of all women with chronic pelvic pain, since psychopathology was found in all women with pain regardless of whether or not they had pelvic pathology. He considers chronic pelvic pain to be a manifestation of psychiatric disturbance (170). Several investigators including Gidro-Frank, Castelnuovo-Tedesco, and Renaer found similar psychopathology in women with pain regardless of the presence of pelvic pathology (169,170,172). Patients with and without pelvic pathology could not be differentiated on the basis of either the nature or the severity of the psychiatric findings.

Castelnuovo-Tedesco concluded that chronic pelvic pain, even in the presence of pelvic pathology was more than pelvic disease. These patients have significant emotional difficulties, generally consisting of major personality disorders of long-standing which are central to the complaint of pain (170).

Walker et al and others have reported similar pelvic pathology in women with and without pain. In this study there was no difference in either the prevalence or the severity of pelvic pathology on laparoscopy between the pain patients and the pain-free gynecologic. They concluded that for most women with chronic pelvic pain, the pathological findings on laparascopy have little or no relevance to the chronic pelvic pain which they feel is due to the past and present psychological problems of these women (psychosomatic effect). Laparoscopy is useful to understand pelvic pathology, but it does not establish a physical cause of pain. The situation is complicated by the fact that psychological problems may arise from chronic pain itself (somatopsychic effect). These authors further hypothesize that chronic pelvic pain may represent chronic psychological pain and may act in a defensive manner to protect the woman from painful memories (173).

Psychiatric Diagnoses

Some investigators have not found psychopathology to differentiate women with and without pelvic pathology, others have. Beard reported higher Neuroticism scores on the Eyseneck Personality Inventory in women with negative laparoscopies as opposed to those with pelvic pathology (187). Magni also reported depression in women who had no pelvic pathology on laparoscopy as compared to women who had pelvic findings (174). The women with pain and no pelvic findings had more depressed mood, clinical depression (i.e., major depression according to DSM-III-R criteria), somatic symptoms associated with depression, a past history of depression, and a family history of depressive spectrum disorders (depression, alcoholism, sociopathy) as compared with women with pain and pelvic pathology (188). Somatic symptoms included headache, anorexia, insomnia, constipation, fatigue, and sexual problems.

Other chronic pain patients have also shown high rates of depression (189-192). And patients with depression may experience guilt and pain as well. Beresin reports a case which responded to tricyclic antidepressant therapy (193).

Chronic pain has also been conceptualized as a Conversion Disorder or a Somatoform Disorder. Castelnuovo-Tedesco concluded that chronic pelvic pain was a symptom, not a diagnosis, and remains a poorly defined entity (170).

Sexual Abuse

Walker et al reported psychopathology and a past history of sexual abuse in women with chronic pelvic pain as compared to other gynecologic patients. Patients with chronic pelvic pain were younger, single, and had lower occupational status than gynecologic patients. In particular, these investigators found major depression, substance abuse, sexual dysfunction, and somatization in addition to a past history of sexual abuse both in childhood and adulthood. Major depression was present in 62% of this sample, and drug dependence or abuse in 52%. In most cases, the psychopathology (depression or drug abuse) antedated the onset of the pelvic pain. Multiple somatic complaints were also common among chronic pelvic pain patients as compared with gynecologic patients. A past history of childhood sexual abuse was associated with an increased incidence of sexual dysfunction, depression, and drug abuse in women with chronic pelvic pain. for women with the most severe sexual abuse in childhood, chronic pelvic pain and major depression were associated (173). They hypothesize that as a result of childhood sexual traumatization and adult sexual dysfunction, the pelvis is selected in depression-prone individuals as the site of the pain (psychosomatic effect). Based on the criterion of chronic pelvic pain of a duration of three months, a rate of negative findings on laparascopy was 48% and was not different from that of the comparison group.

EVALUATION

The medical work-up for chronic pelvic pain consists of a

pelvic examination and often laparoscopy. Levitan recommends a 3 stage approach: 1) extensive medical work-up, 2) psychological treatment, and 3) laparoscopy. He recommends an extensive medical work-up consisting of complete blood count, urinalysis and culture, vaginal smear, upper gastrointestinal series and barium enema, intravenous pyelography, cholecystogram, plasma fibrinogen (familiar Mediterranean fever is a common cause of abdominal pain in Israel where this was done), lumbosacra spine x-rays, and orthopedic examination (176). If the work-up is completely negative and significant orthopedic, gastrointestinal, and urinary disorders are ruled out, he recommends laraposcopy. He feels that laparoscopy should be reserved for patients who do not respond to psychologic treatment. A cost effectiveness study of the expense saved by not performing laparoscopy, as compared to the cost of psychologic treatment, has not yet been done, however.

TREATMENT

The treatment of chronic pain is problematic for the gynecologist when the organic work-up is carried out, physical treatment is offered, and pain remains. To the extent that these patients seek to form human relationships through pain, the feelings associated with the underlying conflicts may be too overwhelming, the patient may refuse a referral to a psychiatrist. In such a case, the gynecologist must use himself or herself to form a relationship with the patient as a first step. The patient may eventually accept psychiatric referral later.

The non-psychiatric physician can get useful information about the patient by first asking concrete, simple, yes-and-no questions followed by open-ended questions in the context of taking an obstetrical, gynecologic, and sexual history. For example: "How old were you when you got your first period?" "Did you know what it was?" "What was your reaction to it?" This may give information about puberty and about how sexual information was communicated in the woman's family. A sexual history should include such questions as: "How did you first learn about sex?" "Have you ever had trouble with your periods?" "At what age did you become sexually active?" "Are you sexually active now?" "Do you have any sexual problems?" "Have you ever had an adverse sexual experience where someone touched you or tried to have sex with you against your will?"

Another important focus of the history is learning why the pain is appearing now. What is the precipitant? Have ther been any changes in the family, job, community? As with other chronic pain patients, the best strategy for the non-psychiatric physician is to try and establish a relationship with the patient over a period of weeks or months. Each visit need not be long, but the physician communicates his or her interest in the patient and the fact that she is being taken seriously. The physician is recommended not to offer advice or medication until a relationship has been formed with the patient. Speaking briefly about some of the patients life problems may be therapeutic, even if it is not stated overtly that the problems are connected to the pain. (An analogus situation occurs with children in play therapy. They may act out family situations with dolls, yet never admit that they are talking about their own families. Yet talking about the dolls helps them master their own problems.) If the physician recognizes that the woman is seeking a relationship, he or she will not feel guilty about not relieving the pain. In addition, it is important to recognize that the pain may be protecting the woman from more serious symptoms of depression, including suicide, so that it serves a useful function. Just as narcotics do not eliminate pain, but take the edge off it, so a relationship may not remove the pain, but make it bearable. The challenge for the physician is to form a relationship with the patient and learn something about her in an attempt to relieve her suffering (166).

Castelnuovo-Tedesco commented on the high response rate to nonspecific events such as diagnostic gynecologic procedures and diagnostic interviews. He attributed this placebo response to suggestion and interpersonal factors (170). But this response to nonspecific treatment fits with Engel's formulation of these patients' emotional deprivation and need for interpersonal contact and attention. Castelnuovo-Tedesco noted that these women were usually eager to undergo hysterectomy which relieved their pain which was then frequently replaced by other symptoms, frequently psychological ones (170).

Pearce reported therapeutic effects of counselling in chronic pelvic pain patients as compared with a control group who did not receive counselling (194).

Benson studied 35 women with chronic pelvic pain without physical findings and reported that although they rejected the notion that their symptoms had an emotional basis, 50% were amenable to short-term psychotherapy, and that of these, 50% definitely benefited. He diagnosed 83% as hysterical neurosis and 17% as schizophrenic and found that making a psychiatric diagnosis was helpful in the management of these patients (195).

CONCLUSION

The fields of obstetrics/gynecology and psychiatry provide many opportunities for collaboration. Unravelling the mysteries of mind-body interaction continues to be a fascinating dilemma. In addition, a number of critical issues are raised by the topics selected in this review.

In addition to the four syndromes reviewed here, there are other important areas which equally deserve attention. Psychiatric implications of pregnancy, including normal anxiety and ambivalence, teenage pregnancy, and psychiatric disorders other than depression associated with pregnancy are examples. Gynecologic surgery, especially oncology highlight the problems of the psychological aspects of surgery and the psychology of illnesses related to sexual organs and function.

The problem of mind-body interaction, the spectrum of changes from normal to pathological, the strain on the doctor-patient relationship, the inability of many of these patients to accept psychiatric consultation, and the need for a biopsychosocial model of both treatment and research characterize many of the syndromes selected for review.

In addition, postpartum depression represents a problem in the detection of treatable mental disorders among non-psychiatric patients. It also provides a paradigm to understand the psychological and somatic aspects of a much wider range of psychiatric disorders. Pseudocyesis dramatizes the extent of central nervous system influence on ovarian function. Vomiting during pregnancy represents a spectrum of changes from normal to pathological and emphasizes the importance of ruling out physical disorders before assuming symptoms are of psychological origin. Chronic pelvic pain is an example of a common yet poorly understood disorder which has been difficult to study. The meaning of the pain must be integrated with the latest techniques of physical diagnostic procedures to arrive at an integrated treatment approach.

This chapter is intended to review what is known about these four syndromes as a basis for better clinical understanding as well as future research.

References

1. Hamilton J: Postpartum Psychiatric Problems, CV Mosby, St. Louis, Mo, 1962.

2. Weiner A: Childbirth related psychiatric illness. Compr Psychiatry 23: 143-154, 1982.

3. Weissman M, Paykel E: The depressed woman: a study of social relationships. The University of Chicago, Ill, 1974.

4. Dunner D, Patric V, Fieve R: Life events at the onset of bipolar affective illness. Am J Psychiatry, 136:508-511, 1979.

5. Notman M, Nadelson C: Rep roductive crisis. In A Brodsky, R Hare-Mustin (Eds): Women and Psychotherapy. Guilford Press, NY, NY 1980.

6. Uddenberg N, Englesson I; Prognosis of postpartum mental disturbance. A prospective study of primiparous women and their 4 1/2 year old children. Acta Psychitr Scand 58:201-212, 1978.

7. Gise L: Psychiatric Implications of Pregnancy, In S Cherry, R Berkowitz, N Kase (Eds), Medical, Surgical, and Gynecologic Complications of Pregnancy, Third Edition, Williams and Wilkins, Baltimore, Md, 1984.

8. Hoffman L: Maternal employment. American Psychologist, 34:859-865, 1979.

9. Vickery C: Women's economic contribution to the family. In RE Smith (ED), The subtle revolution: Women at work. Washington DC: The Urban Institute 68-89. 1979.

10. Hopkins J, Marcus M, Campbell S: Postpartum depression: a critical review. Psychological Bulletin, 95:498-515, 1984.

11. Kendell R: Emotional and Physical Factors in the Genesis of Puerperal Mental Disorders. J Psychosom Res 29:3-11, 1985.

12. Myers J, Weissman M. Tischler G et al: Six-month prevalence of psychiatric disorders in three communities. Arch Gen pSychitry 41:959-967, 1984.

13. Weissman M, Leaf P, Tischler G et al: Affective disorders in five United States communities. Psychological Medicine 18: 141-153, 1988.

14. Hankin J, Locke B: The persistence of depressive symptomatology among prepaid group practice enrollees: An exploratory study. Am J Public Health 72:1000-1009, 1984.

15. Nielson A, Williams T: Depression in ambulatory medical patients. Arch Gen Psychiatry 37:999-1004, 1980.

16. Katon W: Depression: Relationship to somatization and chronic medical illness. J Clin Psychiatry 45:4-11, 1984.

17. Report to the President from the President's Commission on Mental Health, Volume 1, Washington, DC, 1978.

18. Regier D, Goldberg I, Taube C et al: DeFacto US Mental Health Services System. Arch Gen Psychitry 35:685-693, 1978.

19. Hoeper E et al: Estimated prevalence of ΓDC mental disorder in primary medical care. Int J Ment Health 8:6-15, 1979.

20. Wheatly D: Psychopharmacology in Medical Practice, New York, Appleton-Century-Crofts, 1973.

21. Balter M: An analysis of psychotherapeutic drug consumption in the United States, in Bowen R (ed), Proceedings of the Anglo-American Conference on Drug Abuse: Etiology of Drug Abuse, vol 1, London, Royal Society of Medicine, pp 58-65, 1973.

22. Goldberg D: Mental health priorities in a primary care setting. An NY Acad Sci 310:65-68, 1978.

23. Cox J. Connor Y, Henderson I, McGuire R, Kendell R: Prospective study of the psychiatric disorders of childbirth by self report questionnaires, J Affective Disorders, 5:1-7, 1983.

24. Kumar R, Robson K: Neurotic disturbance during pregnancy and the puerperium - preliminary report of a prospective survey of 119 primiparae, In: M Sandler (Ed), Mental Illness in Pregnancy and the Puerperium, Oxford Univ Press, London, 1978.

25. Cos J, Connor Y, Kendell R: Prospective study of the psychiatric disorders of childbirth, Brit J Psychitry, 140:111-117, 1982.

26. Cos J, Holden J, Sagovsky R: Detection of postnatal depression: Development of the 10-item Edinburgh Postnatal Depression Scale. Brit J Psychitry 150:782-786, 1987.

27. Dalton K: Prospective study into puerperal depression. Brit J Psychiatry 118:689-692, 1971.

28. Handley S, Dunn T, Waldron G et al: Tryptophan, cortisol and puerperal mood.   Brit J Psychiatry, 136:498-506, 1980.

29. Treadway C, Kane F, Jarrahi-zadeh A Et al: A psychoendocrine study of pregnancy and puerperium.   Am J Psychiatry, 125:1380-1386, 1969.

30. Nott P, Franklin M, Armitage C et al: Hormonal change in the puerperium.   Brit J Psychiatry, 128:279-283, 1976.

31. Steiner M: Psychobiology of mental disorders associated with childbearing.   Acta Psychiatrica Scandinavica, 60:449-464, 1979.

32. Schopf J, Bryois C, Jonquiere M et al: On the nosology of severe psychiatric post-partum disorders, Eur Arch Psychitr Neurol Sci 234:54-63, 1984.

33. Frank E, Kupfer D, Jacob M et al: Pregnancy-related affective episodes among women with recurrent depression.   Am J Psychiatry 144:288-293, 1987.

34. Glick I, Bennett S: Psychiatric complications of progesterone and oral contraceptive,   J Clin Psychopharmocal. 1:350-367, 1981.

35. Cheetham RW, Rzadkowolski A, Rataemane S: Psychiatric disorders of the puerperium in South African women of Nguni origin.   A pilot study.   S Afr Med J 60:502-506, 1981.

36. George AF, Wilson KC: Monoamine oxidase activity and the puerperal blues syndrome,   J psychosom Res 25:409-413, 1981.

37. Gupta BK: Depression after childbirth, Br Med J 284:980-981, 1982.

38. Harris B; "Maternity blues" in East African clinic attenders.   Arch Gen Psychiatry 38:1293-1295, 1981.

39. Karacan I, Williams RL: Current advances in theory and practice relating to postpartum syndromes.   Psychiatr Med 1:307-328, 1970.

40. Stein GS: Headaches in the first postpartum week and their relationship to migraine.   Headache 21:201-205, 1981.

41. Asch SS, Rubin LF: Postpartum reactions: some unrecognized variations. Am J Psychiatry 131:870-874, 1974.

42. Stern G, Kruckman, L: Multi-disciplinary perspectives on post-partum depression: an anthropological critique. So Sc: Med. 17: 1027-1041, 1983.

43. Cox J: Postnatal depression: a comparison of African and Scottish women. Soc Psychiatry 18:25-28, 1983.

44. Pitt B: Maternity blues. Brit J Psychiatry, 122:431-433, 1973.

45. O'Hara M, Rehm L, Campbell S: Postpartum depression: a role for social network and life stress variables. J Nerv Met Dis, 171:336-341, 1983.

46. Kau: In Owels J (ed): Modern Perspectives in Psycho-Obstetrics. New York, Brunner/Mazel, 1972.

47. Fegetter G, Cooper P, Gath D: Non-psychiatric disorders in women one year after childbirth. J Psychosom Res, 25:369-372, 1981.

48. Kendell R, McGuire R, Connor Y: Mood changes in the first three weeks after childbirth. J Affect Disord, 3:317-326, 1981.

49. Codon J, Watson T: The maternity blues: exploration of a psychological hypothesis. Acta Psychiatria Sc and, 76:164-171, 1987.

50. Herzog A, Detre T: Psychotic reactions associated with childbirth. Dis Nerv System, 37:229-235, 1976.

51. American Psychiatric Association: Diagnostic and Statistical Manual of Mental Disorders, Third Edition, Revised. Washington DC, American Psychiatric Association, 1987.

52. Paffenbarger R: Epidemiological aspects of postpartum mental illness, Br J Prev Soc Med 18:189-195, 1964.

53. Brook N, Cookson I: Bromocriptine-induced mania? Br Med J 1:790, 1978.

54. Vlissides D, Gill D, Castelow J: Bromocriptine-induced mania? Br Med J 1:510, 1978.

55. Baker M, Dorzab J, Winokur G et al: Depressive disease: the effect of the postpartum state, Biol Psychiatry 3:357-365, 1971.

56. Davenport Y, Adland M: Postpartum psychosis in female and male bipolar manic depressive patients. Am J Orthopsychiatry 52:288-297, 1982.

57. Nadelson C: "Normal" and "Special" Aspects of Pregnancy: a psychological approach. In Nadelson CC, Notman MT (eds): The Woman Patient, Medical and Psychological Interfaces: Vol 1. Sexual and Reproductive Apects of Women's Health Care. New York, Plenum, 1978.

58. Hayworth J, Lettle B, Carter S et al: A predictive study of postpartum depression: some predisposing characteristics. Br J Med Psychol 53:161-167, 1980.

59. Watson J, Elliot S, Rugg A et al: Psychiatric disorder in pregnancy and the first post-natal year. Brit J Psychiatry 144:453-462, 1984.

60. O'Hara, M: Psychological factors in the development of postpartum depression. In Inwood D (ed): Recent Advances in Postpartum Psychiatric Disorders, Washington DC, American Psychiatric Press, Inc. 1985.

61. Saks B, Frank J, Lowe T et al: Depressed mood during pregancy and the puerperium: clinical recognition and implications for clinical practice. Am J Psyciatry 143:728-731, 1985.

62. Kane F: Psychiatric Reactions to oral contraceptives. Am J Obstet Gynecol. 102:105-133, 1968.

63. Brixen-Rasmussen L, Halgrener J, Jorgensen A: Amitriptyline and notriptyline excretion in human breast milk. Psychopharmacology 76:94-95, 1982.

64. Normand WC: Postpartum disorders. In Freedman AM, Kaplan IH (eds): Comprehensive Textbook of Psychiatry. Baltimore, Williams and Wilkins, 1967.

65. Paffenbarger, RS: The picture puzzle of the postpartum psychosis. J Chronic Dis 13:161-173, 1961.

66. Protheroe, C: Psychiatric illness associated with childbirth Practitioner 225:1245-1251, 1981.

67. McNeil, T: A prospectively study of postpartum psychosis in a high-risk group. Acta psychiatr scand 75:35-43, 1987.

68. Hall R, Popkin M, Stickney S, et al: Presentation of the steroid psychosis. J Nerv Ment Dis 167:229-236, 1979.

69. Kendell R, Wainwright S, Hailey A, et al: The influence of childbirth on psychiatric morbidity. Psycho Med 6:297-302, 1976.

70. Melges F: Postpartum psychiatric syndromes. Psychosom Med 30:95-108, 1968.

71. Reich T, Winokur G: Postpartum Psychosis in patients with manic-depressive disease. J Nerv Ment Dis 151:60-68, 1970.

72. Nurnberg H, Prudic J: Guidelines for treatment of psychosis during pregnancy. Hosp Community Psychiatry 35:67-71, 1984.

73. Gruenbaum H, Weiss J: Psychotic mothers and their children: joint admission to an adult psychiatric hospital. Am J Psychiatry 119:927-933, 1963.

74. Luepker E: Joint admission and evaluation of postpartum psychiatric patients and their infants. Hosp Community Psychiatry 23:284-286, 1972.

75. Sobel D: Fetal damage due to ECT, insulin, coma, chlorpromazine or reserpine. Arch Gen Psychiatry 2:606-611, 1960.

76. Hamilton J: Guidelines for therapeutic managment of postpartum disorders. In Inwood D (ed): Recent Advances in Postpartum Psychiatric Disorders, Washington DC, American Psychiatric Press, Inc., 1985.

77. Gabriel A: Unpublished report (personal communication), 1983.

78. Ballinger C: Emotional disturbance during pregancy and following delivery. J Psychosom Res, 26:629-634, 1982.

79. Bridge L, Little B, Hayworth J et al: Psychometric ante-natal predictors of post-natal depressed mood. J Psychosom Res, 29:325-331, 1985.

80. Buesching D, Glasser M, Frate D: Progression and Depression in the Prenatal and Postpartum Periods. Women and Health, 11:61-78.

81. Casiano M, Hawkins D: Major Mental Illness and Childbearing: A Role for the Consultation-Liaison Psychiatrist in Obstetrics in Psychiatric Clinics of North America 10:35-51, 1987.

82. Targum S, Davenport Y, Webster M: Postpartum mania in bipolar depressive patients withdrawn from lithium carbonate. J Nerv Ment Dis 167:572-574, 1979.

83. Schou M: What happened to the lithium babies? A follow-up study of children born without malformations. Acta Psychiatr Scand 54:193-197, 1976.

84. Donalson J: Neurology of pregnancy. Philadephia. WB Saunders, 1978.

85. Goldberg H, Diamscia A: Psychotropic drugs in pregnancy. In Lipton M, Dimascio A, Killam K (eds): Psychopharmacology: A generation of progress. New York. Raven Press. 1978 pp 1047-1055.

86. Karlsson R, Lindstedt G, Jundberg P et al: Transplacental lithium poisoning: reversible inhibition of fetal thyroid. Lancet 1:1295, 1975.

87. Cogill S, Caplan H, Alexandra H, Robson K, Kumar R: Impact of maternal postnatal depression on cognitive development of young children, Brit Med J, 292:1165-1167, 1986.

88. Cohn J, Tronick E: Three-month old infants' reaction to simulated maternal depression. Child Development, 54:185-193, 1983.

89. Trause M, Kramer L: Preterm birth: effects on parents. Paper presented at the Society for Research in Child Development, Boston, MA, April, 1981.

90. Richman N: Depression in mothers of preschool children. J Child Psychology and Psychiatry, 17:75-78, 1976.

91. Livingood A, Daen P, Smith B: The depressed mother as a source of stimulation for her infant. J Clin Psychology 39:369-375, 1983.

92. Persson-Blennow I, Naslund B, McNeil T, et al: Offspring of women with nonorganic psychosis: mother-infant interaction at three days of age. Acta psychiatr Scand 70:149-159, 1984.

93. David H: Post-abortion and post-partum psychiatric hospitalization. Abortion: medical progress and social implications, Pitman, London (Ciba Foundation Symposium 115) 150-164, 1985.

94. Davidson J, Robertson E: A follow-up study of post-partum illness, 1946-1978. Acta Psychiatr Scand 71:451-457, 1985.

95. Resnick P: Murder of the newborn: a psychiatric review of neonaticide. Am J Psychiatry 126:1414-1420, 1970.

96. Brozovsky M, Falit H: Neonaticide: clinical and psychodynamic considerations. J Am Acad Child Psychiatry 10:673-683, 1971.

97. Beattie J: Observations on post-natal depression and a suggestion for its prevention. Int J Soc Psychiatry 24:247-249, 1978.

98. Gordon R, Kapostins E, Gordon K: Factors in postpartum emotional adjustment. Obstet Gynecol 25:158-166, 1965.

99. Knight J: Falso pregnancy in a male. Psychosom Med 22:260-266, 1960.

100. Moulton R: The psychosomatic implication to pseudocyesis. Psychosom Med 4:376-389, 1942.

101. Kroger W: Psychosomatic Obstetrics, Gynecology and Endocrinology. Springfield Il. Charles C. Thomas, 1962.

102. Good J: Psychological System of Nosology with Corrected and Simplified Nomenclature. Wells and Lilly, Boston, 1823.

103. Murray J, Abraham G. Pseudocyesis: a review. Obstet Gynecol 51:627-631, 1978.

104. Cohen L: A current perspective of pseudocyesis. Am J Psychiatry 139:1140-1144, 1982.

104a. Small G: Pseudocyesis: An Overview. Can J Psychiatry 31:452-457, 1986.

105. Christodoulou G: Pseudocyesis. Acta Psychiatr Belg 78:224-234, 1978.

106. Barglow P: Pseudocyesis and psychiatric sequelae of sterlization. Arch Gen Psychiatry 11:571, 1967.

107. Hardwick P, Fitzpatrick C: Fear, folie and phantom pregnancy: Pseudocyesis in a fifteen-year-old-girl. Br J Psychiatry 139:558-560, 1981.

108. Barglow P: Pseudocyesis: to be and not to be pregnant: a psychosomatic question. In Howells J (ed): Modern Perspectives in Psycho-Obstetrics. New York. Brunner Mazel. 1972.

109. Evans D, Seely T: Pseudocyesis in the male. J Nerv Ment Dis 172:37-40, 1984.

110. Evans W: Simulated pregnancy in a male. Psychoanal Q 20:165-178, 1951.

111. Aronson G: Delusion of pregnancy in a male homosexual with an abdominal cancer. Bull Menninger Clin 16:159-166, 1952.

112. Fischer I: Hypothalmic amenorrhea: pseudocyesis. In Kroger W (ed): Psychosomatic Obstetrics, Gynecology and Endocrinology. Springfield, Il. Charles C. Thomas. 1962, p 291.

113. Bivin G, Klinger M: Pseudocyesis. Bloomington Il. Principia Press. 1937.

114. d'Orban P: Child stealing and pseudocyesis. B J Psychit 141:196-198, 1982.

115. Guzinak G, Conrad S: Pseudocyesis and Sonography. Am J Obstet Gynecol. 138:230-232, 1980.

116. Daw E: Pseudocyesis. Br J Clin Pract 27:181-183, 1973.

117. Williams R (ed): Textbook of Endocrinology; ed 6. Philadelphia, WB Saunders, 1981.

118. Fried P, Rakoff A, Schopbach R et al: Pseudocyesis; A psychosomatic study in gynecology. JAMA 145:1329-1335, 1951.

119. LaFerla J, Anderson D, Schalch D: Psychoendocrine response to sexual arousal in human males. Psychosom Med 40:166-172, 1978.

120. Pawlowski E, Pawlowski M: Unconscious and abortive aspects of pseudocyesis. Wis Med J 57:437-440, 1958.

121. Brown E, Barglow P: Pseudocyesis: A paradigm for psychophysiological interactions. Arch Gen Psychiatry 24:221-229, 1971.

122. Starkman M, Marshall J, LaFerla J, et al: Pseudocyesis, psychologic and neuroendocrine interrelationships. Psychosom Med 47:46-56, 1985.

123. Cramer B: Delusion of pregnancy in a girl with drug-induced lactation. Am J Psychiatry 127:960-963, 1971.

124. Taylor J: Recurrent pseudocyesis and hypomania. Brit J Psychiatry 151:120-122, 1987.

125. Ayers J, Seiler J: Neuroendocrine indices of depression in pseudocyesis: a case report. J Reprod Med 29:67-69, 1984.

126. Forsbach G, Guitron A, Munoz M et al: pituitary hormone secretion in patients with pseudocyesis. Fertility and Sterility 40:637-641, 1983.

127. Tulandi T, McInnes R, Lal S: Altered pituitary hormone secretion in patients with pseudocyesis. Fertility and Sterility 40:637-641, 1983.

128. Devane G, Vera M, Buhi W et al: Opioid peptides in pseudocyesis. Obstet and Gynecol 65:183-188, 1985.

129. Yen R, Quesenberry N: Pituitary function in pseydocyesis. J Clin Endocrinol Metab 43:132-136, 1976.

130. Weddington W, Porter S: Pseudocyesis following sterlization: role of the pseudofather. Psychosomatics 25:563-565, 1984.

131. Starkman M: Impact of psychodynamic factors on the course and management of patients with pseudocyesis. Obstet and Gynecol 64:142-145, 1984.

132. Fairweather D: Nausea and vomiting during pregnancy. Obstet Gynecol Annu 7:91-105, 1978.

133. Dozeman R, Kaiser F, Cass O,, et al: Hyperthyroidism appearing as hyperemesis gravidarum. Arch Int Med 143:2202-2203, 1983.

134. Innerfield R, Hollander C: Thyroidal complications of pregnancy. Med Clin North Am 61:67-68, 1977.

135. Bober S, McGill A, Turn bridge W: Thyroid function in hyperemesis gravidarum. Acta Endocrinologica 111:404-410, 1986.

136. Chertok L: The psychopathology of vomiting of pregnancy. In Howells J (Ed): Modern Perspectives in Psycho-Obstetrics. New York, Brunner/Nazel, 1972 pp 269-282.

137. Taylor H: Nausea and vomiting of pregnancy: hyperemesis gravidarum. In Kroger W (ed): Psychosomatic Obstetrics and Gynecology and Endocrinology. Springfield Il, Charles C. THomas 1962.

138. Depue R, Bernstein I, Ross R et al: Hyperemesis gravidarum in relation to estradiol levels, pregnancy outcome, and other maternal factors: A seroepidemiologic study. Am J Obstet Gynecol 156:1137-1141, 1987.

139. Pearlman W, Crepy O, Murphy M: Testosterone-binding levels in the serum of women during normal menstrual cycle, pregnancy and the post-partum period. J Clin Endocrinal Metab 27:1012, 1967.

140. Bernstein L, Depue R, Ross R, et al: Higher maternal levels of free estradiol in first compared to second pregnancy: a study of early gestational differences, J Natl Cancer Inst 76:1035, 1986.

141. MacMahon B, Trichopolous D, Cole P et al: Cigarette smoking and urinary estrogens. N Engl J Med 307:1062, 1982.

142. Klebanoff M, Kaslow RA, Kaslow R et al: Epidemiology of vomiting in early preganacy. Obstet Gynecol 66:612, 1985.

143. Little E, Hook E: Maternal alcohol and tobacco consumption and their association with nausea and vomiting during pregnancy. Acta Obstet Gynecol Scand 58:15, 1979.

144. Kallen B: Hyperemesis during pregacy and delivery outcome: a registry study. Eur J Obstet Gynecol Reprod Biol 26:291-302, 1987.

145. Schoeneck F: Gonadotropin hormone concentrations in emesis gravidarum. Am J Obstet Gynecol 43:308, 1942.

146. Kauppila A, Keikinheimo M, Lohela H et al: Human Chorionic gonadotrophin and pregnancy-specific beta-1-glycoprotein in predicting pregancy outcome and in association with early pregancy vomiting. Gynecol Obstet Invest 18:49-53, 1984.

147. Soules M, Hughes C, Garcia J et al: Nausea and vomiting of pregnancy: Role of human chorionic gonadotropin and 17-hydroxyprogesterone. Obstet Gynecol 55:

148. Juras N, Banovac K, Sekso M: Increased serum reverse triiodothyronine in patients with hyperemesis graviarum. Acta Endocrinologica 102:284-287, 1983.

149. Jarnfelt-Samsioe A, Eridsson B, Waldenstrom J et al: Some new aspects on emesis gravidarum: Relations to clinical data, serum electrolytes, total protein and creatinine. Gynecol Obstet Invest 19:174-186, 1985.

150. Deutsch H: The Psychology of Women: Vol II. Motherhood. New York. Grune and Stratton, 1945.

151. Uddenberg N, Nilsson A, Almgren P: Pregnancy psychological and psychosomatic aspects. J Psychosom Res 15:269-276, 1971.

152. Katon W, Ries R, Bokan J et al: Hyperemesis gravidarum: a biopsychosocial perspective. Int J Pscyhiatry Med 10:151-162, 1980.

153. Fairweather D: Nausea and vomiting during pregnancy. Am J Obstet Gynec 102:135-175, 1968.

154. Kaltenbach R: Ueber Hyperemesis Gravidarum. Z Geburtschilfe Gynaekol 21:200, 1981.

154a. Long M, Simone S, Tuchner J: Outpatient Treatment of Hyperemesis Gravidarum with Stimulus Control and Imagery Procedures. J Behav Ther & Exp Psychiatr 17:105-109, 1986.

155. Engel G: The need for a new medical model: a challenge for biomedicine. Science 196:129-136, 1977.

156. Robertson G: Nausea and vomiting of pregnancy. Lancet 2:336, 1946.

157. Freud S, Breuer J: Studies on hysteria. In Frued S (ed): Complete Psychological Works. Standard Edition 2. London. Hogarth Press, 1955.

158. Weiss E, English O: Psychosomatic Medicine, ed 3. Philadelphia, WB Saunders, 1957.

159. Palmer R: A psychosomatic study of vomiting of early pregnancy. J Psychosom Res 17:303-208, 1973.

160. Harvey W, Sherfey M: Vomiting in pregnancy. Psychosom Med 16:1, 1954.

161. Tylden E: Hyperemesis and physiological vomiting. J Psychosom Res 12:85, 1968.

162. Wokind S, Zajick E: Psychosocial correlates of nausea and vomiting in pregnancy. J Psychosom Res 22:1-5, 1978.

163. Fairweather D: Hyperemesis gravidarum. MD thesis. University of St. Andrews, 1965.

164. Fitzgerald J: Epidemiolody of hyperemsesis gravidarum. Lancet 1:606-662, 1956.

165. Lavin P. Smith D, Kori S et al: Wernicke's encephalopathy: A predictable complication of hyperemesis gravidarum. Obs & Gyn 62:13S-15S, 1983.

166. Friederich MA: Psychological Aspects of Chronic Pelvic Pain. Clin Obs and Gyn 19:399-406, 1976.

167. Barsky J, Klerman G: Overview: Hypochondriasis, Bodily Complaints, and Somatic Styles. Amer J Psychiatry 140:273:283, 1983.

168. Bonica J: The management of pain. Lea & Febiger, Phila, Pa 1953.

169. Renaer M, Vertommen II, Nijs P et al: Psychological aspects of chronic pelvic pain in women. A J Obstet Gynecol, 134:75-80, 1979.

170. Castelnuovo-Tedesco P, Krout BM: Psychosomatic Aspects of Chronic Pelvic Pain, Int J Psychiatry Med, 1:109-126, 1970.

171. Engel G: Psychogenic pain and the pain-prone patients. Am J Med 26:899-918, 1959.

172. Gidro-Grank L, Gordon T, Taylor HC: Pelvic pain and female identity: A survey of emotional factors in 40 patients. Amer J Obstet Gynec, 79:1184-1202, 1960.

173. Walker E, Katon W, Harrop-Griffiths J et al: Relationship of Chronic Pelvic Pain to Psychiatric Diagnosis and Childhood Sexual Abuse, Am J Psychiatry, 145:75-80, 1988.

174. Magni G, Salmi A, de Leo D et al: Chronic Pelvic Pain and Depression. Psychopathology, 17: 132-136, 1984.

175. Duncan CH, Taylor HC: Psychosomatic study of pelvic congestion. Amer J Obstet Gynce, 64:1-12, 1952.

176. Levitan Z, Eibschitz, de Vries K et al: The Value of Laparoscopy in Women with Chronic Pelvic Pain and a "Normal Pelvis", Int J Gynaecol Obstet, 23:71-74, 1985.

177. Sternbach RA, Wolf SR, Murphy RW et al: Aspects of chronic low back pain, Psychosomatics, 14:52, 1973.

178. Taylor HC: Vascular congestion and hyperemia. Their effect on structure and function in the female reproductive system. Amer J Obstet Gynec, 67:1177-1196, 1954.

179. Lunberg WI, Wall JE, Mathers JE: Laparoscopy in the evaluation of pelvic pain, Obstet Gynecol, 42:872, 1973.

180. Beard RW, Highman JH, Pearce S et al: Diagnosis of pelvic varicosities in women with chronic pelvic pain. Lancet, 2:946-949, 1984.

181. Kresch A, Seiter D, Sachs L, et al: Laparoscopy in 100 Women with Chronic Pelvic Pain. Bos Gyn, 64:672-674, 1984.

182. Semchyhyn S, Strickler RC: Laparoscopy: Is it replacing clinical acumen? Obstet Gynecol, 48:615, 1976.

183. Gillebrand PN: Investigation of Pelvic Pain. Communication at the Scientific Meeting on Chronic Pelvic Pain - A Gynecologic Headache, Royal College of Obstetricians and Gynecologists, May 1981.

184. Pent D: Pent D: Laparoscopy: Its role in private practice. Am J Obstet Gynecol, 113:459, 1972.

185. Snaith L, Ridley B: Gynecological psychiatry. Brit Med J, 2:418-421, 1948.

186. Lock FR, Connelly JF: The incidence of psychosomatic disease from a private referred gynecologic practice. Amer J Obstet Gynec, 54:783-790, 1947.

187. Beard RW, Belsey EM, Liebernab BA et al: Pelvic pain in women. Am J Obstet Gyne, 128:566-570, 1977.

188. Winokur G, Cadoret R, Dorzab J: Depressive disease: a genetic study. Archs Gen Psychit, 24:135-144, 1971.

189. Clouse R, Lustman P: Psychiatric illness and contraction abnormalities of the esophagus. NEJM, 309:1339-1342, 1983.

190. Katon W, Egan K, Miller D: Chronic Pain: Lifetime Psychiatric diagnosis and family history. Am J Psychiatry, 142:1156-1160, 1985.

191. Garvey M, Schaffer C, Tuason V: Relationship of headaches to depression. Br J Psychiatry. 143:544-547, 1983.

192. Young S, Alpers D, Norland C, et al: Psychiatric illness, and the irritable bowel syndrome: practical implications for the primary care physician. Gastroenterology 70:162-169, 1976.

193. Beresin E: Impiramine in the treatment of chronic pelvic pain. Psychosomatics 27:294-296, 1986.

866

194. Pearce S, Knight C, Beard RW: Pelvic Pain: a common gynecological problem, J Psychosom Obstet Gyne, 1:12, 1982.

195. Benson RC, Hanson KH, Matarzzo JD: Atypical pelvic pain in women: Gynecologic psychiatric considerations. Amer J Obstet Gyne, 77:806-825, 1959.

PSYCHOLOGICAL DISTRESS IN ONCOLOGY PATIENTS

Michael E. Stefanek, Ph.D.
Assistant Professor, Oncology and Medical Psychology
Johns Hopkins University School of Medicine
The Johns Hopkins Oncology Center B150
600 North Wolfe Street
Baltimore, MD 21205

CONTENTS:

PSYCHOLOGICAL DISTRESS IN ONCOLOGY PATIENTS
Michael E. Stefanek, Ph.D.

It is reasonable to state that, with the recent exception of AIDS, no disease diagnosis is viewed with as much fear and dread as the diagnosis of cancer. This fear is likely engendered by the awareness of the high incidence of cancer and the fact that it strikes the best and worst of us, both sexes, all ages, ethnic, and economic groups. In addition, cancer is unfortunately typically viewed as a fatal disease, involving intensive, difficult treatment regimens with distressing side effects – in short, a painful, protracted, expensive, and, on occasion, fruitless process. It is not surprising that psychological distress often occurs with the diagnosis and treatment of this illness. This chapter will deal with assessment issues, the prevalence and type of psychological distress among adult cancer patients, variables related to psychological adjustment, sexual concerns/issues of cancer patients and research detailing what we know about adjustment of cancer "survivors".

ASSESSMENT ISSUES

Until recently the literature examining psychological reactions to cancer has relied on assessment instruments developed for use with psychiatric populations rather than the physically ill. This obviously poses diagnostic validity problems. For example, somatic symptoms due to cancer and somatic symptoms of depression may overlap and make assessment a difficult task. Some confounding possibilities which may cloud the diagnostic picture include fatigue and loss of appetite from radiation and/or chemotherapy treatments, anxiety and restlessness as a side effect of antiemetic therapy (e.g. Reglan, Compazine) or a direct result of tumor (e.g., pheochromocytoma), mixed emotional reactions and sleep disturbances as a result of intracranial tumors, steroids, or electrolyte or mineral imbalances.

Fortunately, since Plumb and Holland (1) noted the difficult task of teasing apart psychiatric symptomatology from symptoms resulting from disease itself, some attention has been paid to the development and standardization of instruments for specific populations of medically ill patients.

In terms of multidimensional symptom inventories, the SCL-90-R and Brief Symptom Inventory (BSI) (2,3) have been most extensively utilized with medical/cancer patients (4,5,6). The SCL-90 and BSI report distress on nine clinical scales: Somatization, Obsessive Compulsiveness, Interpersonal Sensitivity, Depression, Anxiety, Hostility, Phobic Anxiety, Paranoid Ideation, and Psychoticism. In addition three summary measures of distress are scored, including the General Severity Index (GSI), the Positive Symptom Distress Index (PSDI), and the Positive Symptom Total (PST). The GSI is the most sensitive of the three global scores and is derived by dividing the grand total by the total number of items (thus providing information on frequency and severity). The PST is derived by counting all non zero symptoms responses (frequency), while the PSDI is calculated by dividing the grand total by the PST (severity per item endorsed). The patient rates each item on a 5-point scale. These instruments have proven sensitive to psychological distress in oncology patients (7,8) and also have established norms for psychiatric outpatients, psychiatric inpatients, and nonpatients, with separate norms available for men and women. Added strengths include the distinct measure of nine primary symptom dimensions, three global summary scores, and brevity of administration (approximately 10 and 20 minutes for the BSI and SCL-90-R, respectively).

In terms of affect and mood measures, there are two measures with much to recommend them. The POMS (Profile of Mood States) is a 65-item adjective checklist utilized frequently in psychosocial oncology research assessing six primary mood states, including tension-anxiety, depression-dejection, confusion, anger-hostility, vigor, and fatigue (9). The scale is brief (10-15 minutes) to complete, has acceptable internal consistency and test-retest reliability at one month (10), and has demonstrated predictive validity in psychotherapy (11) and psychopharmacology (12) change studies. The Affect Balance Scale (ABS) (13) is a 40-item instrument assessing four negative dimensions (anxiety, dimension, guilt, hostility) and four positive dimensions (joy, contentment, vigor, affection), and includes an overall difference score between positive and negative affect. This scale is also brief, taking 5-10 minutes to complete, and has norms on psychiatric inpatients, psychiatric outpatients and nonpatient normals. In addition, some evidence of predictive validity exists, including an investigation with a breast cancer population (14). The distinction between negative and positive affect and the difference between these dimensions presented as a summary score is a core feature of this instrument and makes it an attractive one in psychosocial oncology research.

Depression is a common feature among oncology patients and is perhaps the affective state which has prompted the most assessment instruments. There appears to be a great deal of overlap across self report/observer measures of this symptom. In a recent review (15), correlations between the Beck Depression Inventory (16) and a variety of other measures of depression including clinical ratings were reported across 35 studies. Concurrent validity with the Hamilton Rating Scale for Depression, Zung and MMPI-D Scale across different samples including depressed, alcoholic, drug abusers, college undergraduates, cardiac patients and chronic pain patients have been rather consistenty high.

Generally, correlation coefficients have ranged from .60 to .80. It has also demonstrated concurrent validity with the SCL-90-R (2). It is clear that the Beck Depression Inventory (BDI) has become one of the most widely used instruments for assessing depression (15). However, as with other depression scales, somatic items are included which are potentially confounded with medical illness in a population such as cancer patients. In two related reports (17,18) the BDI was administered to medically ill inpatients (n=335), depressed patients (n-101), and normal controls (N=104) in an attempt to determine those items which discriminate depression in the medically ill. The medical patients reported each of the somatic symptoms (work inhibition, sleep disturbance, fatigue, anorexia, weight loss, health worries, decreased interest in sex) except decreased interest in sex, between 50% and 75% of the time. Thus, these symptoms are very prevalent among the medically ill regardless of mood state. Several other interesting findings emerged. Items that discriminated for depressive severity in the psychiatric and normal sample, but not in the medical sample included hopelessness, guilt, self-hate, self-blame, irritability, poor body image, work inhibition, and fatigue. That is, severity of depression among the medically ill sample could not be predicted by the presence of these symptoms. One item which discriminated depressive severity in the medical sample, but not the other samples, was crying. This finding suggests that tearfulness should be assessed carefully as a sign of concurrent depression. Symptoms that discriminated for severity of depression in the medical sample and the psychiatric-normal samples were: dissatisfaction, loss of social interest, indecision, sense of failure, sense of punishment, and suicidal thoughts, with the best discriminants including dissatisfaction and loss of social interest. Among medical patients, scores on the somatic items increased only minimally as depression worsened. Thus, in the medical population, specific cognitive/affective symptoms may be the best indicators for severity of depression, while somatic symptoms are not indicative of depression.

An investigation specifically assessing depressive symptoms in cancer patients vs. physically healthy suicide attempters (n=99) utilizing the BSI supports this notion (1). While mean BDI scores among the cancer patients placed them in the not-depressed range, cancer patients and physically healthy suicide attempt patients had nearly identical means for physical items. Thus physical symptoms, while critical in the assessment of depression among healthy individuals, do not appear to discriminate very efficiently among medically ill or cancer patients. More specifically, the presence of mild work inhibition, sleep disturbance, fatigue, anorexia, weight loss, and worry about health should not be considered as evidence of depression among oncology patients. However, if these symptoms are severe and out of proportion to what is known about the physical illness and appear in tandem with cognitive/affective symptoms, they may certainly be viewed as supportive of the diagnosis of depression.

Thus, given the history and psychometric properties of the Beck Depression Inventory, its use is recommended with the caveat noted above regarding reliance on somatic symptoms. Other assessment instruments such as the Raskin Depression Scale and Hamilton Rating Scale for Depression may be too somatically focused for general use among cancer patients without major allowances for confounding of illness-related somatic symptoms.

PREVALENCE OF PSYCHOLOGICAL DISTRESS

As Derogatis et al (4) note, the association between cancer and psychological stress has a long historical base. Galen reported this relationship (19) and a number of 18th and 19th century physicians have indicated a relationship between cancer and psychological disorders (20). However, it is only relatively recently that formal prevalence studies of psychiatric disorder among cancer patients have appeared in the literature (7,21). In one of the first attempts to quantify levels of symptomatology and differentiate symptom patterns beyond global descriptions of emotional distress, Craig and Abeloff (7) utilized a self report 90 item symptom inventory, the SCL-90, which assessed the degree to which the respondent is distressed by each item during a specified time period (usually 1-2 weeks). Results of the Craig and Abeloff investigation indicated that more than half of the patients showed moderate to high levels of depression, and roughly one-third had elevated levels of anxiety. Nearly one-fourth had overall symptom patterns virtually identical to those seen in patients admitted to an emergency psychiatric service. The summary scores noted above were not reported, and other symptom dimensions of the SCL-90 were not elevated beyond those seen in normal populations. Despite the sample size limitations (n=30) this was an important investigation in providing suggestive evidence of the prevalence and type of emotional distress for further investigations and in raising questions about the often-held notion that virtually all cancer patients are suffering significant emotional distress (22). Although other reports followed (1,21), three recent investigations worthy of reviewing in some detail (4,5,6) have utilized a standard psychometric instrument, sampled inpatient and outpatient populations, included series of patients large enough to warrant some degree of generalization, and assessed a wide range of psychiatric disorders.

The first such investigation (4) assessed 215 (inpatient and outpatient) cancer patients at 3 major regional cancer centers. This sample consisted of patients who were new admissions to the inpatient or outpatient facilities of the hospital, at least 19 years old, were engaged in active treatment, and had scores on the Karnofsky Performance Scale (23) of at least 50 ("requires considerable assistance and frequent medical care"). These investigators used a psychiatric interview, observer ratings, and a self report measure, the SCL-90, to determine the level, nature, and prevalence of psychiatric disorders. The observer rating scores consisted of the Raskin Depression Screen (24) and the Global Adjustment to Illness Scale (25). The basic finding of this study indicated that 101 of 215 patients examined were appropriate for a DSM-III psychiatric diagnosis. Thus a prevalence rate for psychiatric disturbance of 47% was reported (see Table 1). Sixty-eight percent (68%) of these diagnoses consisted of adjustment disorders, i.e. 32% across the entire sample. As noted in Table 1, the next most frequent diagnoses involved major affective disorders, with a prevalence rate of 6% (13% of all diagnoses). Focusing upon conditions that feature prominent depression, anxiety or both as a central component, these conditions had a prevalence rate of 40% in the sample, while accounting for 85% of the diagnoses.

A second investigation (5) assessed psychological distress among oncology outpatients, again utilizing the SCL-90-R with 141 oncology outpatients, 70% of whom were receiving active treatment for this illness. Approximately 50% reported no activity limitations as a result of their illness, with approximately 90% of the patients experiencing disease remission or stable disease at the time of SCL-90-R completion. Results revealed that mean psychological distress scores on the SCL-90, although somewhat elevated compared to nonpatient norms, fell within "normal" limits, with the exception, as would be expected with this population, of the Somatization scale. Moderate-high distress was reported by 31% of the sample (GSI summary scale), with 40% reporting moderate-high depression, and 28% reporting moderate-high levels of anxiety. Overall, 34% of the patients had scores on at least one SCL-90 scale (excluding Somatization) two standard deviations or more above the mean of the non-patient norm group.

Finally, a recent investigation (6), assessed the psychological status of 126 oncology outpatients with heterogenous diagnoses and generally normal activity status. Patients completed the Brief Symptom Inventory (BSI) (3) during their initial visit to a major oncology center. The BSI is a 53 item abbreviated version of the SCL-90, measuring identical symptom constructs, and demonstrates excellent correlations with the SCL-90-R across all symptom dimensions. The percentages of patients attaining levels of moderate or high distress on the nine BSI scales and three summary scales are presented in Table 2. The percentages of patients with moderate and high levels of distress range from 38.8% (Somatization) to 15.1% (Interpersonal Sensitivity), based on nonpatient norms, the latter also used for comparative purposes in both the Farber (5) and Derogatis (4) investigations. Of interest was the finding that 19% of the sample had a score on one or more clinical scales (excluding Somatization) equal to or greater than two standard deviations above the mean of the nonpatient norms. Moderate to high levels of depression and anxiety were reported by 32% and 35% of the sample.

In summary, three investigations utilizing (1) relatively large samples, (2) instruments with standardized scores (T-scores) and established reliability validity, and normative groups, and with (3) reasonably high compliance (66%-82%) have been completed to determine prevalence and type of emotional distress among cancer patients (see Table 3). Findings across investigations are generally consistent. Across each investigation, moderately elevated anxiety and depression were commonly reported. Based on the above investigations, and despite differences in patient status (i.e. out/inpatient) and in the timing of assessments (e.g. initial visit vs. later in treatment), it appears that approximately 20-35% of cancer patients warrant, at minimum, evaluation for elevated emotional distress. This is based on the finding by Stefanek et al (6) that 1 in 5 patients scored two or more standard deviations above the nonpatient norms, and the Farber et al (5) finding of approximately 1 in 5 patients scoring in the same range on the Depression (18.8%) and Anxiety (13.4%) subscales, as well as the General Severity Index summary scale (19.1%). It should be noted that patients in both of the investigations above were generally of good performance status, and, as will be discussed in a subsequent section, poor performance status is a variable predictive of emotional distress. In fact, the Derogatis et al (4) investigation found rather widely varying prevalence rates for psychiatric diagnoses across treatment settings, a difference ascribed, in part, to differences in performance status.

These findings indicate that most patients appear to respond to the diagnosis and treatment of cancer without significantly elevated emotional distress. A significant minority of patients do, however, report moderate-severe emotional distress, and, based on the Derogatis investigation, this distress is potentially treatable (adjustment disorders major affective disorders) with psychotherapeutic and/or pharmacological approaches.

. 71

Of interest is the prevalence of psychological distress in cancer patients vs. psychiatric morbidity among general hospital populations. Although difficult to interpret due to definitional and instrumentation problems, along with population heterogeneity, it appears that about one-third of medical inpatients report mild-moderate depression, while perhaps as many as one-fourth suffer with severe depression (26). One recent investigation (27) examined psychological status across five different chronic illnesses including arthritis (n=84), diabetes (n=199), cancer (n=193), renal disease (n=60), and dermatologic disorders (n=122) vs. patients under treatment for depression. Utilizing the Mental Health Index (28) as a dependent measure, no significant differences were found across chronic illness categories, including no differences on depression and anxiety subscales. All chronic illness categories reported less distress than the depression sample. Thus, assumptions of diagnosis-specific emotional responses may be untenable, and a basic similarity in psychological status among patients with different chronic physical illnesses may exist. As will be seen in the following section, variables other than disease type may well be critical in predicting psychological adjustment.

VARIABLES RELATED TO ADJUSTMENT

As noted previously, the negative impact of cancer diagnosis and treatment on psychological distress is quite well documented. There exists a great deal of variation in the degree to which emotional distress is self-reported across cancer patients. One obvious aim is to predict those patients who will report elevated psychological distress, to detect this emerging distress cost-efficiently and facilitate subsequent interventions, particularly since this distress is potentially very treatable. In two of the prevalence investigations previously described in some detail (5,6) predictors were not plentiful. Farber (5) found no differences in distress across sex, treatment (receiving treatment vs. no treatment), status of disease (in remission or not), or performance status variables. Likewise, Stefanek et al (6) found no relationship between depression, anxiety, and overall psychological distress and marital status, sex, or activity status. A caveat is the fact that both samples consisted primarily of ambulatory outpatients with generally good performance/activity status. Derogatis et al (4), on the other hand, found that patients within each treatment setting with lower Karnofsky Performance Scale scores (more physically impaired) had a higher prevalence of diagnosed psychiatric disorders. The study by Cassileth et al (27) investigating the prevalence of psychological distress across chronic illnesses, found a direct relation between declining physical status and psychological distress. Within their cancer subsample, patients capable of normal activity fared significantly better emotionally than symptomatic or bedridden patients. Of interest was this investigation finding that length of time from diagnosis was significantly related to distress. More specifically, patients whose illness had been diagnosed for three months or less had significantly more distress than those diagnosed for longer intervals. This result was not corroborated by the Derogatis et al (4), Farber et al (5) or Stefanek et al (6) investigations. It is possible that time since diagnosis is less sensitive within oncology diagnoses, since recurrences, remissions, and patient uncertainty related to prognosis complicate this variable. Not surprisingly Cassileth et al (27) also found that patients completing their course of therapy had better psychological status than patients under active treatment, and that patients under active treatment reported less distress than patients under palliative care.

Obviously, there is some danger in generalizing findings related to predictor variables in a study incorporating analyses across disease categories, but data exist that lend some support to these latter findings (29). An investigation assessing the relationship between psychological distress, extent of disease, and performance status in patients with lung cancer, utilized the Profile of Mood States (POMS) (10). Consistent with results utilizing the SCL-90 and BSI (5,6), mean subtest and total scores for the entire sample (n=455) fell within the normal (college sample) range. Findings revealed a significant relationship between extent of physical impairment and Total Mood Disturbance score on the POMS, in addition to a main effect for gender (women reporting elevated emotional distress). Extent of disease contributed to psychological distress only with poorer performance status. Of note considering the lack of relationship between physical status and distress in previously discussed investigations (5,6) is the finding that patients with performance status indicating severe (vs. none or moderate) impairment were at risk for high distress. As the authors note (29), there may be a threshold at which physical variables (e.g. performance status, extent of disease) begin to exert an effect on psychological adjustment, and that, prior to reaching this threshold of severity, physical/disease variables may exert little impact on psychological adjustment. Finally, despite these statistically significant findings, extent of disease and performance status predicted only about 10-15% of the variability in POMS scores, thus indicating the importance of other variables in determining the psychological response to cancer.

Weisman and Worden (30) were among the first investigators to attend to discerning variables which might predict emotional distress. One hundred sixty three (n=163) patients across several diagnostic grouping (breast, n=40; GI, n=32; Hodgkins, n=21; lung, n=40; melanoma, n-30) were assessed within 10 days of hospitalization and then followed at 4-6 week intervals for a 6-month period. Specifically, patients were assessed with 2-hour semistructured interviews, and a number of psychological inventories and rating scales including the MMPI, Thematic Apperception Test (TAT), POMS, and Inventory of Predominant Concerns. The latter is a list of 72 concerns related to illness, including health, work/finances, religion, family, friends, self appraisal, and existential concerns. While the modal staging category was regional spread of disease, staging ranged from local (19%-67% across diagnostic groupings) to distant metastases (6%-35% across diagnoses). From initial evaluation through follow-ups, eighty-one percent (81%) of all patients received surgery, 37% of all patients received radiation and 15% received chemotherapy. Males (44%) and females (56%) were equally represented, although, as expected, all of the breast cancer sample was female, while all of the lung cancer sample was male. Emotional distress at each assessment was based upon the combination of the Total Mood Disturbance scale of the POMS and a Vulnerability scale, derived from ratings during the semistructured interview (4 point scale) on variables such as Hopelessness, Frustration, Denial, etc (30,31). Table 4 displays a predictive profile that differentiates patients reporting low emotional distress vs. those reporting high emotional distress at follow-up intervals. Multiple regression analysis indicated that at any one assessment, 40-60% of emotional distress could be attributed to medical factors. In addition, on the Inventory of Predominant Concerns, the rank order of concerns did not change with time, with existential (e.g. concerned about future, taking things too seriously) and work-finance being paramount. While there was a tendency for frequency of problems to diminish after the first 8-10 weeks, level of distress did not follow this pattern. In fact, 60% of patients reported maximum emotional distress at some point beyond the first ten weeks of illness. Obviously, cancer progression or side effects of treatment play a role in this increased distress; however, noting the findings that only 40-60% of distress was related to medical factors, it appears that some psychosocial variables persist at least partly independent of physical status. Non-medical problems predominated when patients were asked to rate the most urgent problems at peak psychological distress. Consistent with this is a recent finding that worry among cancer patients is dominated by such issues as family coping with a patient's illness, emotional impact of the illness on family/friends, finances, and returning to normal activity level, in addition to worries such as survival and efficacy of treatment (32). Finally, all patients reported periodic psychosocial concerns and episodes of distress, although, not unexpectedly, peak levels of emotional distress fluctuated widely.

Overall, the investigators found that the most vulnerable patients were pessimistic, with regrets about the past, a history of depression, from multi-problem families, with current marital problems. These patients reported little anticipation of emotional support, and were of lower socioeconomic status (Table 4).

Of some interest is the use of psychological testing to predict postdiagnosis psychosocial adjustment. Sobel and Worden (33) administered the MMPI to patients with five different neoplastic diseases (breast, n=34; colon, n=23; lung, n=28; malignant melanoma, n=28) and Hodgkins disease (n=20) to determine the extent to which MMPI scales could differentiate cancer patients who report low distress versus those who cope poorly with the disease.

Assessment following MMPI administration occurred every 4-6 weeks for a total of five follow-up assessments. Dependent measures of adjustment included a composite emotional distress indicator consisting of the POMS and Index of Vulnerability, percentage of problems in six psychosocial areas (Inventory of Predominant Concerns), and actual problem resolutions, i.e. patients effectiveness in solving specific illness-related problems. A multiple regression analysis showed that significant amounts of variance could be accounted for based solely upon the MMPI Scales, including 51% of the variance of the Inventory of Predominant Concerns, and 41% of the variance of the composite emotional distress variable. Specifically, statistically significant mean differences on 8 of the 14 scales were found, including a significant difference between the low distress and high distress groups on the three "neurotic" triad scales (Hs, D, Hy). A further discriminant analysis correctly categorized 75% of the cancer patients into the high or low distress group. Although the MMPI is obviously not practical for all cancer patients, the fact that it accounts for significant amounts of variance in predicting psychological distress, in addition to the previously mentioned mixed results relating disease variables to distress, emphasizes the importance of looking beyond purely disease/physical status variables in predicting patients who may fall into the "high distress" category following diagnosis.

In summary, the investigations reviewed above emphasize the complexity of predicting emotional distress among cancer patients. While studies indicate a significant minority of cancer patients report significant distress, it is apparent that the diagnosis and/or treatment of these illnesses in and of themselves do not prompt high distress, either during the early stages related to diagnosis (6) or months post-diagnosis (30,31). In Weisman and Wordens work (30), 25%-38% of the variance in emotional distress was unaccounted for across follow-ups (i.e. 25-38% of distress unexplained by the variables examined). Therefore, identifying psychosocial variables, particularly those potentially modifiable (Table 4) continues to be a critical need in the area of psychosocial/behavorial oncology.

PSYCHOLOGICAL DISTRESS: SITE-SPECIFIC DATA

Due to criticisms that generalizations across cancer sites may be untenable as a function of differing treatments, side effects, and prognoses, among other factors, a number of investigators have focused upon specific diagnostic groups to determine the type, prevalence, and course of psychological distress. For example, in two investigations examining depressive illness and lung cancer (34,35), 16% of a total 134 patients manifested major depressive illness, with a past history of psychiatric illness and presence of metastatic disease the most significant correlates of depression. The emotional impact/psychological problems associated with a diagnosis of lymphoma has also been addressed (36,37,38). These investigations have involved prospective (37,38) and retrospective studies (36) with findings indicating a prevalence rate of significant anxiety and/or depression of 22%-38%. In one of the more systematic investigations (37), albeit without a control group comparison, 120 patients newly diagnosed with Hodgkins and non-Hodgkins lymphoma were interviewed using a brief version of the Present State Examination at diagnosis, two, six, and twelve months post diagnosis. While psychiatric morbidity was greatest between diagnosis and treatment and early in the course of treatment (48% and 73% of depressive illnesses and anxiety states occurred initially during months 1-3), anxiety and depressive episodes did continue to develop throughout the 12 month follow-up. Of interest, and an area to be discussed in a later section of this chapter, although most patients were finished treatment and free of disease at the one year follow-up, significant morbidity remained. Approximately 40% of patients continued to report loss of energy, 15-20%, loss of libido and irritability, and 10-15% of poor concentration and memory impairment, respectively.

An investigation assessing the prevalence of major depression found that 19 of 83 (23%) patients with cervical, endometrial, or vaginal cancer being evaluated for cancer staging and for initial cancer treatment met DSM III Criteria by psychiatric interview, and Hamilton Rating Scale for major depression (39). This result is not significantly different from the higher range of prevalence rates found in investigations of hospitalized cancer patients (7,40).

Although investigations across other diagnostic groups have been reported (41), in terms of sheer frequency of research reports related to psychological distress, breast cancer patients have been most extensively assessed.

BREAST CANCER

Psychological Distress

Breast cancer strikes approximately 120,000 women in this country annually, accounts for more than one-fourth of all women's cancers, and will develop in roughly 1 of every 10 women in their lifetime (42). There is little question that breast cancer and its treatment impact upon a woman's psychological, social, and sexual world. Meyerowitz (43) provided an initial review of research prior to 1980 describing psychosocial correlates of breast cancer in an attempt to organize a large but relatively unstructured body of literature. In terms of psychological discomfort, consistent findings included a moderate-high level of depression, anxiety and/or anger, similar to levels found in studies assessing psychological distress across diagnoses (4,6). Disruption in everyday life patterns was common, including marital/sexual relationships. In one investigation, 40% of breast cancer patients having undergone mastectomy reported sexual difficulties at a 4-month follow-up compared to 11% of control group of benign breast tumor biopsy patients (44). Overall, methodological problems of these earlier studies precluded definitive statements regarding the prevalence and type of psychosocial consequences of the diagnosis, hospitalization, surgery and follow-up treatment of breast cancer. Unfortunately, researchers most often did not control for such variables as spread of disease, type of treatment received, or age at diagnosis, nor was information typically reported on the reliability or validity of assessment instruments. However, despite the lack of specific findings based upon reasonably rigorous studies, there is a rather striking consistent trend. Virtually all of these early investigations reported common psychological discomfort involving depression, anxiety and hostility, often extending well beyond physical recovery from surgery. Changes in life patterns reflected by physical discomfort, marital/sexual changes, activity level reductions, fears and concerns revolving around issues of recurrence, death, mutilation, and loss of feminity were common findings reported. A number of investigations have followed, often specifically addressing differences in adjustment across different treatment regimens or following breast cancer patients longitudinally to assess psychosocial impact. McArdle et al (45) assessed social, emotional, and financial implication of adjuvant chemotherapy.

Chemotherapy consisted of Cyclophosphamide, Methotrexate, and 5-FU (CMF) beginning 4-6 weeks post surgery for 1 year given days 1 and 8 of 28-day cycles. Utilizing the General Hospital Questionnaire psychiatric morbidity was present in 36% of the patients (n=107 stage II patients) post diagnosis but pre-mastectomy. Measurements at 1,3 and 6 months post-mastectomy showed no difference in morbidity across three treatment groups (radiation alone, chemotherapy alone, radiation plus chemotherapy). However, at 12 months (completion of chemotherapy) depression was significantly higher in the chemotherapy groups (38%) vs. radiation alone (6%). At 18 months, the pattern was similar, with less morbidity. In a similar investigation by the same authors (46), psychological symptoms were assessed over 2 years in a randomized trial of 3 forms of treatment administered after mastectomy for stage II patients. The treatments were identical to those noted in the previous study, and involved follow-up at 1,3, 6, 13, 18, and 24 months post-simple mastectomy with the General Health Questionnaire. While emotional distress decreased in the radiotherapy group from a high of 39% at 3 months to 16% and 14% at 13, and 24 months respectively, chemotherapy only patients reported distress in the 20-30% range through month 13, decreasing to 5% at months 18 and 24. Finally, the prevalence of emotional distress in the combined treatment group ranged from 26-41% through month 13, decreasing to 15% at months 18 and 24. Thus, of patients receiving combined treatment, the duration of which exceeded the other two treatment groups, psychiatric morbidity decreased significantly at the end of treatment across measures. Specifically, severe depression was reported by only 10-15% of patients in the combined group at 18 and 24 months respectively on the General Health Questionnaire. In both investigations, survival was significantly greater for patients in the chemotherapy groups by the 24 month follow-up (38% of patients undergoing radiotherapy had died vs. 12% in the chemotherapy groups). Thus, the benefit of these studies lie not in treatment decision making but in assessing the distress associated with the more effective adjuvant chemotherapy regimens for premenopausal and postmenopausal women with positive axillary lymph nodes. Other investigations have found increased psychiatric morbidity in women receiving multiple agent adjuvant therapy vs. mastectomy or single agent adjuvant treatment (47). Meyerowitz, in an uncontrolled interview assessment, reported that all women (n=50 stage II patients) experienced adverse changes during adjuvant chemotherapy, with 88% reporting decreased activity. However, 74% of these women indicated they would recommend adjuvant treatment. In the Knobf study, utilizing among other instruments the Psychiatric Status Schedule (48), diagnosis was perceived as the most stressful event, followed by loss of the breast and uncertainty of survival. Depression and anxiety were significantly correlated with change in appearance, feelings about uncertainty of survival, and pessimism regarding treatment. Distress was found to persist beyond therapy proper, consistent with other investigators (49), with 35% of women expressing mixed or insecure feelings about the termination of adjuvant therapy. Again, the findings of the majority of these studies are limited, due to differing sensitivities of the instruments utilized (General Health Questionnaire, Psychiatric Status Schedule) or nonrandom samples (50). However, implications for clinical practice would indicate the need to follow women throughout adjuvant therapy and beyond, since some women (10-15%) continue to report significant psychiatric distress at 6-12 months post-chemotherapy treatment.

Postmastectomy Adjustment

The psychosocial impact of mastectomy has been a relatively well-researched area within psychosocial oncology. One of the earlier important and systematic investigations in this area (51) compared 40 newly diagnosed post-mastectomy patients with 50 women with other types of cancer using the MMPI Depression Scale, POMS, observer ratings, and the Inventory of Predominant Concerns (30). Findings indicated no differences on measures of depression or self esteem between the diagnostic groupings, with about 20% of women reporting problems in these areas across the five assessments completed at 4-6 week intervals. Consistent with this was a subsequent investigation (52) in which 60% of women with a mean post-mastectomy interval of 22 months rated their adjustment as "very good", 23% "good", 7% "adequate" and 10% "not good". Those reporting better adjustment were older, married longer, and reported more emotional support from physicians, nurses, spouses, and children. The most emotionally distressing period reported was the time immediately after finding the lump (42%), while approximately 1 in 4 women reported suicidal ideation after mastectomy.

Other studies support the findings that mastectomy need not have a long term effect on psychological functioning (53,54). Schottenfeld and Robbins (53) found 84% of patients reporting a return to preoperative employment and functioning 5 years post-surgery. Craig et al (54) with breast cancer patients diagnosed more than 5 years previously, found no differences between this group and two population control groups (matched for age, sex, and neighborhood) other than a small increase in overall disability in the patient group.

A large (n=412) prospective study (55) of patients with modified radical mastectomies for stage I and II breast cancer (n=145) compared this group with samples of patients treated with cholecystectomy for gall bladder disease (n=90), biopsies for benign breast disease (n=87) and healthy women (n=90). All were between 30-70 years of age without pre-existing psychiatric illness and absence of current physical illness, seen within 3 months of surgery and assessed every 4 months for 1 year with a number of instruments, including the Brief Symptom Inventory to determine presence and severity of psycho-pathological symptoms, mood, physical complaints, self esteem, and quality of interpersonal relationships. The findings indicated the mastectomy group did not show psychopathology severe enough to warrant psychiatric intervention more than the other groups over the year period, although they did report more psychosocial, somatic distress, and irritability than the cholecystectomy, biopsy groups or the healthy women. Thus, consistent with other research reported above, while women with breast cancer undergoing mastectomy experience moderate psychological symptomatology and disruption in their daily lives, as a group they do not appear to evidence severe psychiatric sequelae of their surgical procedures. Of interest in this area is a recent investigation (56) contrasting the psychological outcome of lumpectomy and radiation versus mastectomy in stage I or II breast cancer. Fourteen (14) months after surgery these two groups did not differ on the POMS or on the Beck Depression Inventory total score. Lumpectomy patients did report fewer problems with feelings of attractiveness/femininity, less self-consciousness about their appearance, and less restriction on certain tasks (work, leisure activities, shopping, laundry).

In summary, despite methodological shortcomings, particularly in the earlier investigations assessing the psychological impact of breast cancer, several conclusions can be tentatively drawn: 1) breast cancer and its treatment does indeed cause moderate-high emotional distress in a significant minority of women, with estimates ranging from 20-40%; 2) this distress, although often decreased, frequently extends during and after treatment for up to 1-2 years (53,57); 3) multiple treaments (e.g. chemotherapy and radiation) may exacerbate distress, although time in treatment may be the more critical variable; 4) across types of assessment (interview, self report, patients verbal report, observer ratings) although psychosocial sequelae are certainly common, the majority of patients do not experience severe psychopathology or mood disturbance following the diagnosis or treatment of breast cancer.

Predictors of Adjustment to Breast Cancer

Predictors of emotional distress among cancer patients in general have been addressed (see Variables Related to Adjustment) and patient samples in these studies have included breast cancer patients. However, two investigations have specifically targeted adjustment to breast cancer (58,59) and warrant mention. Bloom (58) assessing 133 women with non-metastatic breast cancer from 1 week to 2 1/2 years post surgery, found social support to have direct effects on emotional distress, although information on reliability and validity of the dependent measures selected was not provided. Social support, specifically perception of family cohesiveness and amount of social contact had direct effects on coping; social status and being employed also impacted upon self report ratings of psychological distress. Taylor et al (59) assessed attributions for cancer and beliefs about control over cancer as they relate to adjustment to breast cancer. The sample (n=78) included women who had been treated surgically for breat cancer (status-post lumpectomy or mastectomy 1-60 months), and consisted of 38% stage I cancers, 45% stage II cancer, with 18% of the women having distant sites of metastases . Assessment included interview and self report data (e.g. POMS). Findings indicated that no particular attribution for cancer (e.g. self-blame, external factors, chance, etc.) was related to good psychological functioning. Only blame of another person (e.g. doctors, spouse for creating stress) was related to poor adjustment. Self blame bore no relation to adjustment. The perception that one or others can control ones cancer were both significantly related to good adjustment. Finally, construing benefit from the cancer experience significantly predicted good adjustment, while information control, i.e. cancer related information seeking behavior showed a nonsignificant curvilinear relation to adjustment. Thus, information without control or too much reading about cancer without a direct way of control may predict poor adjustment.

These investigators are important beginning steps in continuing to pinpoint predictors of psychological distress. As previously noted (30), at repeated follow-up assessments of psychological distress throughout the illness process, 25-38% of the variance in distress is unexplained, even when medical treatment variables are included. Thus, the search for variables, including cognitive-social ones, to predict distress continues to be needed, and it certainly seems reasonable to target specific diagnoses/stages of disease initially before testing models across cancers.

EFFECTS OF CANCER ON SEXUAL ACTIVITY

The issue of sexual functioning and cancer is a very complicated one, and, unfortunately, one which still remains in its infancy. There are a complexity of variables which potentially impact upon the physiology, psychology, and interpersonal nature of the sexual response, including the effect of cytotoxic therapy and radiation on gonadal function, performance anxiety due to disrupted body image, decreased energy due to the disease and/or treatment, loss of self esteem, perception of the spouses rejection, and premature menopause induced by treatment, among other factors. In research looking specifically at prevalence of sexual difficulties (60,61) results consistently indicate sexual problems to be more frequent among breast cancer and gynecological cancer patients vs. other female cancer patients. Twenty to thirty-five percent (20-35%) of women report difficulties with sexual relations postmastectomy, and these difficulties do not necessary resolve even by 2 year follow-up (62). Interestingly, the adjuvant breast cancer studies reviewed earlier in terms of increased emotional distress (43,50) indicate a high rate of sexual difficulty. More specifically, Meyerowitz et al (43) reported a 40% rate of disruption of sexual activities in 50 women on adjuvant CMF. In the Knobf report (50), 56% of the premenopausal women reported a change in the frequency and quality of their sexual relationship, with menopausal symptomatology experienced by 72% of the premenopausal subjects. Not surprisingly, more women with these symptoms reported a change in their sexual relationship.

In an excellent review of the effects of gynecological cancers on female sexuality (63), findings controlling for stage of disease and other variables prospectively indicated that approximately 30% of radiation and hysterectomy patients reported sexual difficulties ranging from diminished to completely disrupted sexuality.

Unfortunately, the area of sexual adjustment as it relates to psychosocial adjustment is limited to primarily descriptive data and by the fact that many health care professionals lack knowledge or are uncomfortable in the area of sexual functioning. As a rare clinical note, it has been my experience that it is the very unusual patient who has been asked or has discussed sexual difficulties with his/her physician or nurse, including specifics about the impact of their illness on sexual functioning, realistic expectations, or availability of treatment options (e.g. penile implants for prostatectomy patients). It is clear that attention to sexual issues in cancer and other chronic illnesses is woefully neglected, and the need for multidisciplinary research is sorely needed.

CANCER SURVIVORS

Until very recently, the psychosocial adjustment of cancer survivors has not been critically assessed. Fortunately, with early detection and multimodal treatment approaches, the number of cancer survivors is growing, with estimates indicating that as many as 3,000,000 Americans have survived more than 5 years, with many of these considered cured (64). Thus, the need to determine the answer to the question "at what cost survival" has been raised. One recent investigation (65) assessed the adaptation of adult bone marrow transplant patients who were an average of 42 months post-transplant. About 25% reported ongoing medical problems, and 15-25% reported significant emotional distress (POMS), low self esteem, and less than optimal life satisfaction. Interestingly, the patients current quality of relationship with their donors was highly correlated with many measures of psychological functioning. Although the sample size was small (n=26) it provides some support for the notion that most (75-85%) transplant patients perceive themselves as having a satisfactory level of functioning.

Fabair et al (66) examined psychosocial problems among survivors of Hodgkins Disease in a cross-sectional study of 403 patients, with an average age of 36 years, 9 years post-treatment (median). Sixty (60%) were stage I or II, with 98% free of disease at time of interview. Self report of depression as measured by the CES-D (67), a 20-item standardized scale excluding symptoms of physical illness, was not significantly different from that of community norms. Results indicated that energy had not returned to pre-morbid (per patients report) levels among 37% of the sample. Moderately-high divorce rates (32%), problems with infertility (18%), less interest in sexual activity (20%) and difficulties at work (42%) were reported. Unfortunately, no control group comparison was utilized and the significance of the frequency of these problems vs. other cancer survivors, other illnesses, or healthy, individuals is left unclear. An excellent, well-controlled study investigating psychosocial sequelae of cancer and its treatment has been conducted recently by Cella and Tross (68) with this same population (Hodgkin's disease). Sixty (60) male Hodgkin's disease survivors (age 20-47) free of disease and off treatment for a minimum of six months (mdn=2 years) were compared with an age matched sample of 20 physically healthy men. A number of self-report assessment instruments were utilized, including the BSI, Derogatis Sexual Functioning Inventory (69), Impact of Event Scale (70) which taps coping styles, Rosenberg Self Esteem Scale (71) and Death Anxiety Questionnaire (72). In addition, the modified Problem-Oriented Record (73), a semi-structured interview related to adjustment to illness was completed. Finally, interview ratings were included in the form of the Global Assessment Scale (74). Overall, on most measures of psychological functioning, survivors were not significantly different from nonpatients. There was evidence of increased avoidant thinking about illness, diminished work capacity, and subjective somatic distress. Patients with late stage disease (IIB, IIIB, IVA, IVB) and less time since treatment (6-24 months) showed significantly more distress on a number of measures compared to early stage patients further from treatment (30-140 months). Specifically, compared to other patient groups, this late stage, recent treatment group reported more global distress, elevated anxiety, more illness-related intrusive thinking, and reduced work adjustment. Several important findings tentatively emerge from this well-controlled investigation: 1) survivors may not differ from healthy age-matched controls on most measures of psychopatholoy or adjustment although reduced work status and elevated somatic distress were common sequelae; 2) among survivors, distress is related to disease severity (stage) and time since treatment, with late stage, less elapsed time since treatment predictors of increased distress; 3) interview data indicated that many survivors felt resentment related to being deprived of interpersonal/occupational facets of their lives with decreased stamina and heightened health awareness; 4) increased appreciation of life's pleasures was often reported as a positive aspect of the cancer experience, consistent with other findings (75). In fact, more patients reported a positive (vs. negative) effect of the illness on relationships with significant others after treatment, including friends and family compared to pre-diagnosis. Table 5 indicates psychosocial categories of potential adjustment problems and summaries within these categories. As a caveat, it should be kept in mind that measures of these areas (e.g. psychological symptoms) may not be sensitive enough to detect low grade distress among survivors. Also, reliable, valid measures of some variables may still be in the developmental process (e.g. motivation to form intimate relationships). Finally, Cella (76) notes quite accurately that the difficulties experienced by the cancer "survivors" are more likely to be intrapersonal and interpersonal ones and less likely purely medical. It is clear that, as Table 5 indicates, there is a need for more specific information regarding sequelae, across realms of functioning specifically focusing upon delineation of variables predictive of "survival problems". In addition, increased focus upon improving the qualtiy of life for the relative minority of cancer survivors experiencing significant intrapersonal, interpersonal, or occupational problems is needed.

CONCLUSION

Cancer affects as many as one in every four individuals. This fact, coupled with aggressive treatments and the prolonged lifespan of many cancer patients, emphasizes the need for understanding their psychological/ psychosocial experience. The three prevalence studies described earlier in this chapter find that at least 1 in 5 cancer patients warrant systematic formal evaluation for psychological distress related to their cancer experience, and 1 in 3 may benefit from some mental health intervention. With the inclusion of long standing personality disorders and impaired cognitive states, almost half can be categorized with a DSM III diagnosis.

Predictors of psychological distress have included prognosis, physical status and tumor status with contributions by a number of psychosocial variables (see Table 4). Physical status has been inconsistently predictive of psychological distress. It appears that a "threshold effect" may be operative, with contributions by physical status apparent when samples exhibit a full performance range (normal to bedridden). Findings have not supported a major role for tumor site, treatment modalities, or demographic variables such as sex, age, race, or marital status. Notably, across time intervals, only 40-60% of the variance associated with psychological distress is explained by purely medical factors (30).

Thus, there remains the need for specifying predictors of psychological distress along with continued need to assess sexual dysfunction and family relationships, which have not been satisfactorily examined. Cella et al (68) present a model for examining the long-term impact of cancer on the quality of patients lives. This area also needs continuing assessement and intervention, particularly with that subset of survivors who report significant problems with self esteem and family/marital relationships.

Table 1

RATES OF DSM-III PSYCHIATRIC DISORDERS OBSERVED IN 215
CANCER PATIENTS FROM THREE CANCER CENTERS*

DIAGNOSTIC CATEGORY	DSM-III CODE	SPECIFIC CATEGORY, No.(%)	DIAGNOSTIC CLASS, No.(%)	% OF, PSYCHIATRIC DIAGNOSIS
Organic mental disorders				
Presenile dementia	290.10	1(0.5)	8(4)	8
Dementia with depression	290.21	1(0.5)		
Organic affective syndrome	293.83	2(1.0)		
Dementia	294.10	1(1.0)		
Atypical organic brain syndrome	294.80	2(1.0)		
Organic personality syndrome	310.10	1(0.5)		
Major affective disorders				
Major affective disorder--unpolar depression	296.20	8(4.0)	13(6)	13
Major affective disorder--bipolar depression	296.50	1(0.5)		
Major affective disorder--atypical depression	296.82	3(1.5)		
Dysthymic disorder	300.40	1(0.5)		
Adjustment disorders				
Adjustment disorder with depressed mood	308.00	26(12.0)	69(32)	68
Adjustment disorder with mixed emotional features	309.28	29(13.0)		
Adjustment disorder with anxious mood	309.24	12(6.0)		
Adjustment disorder with emotion and conduct	309.40	2(1.0)		
Anxiety disorders				
General anxiety disorder	300.02	1(0.5)	4(2)	4
Simple phobia	300.29	1(0.5)		
Obsessive-compulsive disorder	300.30	2(1.0)		
Personality disorders				
Schizoid personality disorder	301.20	1(0.5)	7(3)	7
Compulsive personality disorder	301.40	2(1.0)		
Histrionic personality disorder	301.50	1(0.5)		
Dependent personality disorder	301.60	1(0.5)		
Other personality disorder	301.89	1(0.5)		
Alcohol abuse (in remission)	305.03	1(0.5)		
Total psychiatric diagnoses			101(47)	
Psychiatric diagnosis absent			114(53)	

*Rates given are for principal diagnoses only.

Reprinted with permission from Derogatis, LR, Morrow, GR, Fetting, J et al.
JAMA 249(6): 751-757, 1983.

Table 2

NUMBER AND PERCENTAGE OF PATIENTS WITH MODERATE AND HIGH
DISTRESS ON ITEMS OF THE BRIEF SYMPTOM INVENTORY[*]

BSI SCALE	MODERATE DISTRESS		HIGH DISTRESS		TOTAL	
	N	%	N	%	N	%
Somatization	42	33.3	7	5.6	49	38.8
Obsessive Compulsiveness	21	16.7	6	4.8	27	21.5
Interpersonal Sensitivity	15	11.9	4	3.2	19	15.1
Depression	30	23.8	11	8.7	41	32.5
Anxiety	33	26.2	12	9.5	45	35.7
Hostility	23	18.3	0	0.0	23	18.3
Phobic Anxiety	28	22.2	5	4.0	33	26.2
Paranoid Ideation	19	15.1	1	0.8	20	15.9
Psychoticism	13	10.3	8	6.3	21	16.6
General Severity Index	26	20.6	9	7.1	35	27.7
Positive Symptom Distress Index	35	27.8	5	4.0	40	31.8
Positive Symptom Total	21	16.7	6	4.8	27	21.5

[*]Moderate distress = scores between one and two SD above the mean of nonpatient norm group. High distress = scores two or more SD above the mean.

From Stefanek, ME, Derogatis, LP, Shaw A. Psychological distress among oncology outpatients. Psychosom 28(10):530-538, 1987.

Table 3

STUDIES OF PSYCHOLOGICAL DISTRESS AMONG CANCER PATIENTS

INVESTIGATOR	PATIENT STATUS AND SEX (n,%)	MAJOR SITES (%)	DISEASE SITES (%)	PERFORMANCE STATUS	TREATMENT STATUS	ASSESSMENT	RESULTS
Derogatis, Morrow, Fetting, Penman, Piasetsky, Schmale, Henrichs, and Carnicke, 1983 (n=215)	Inpatient 131(61) Outpatient 34(39) Male 105(49) Female 110(51)	Lung 20% Breast 18% Lymphomas 11%	Distant metastases, multiple sites – 32.6% Distant metastases, single sites – 11.6%	Karnofsky, $\bar{x}$=74.7, sd=17.2 (exclusions <50)	All receiving active treatment	1)Psychiatric interview 2)SCL-90-R 3)Rankin Depression Screen 4)Global Adjustment to Illness Scale (GAIS)	1)47% received DSMIII diagnosis (68% of diagnosed adjustment disorders) 2)Elevated SCL-90-R scores among those with DSMIII diagnoses: SOM, OC, DEP, ANX, PHOB, PSY, GSI, PSDI
Stefanek, Derogatis, and Shaw, 1987 (n=126)	Outpatient sample Males 55(44) Females 71(56)	Breast 26% Lung 21% Colon 10%	Not available*	Normal activity-36% Some limitations-50% Significant limitations-14%	No treatment (at time of assessment)	Brief Symptom Inventory (BSI)	1)Subscale profile within normal limits (nonpatient norms) 2)Peak elevations on Depression, Somatization, Anxiety 3)28% report overall moderate-high emotional distress (GSI) 4)81% of patients report no clinical scales >2 standard deviations above nonpatient norms (i.e. high distress)
Farber, Weinerman, and Kuypers (1985) (n=141)	Outpatient sample Males 40(28.4) Females 101(71.6)	Breast 47% Hemopoietic 26%	In remission, 58% Stable Disease 34.0% Progressive Disease 8%	Normal activity-48% Some limitations-35% Bedridden-16%	No treatment-33% Hormonal treatment-13% Multiple cytotoxic agents-34.0%	SCL-90	1)Subscale profile within normal limits (nonpatient norms) 2)Peak elevations on Depression, Somatization, Psychoticism** 3)31% report overall moderate-high emotional distress (GSI) 4)66% of patients report no clinical scales >2 standard deviations above nonpatient norms (i.e. high distress)

* Patients assessed at first visit; disease status not available; treatment not initiated.
** Psychoticism Scale also indicator of feelings of withdrawal, isolation, interpersonal alienation vs. frank psychosis.

Table 4

PREDICTORS OF EMOTIONAL DISTRESS

HIGH EMOTIONAL DISTRESS (HED)	LOW EMOTIONAL DISTRESS (LED)
1. More pessimistic, including outcome of illness	1. More optimistic
2. More regrets about past life	2. Fewer regrets about past life
3. History of psychiatric treatment or suicidal ideation	3. Less psychiatric treatment
4. High anxiety, low ego strength (MMPI)	4. Low anxiety, high ego strength (MMPI)
5. More marital problems before cancer	5. Few marital problems before cancer
6. Lower SES	6. Higher SES
7. More ETOH abuse (not use)	7. Less abuse
8. More multiproblem backgrounds	8. Fewer multiproblem backgrounds
9. Less church attendance	9. More church attendance
10. More physical symptoms	10. Fewer physical symptoms
11. Advanced staging	11. Less advanced staging
12. Expects little support from family	12. Expects adequate support
13. Doctor seen as less helpful	13. Doctor is helpful enough
14. More concerns on Inventory of Predominant Concerns, all types	14. Fewer concerns, all types
15. Poorer problem resolution	15. Better problem resolution
16. Feels like giving up	16. Less giving up
17. Use coping strategies of: - Suppression and passivity - Fatalistic submission - Social withdrawal - Blame others - Blame self	17. Use coping strategies of: - Confrontation - Redefinition (i.e. finding something positive in the situation) - Compliance (compliance, cooperation with medical team)

Reprinted with permission from Weisman, AD and Worden, JW. Coping and Vulnerability in Cancer Patients: Research Report. Project Omega, Massachusetts Hospital, Boston, MA 1977.

Table 5

PSYCHOSOCIAL SEQUELAE OF ADULT SURVIORS*

Adjustment Areas	Findings
1. Intrapersonal	
- Mood	Mixed, with self report data indicating less disruption vs. projective or interview assessments; overall, level of mood disruption not found to consistently impact on psychosocial functioning
- Psychological Symptoms	Survivors not found to differ significantly from comparison groups
- Self Esteem	Mixed, with great variability across survivors, including subsets of cancer patients with both increased and decreased self esteem
- Somatic Distress	Fatigue, general health worries, body-oriented distress increased over comparison groups; physical impairment not significantly associated with extent of psychosocial maladjustment
- Cognitive Dysfunction	Long term effects, most often reported as function of intrathecal methotrexate and whole brain radiation (childhood acute lymphocytic leukemia); other treatment effects (e.g. chemotherapy) typically result in acute, reversible changes
2. Interpersonal	
- Family Adjustment	Data sparse; 10-15% report negative impact post-treatment, and typically in first 1-2 years after treatment; 20-25% report beneficial effect of cancer experience
- Marital Adjustment	Data on impact of cancer on ability to form intimate relationships sparse; among married, reports of both improvement of relationship (35%) and worsening (22%)
- Sexual Adjustment	Chemotherapy (e.g. MOPP), surgery for urogenital cancers may impact sexual functioning significantly; distress significant among those reporting infertility
- Social Relationships	Little data; approximately one-third of survivors report problem with a friend during post-treatment period, related to the illness; frequent reports of mixed response (increased emotional ties with some friends, distancing from others)

Table 5 (continued)

PSYCHOSOCIAL SEQUELAE OF ADULT SURVIORS*

Adjustment Areas	Findings
3. Occupational	
- Work Performance	Blue collar workers report more difficulty with job re-entry (perhaps due to physical sequelae); objectively, survivors no less productive; subjectively, 15-40% of survivors report reduced work status
- Work Discrimination	Difficult to measure, especially subtle maltreatment (e.g. non-promotion); results mixed; likely disease site and work-site dependent

*This table is based upon Cella, D., Cancer Survival: Psychosocial and Public Issues. Cancer Investigation, 5(1):59-37, 1987.

REFERENCES

1. Plumb, MM, Holland, J. Comparative Studies of Psychological Functions in Patients with Advanced Cancer: I. Self reported depressive symptoms. Psychosom Med 39:264-276, 1977.

2. Derogatis, LR. The SCL-90-R Administration, Scoring and Procedures Manual I. Baltimore, Clinical Psychometric Research, 1977.

3. Derogatis, LR, Spencer, PM. The Brief Symptom Inventory (BSI): Administration, Scoring and Procedures Manual I. Baltimore, Clinical Psychometric Research, 1982.

4. Derogatis, LR, Morrow, GR, Fetting, J, et. al. The Prevalence of Psychiatric Disorders Among Cancer Patients. JAMA 249(6):751-757, 1983.

5. Farber, DM, Weinerman, BH, Kuypers, JA. Psychosocial Distress in Oncology Outpatients. J Psychosoc Oncol 2:109-118, 1984.

6. Stefanek, ME, Derogatis, LP, Shaw, A. Psychological Distress Among Oncology Outpatients. Psychosom 28(10):530-538, 1987.

7. Craig, TJ, Abeloff, MD. Psychiatric Symptomatology Among Hospitalized Cancer Patients. Am J Psych 141:1323-1327, 1974.

8. Derogatis, LR, Abeloff, MD, McBeth, CD. Cancer Patients and their Physicians in the Perception of Psychological Symptoms. Psychosomatics 17:197-201, 1976.

9. McNair, DM, Lorr, M, and Droppleman, LF. EIPS Manual for the Profile of Mood States. San Diego, CA: Educational and Industrial Testing Service, 1971.

10. McNair, DM, Lorr, M and Droppelman, LF. Profile of Mood State. San Diego Educational and Industrial Testing Service, 1971.

11. Imber, SD. Patient Direct Self-Report Techniques in I.E. Waskow and MB Parloff (eds.). Psychotherapy Change Measures. Rockville: National Institute of Health, 1975.

12. McNair, DM. Self-Evaluations of Antidepressants. Psychopharma Cologia 37:281-302, 1974.

13. Derogatis, LR. The Affects Balance Scale. Baltimore, Clinical Psychometric Research, 1975.

14. Derogatis, LR, Abeloff, MD, Melisaratos, N. Psychological Coping Mechanisms and Survival Time in Metastatic Breast Cancer. JAMA 242:1504-1508, 1979.

15. Beck, AR, Steer, RA, Garbin, MG. Psychometric Properties of the Beck Depression Inventory: Twenty Five Years of Evaluation. Clin Psych Rev 8:77-100, 1988.

16. Beck, AT, Rush, AJ, Shaw, BF et al. Cognitive Therapy of Depression. New York, Guilford Press, 1979.

17. Cavanaugh, S, Clark, DC, Gibbons, RD. Diagnosing Depression in the Hospitalized Medically ill. Psychosomatics 24(9):809-815, 1983.

18. Clark, DC, Cavanaugh, SV, Gibbons, RD. The Core Symptoms of Depression in Medical and Psychiatric Patients. J Nerv Mental Dis 171:705-713, 1983.

19. Goldfarb, C, Driesen, J, Cole, D. Psychophysiologic Aspects of Malignancy. Am J Psych 123:1545-1552, 1967.

20. Guy, R. An Essay on Scirrhus Tumors and Cancers. London, J and A Churchill, 1759.

21. Levine, PM, Silverfarb, PM, Lipowski, ZJ. Mental Disorders in Cancer Patients. Cancer 42:1385-1391, 1978.

22. Peck, A. Emotional Reactions to Having Cancer. Am J Roentgenol 114:591-599, 1972.

23. Karnofsky, DA, Burchenal, JH. A Clinical Evaluation of Chemotherapeutic Agents in Cancer, In Mac Lead CM (ed): Evaluation of Chemotherapeutic Agents. New York, Columbia University Press, 1949.

24. Raskin, A, Schulterbrandt, J, Reatig, N, et. al. Factors of Psychopathology in Interview Ward Behavior and Self Report Ratings of Hospitalized Depressives. J Consult Psychol 31:270-278, 1967.

25. Derogatis, LR. Global Adjustment to Illness Scale. Baltimore, Clinical Psychometric Research, 1975.

26. Rodin, G, Vochart, K. Depression in the Medically Ill: An Overview. Am J Psychiatry 143:696-705, 1986.

27. Cassileth, BR, Lusk, EJ, Strouse, TB, et al. Psychosocial Status in Chronic Illness. N Engl J Med 311:506-11, 1984.

28. Goldberg, DP. The Detection of Psychiatric Illness by Questionnaire. London: Oxford University Press, 1972.

29. Cella, DF, Orofiamma, B, Holland, JC et al. The Relationship of Psychological Distress, Extent of Disease, and Performance Status in Patients with Lung Cancer. Cancer 60:1661-1667, 1987.

30. Weisman, AD, Worden, JW. Coping and Vulnerabilty in Cancer Patients: Research Report. Project Omega, Mass Genl Hosp, Boston, MA, 1977.

31. Weisman, AD. Early Diagnosis of Vulnerability in Cancer Patients. Amer J Med Sci 271(2):187-196, 1976.

32. Stefanek, ME, Shaw, A, DeGeorge, D et al. Illness-Related Worry Among Cancer Patients: Prevalence, Severity, and Content. Cancer Invest (In press).

33. Sobel, HJ and Worden, JW.   The MMPI as a Predictor of Psychosocial
    Adaptation to Cancer. J Cons Clin Psy 47(4):716-724, 1979.

34. Hughes, JE. Depressive Illness in Lung Cancer. I. Depression Before
    Diagnosis. Eur J Surg Onc 11:15-20, 1985.

35. Hughes, JE.   Deppressive Illness in Lung Cancer. II. Follow-up of
    Inoperable Patients. Eur J Surg Onc 11:21-24, 1985.

36. Devlin, J, Maguire, P, Phillips, P: Psychological Problems Associated with
    Diagnosis and Treatment of Lymphomas. I: Retrospective Study. Brit Med J
    295(17):953-954.

37. Devlin, J, Maguire, P, Phillips, P. Psychological Problems Associated with
    Diagnosis and Treatment of Lymphomas. II: Prospective Study. Brit Med J
    295(17):955-957.

38. Lloyd, GG, Parker, AC, Ludlam, CA et al. Emotional Impact of Diagnosis and
    Early Treatment of Lymphomas. J Psychos Res 28(2):157-162, 1984.

39. Evans, DL, McCartney, CF, Nemeroff, CB, et al. Depression in Women Treated
    for Gynecological Cancer: Clinical and Neuroendocrine Assessment. Am J
    Psych 143(4):447-452, 1986.

40. Bukberg, J, Penman, D, Holland, J. Depression in Hospitalized Cancer
    Patients. Psychosom Med 46:199-212, 1984.

41. Davies, AD, Davies, C, and Delbo, MC. Depression and Anxiety in Patients
    Undergoing Diagnostic Investigations for Head and Neck Cancers. Brit J
    Psych 149:491-493, 1986.

42. The Breast Cancer Digest. US Department of Health and Human Services. 2nd
    Edition. NIH Publication No. 841691, April 1984.

43. Meyerowitz, B. Psychosocial Correlates of Breast Cancer and its
    Treatments. Psychol Bull 87(1):108-131, 1980.

44. Maguire, P. Psychological and Social Consequences of Breast Cancer. Nurs
    Mirror 140(14):54-57, 1975.

45. McArdle, CS, Coleman, KC, Cooper, AF et al. The Social, Emotional and
    Financial Implications of Adjuvant Chemotherapy in Breast Cancer. Br J
    Surg 68:261-264, 1981.

46. Hughson, AV, Cooper, AF, McArdle, CS. Psychological Impact of Adjuvant
    Chemotherapy in the First Two Years After Mastectomy.   Brit Med J
    293(15):1268-1271, 1986.

47. Maguire, GP, Tate, A, Brooke, M et al. Psychiatric Morbidity and Physical
    Toxicity Associated with Adjuvant Chemotherapy After Mastectomy. Br Med J
    281:1179-1180, 1980.

48. Spitzer, RL, Endicott, J, Fleiss, JL et al. The Psychiatric Status
    Schedule. Arch Gen Psych 23:41-55, 1970.

49. Holland, JC, Roland, J, Lebowitz, A. Reactions to Cancer Treatment. Assessment of Emotional Response to Adjuvant Radiation as a Guide to Planned Intervention. Psychiatr Clin North Am 2:347-358, 1979.

50. Knopf, MT. Physical and Psychologic Distress Associated with Adjuvant Chemotherapy in Women with Breast Cancer. J Clin Oncol 4:678-684, 1986.

51. Worden, JW, Weisman, AD. The Fallacy of Post-Mastectomy Depression. Amer J Med Sci 273(2):169-175, 1977.

52. Jamison, KR, Wellisch, DK, Pasnau, RO. Psychosocial Aspects of Mastectomy: I. The Woman's Perspective. Am J Psych 135:432-436, 1978.

53. Schottenfeld, D, and Robbins, GF. Quality of Survival among Patients who have had Radical Mastectomy. Cancer 26:650-654, 1970.

54. Craig, TJ, Comstock, GW, and Geiser, PB. The Quality of Survival in Breast Cancer: A Case-Control Comparison. Cancer 33:1451-7, 1974.

55. Bloom, JR, Cook, M, Fotopoulis et al. Psychological Response to Mastectomy. Cancer 59:189-196, 1987.

56. Steinberg, MD, Julano, MA, Wise, L. Psychological Outcome of Lumpectomy vs. Mastectomy in the Treatment of Breast Cancer. Am J Psych 142(1):34-39, 1985.

57. Morris, T, Greer, HS, White P. Psychological and Social Adjustment to Mastectomy: A Two-Year Follow-up Study. Cancer 40:2381-2387, 1977.

58. Bloom, JR. Social Support, Accommodation to Stress and Adjustment to Breast Cancer. Soc Sci Med 16:1329-1338, 1982.

59. Taylor, SE, Lichtman, RR, Wood, JV. Attributions, Beliefs about Control, and Adjustment to Breast Cancer. J Pers Soc Psych 46(3):489-502, 1984.

60. Abeloff, MD, Derogatis, LR. Psychological Aspects of the Management of Primary and Metastatic Breast Cancer. In Stonesifer, Breast Cancer, 505-516, Johns Hopkins University Press, Baltimore, 1977.

61. Amberger, H, Henningsen, B. and Fey, K. Rehabilitation after Radical Mastectomy. In Lewison, Breast Cancer, 543-544, Allen R. List Inc., New York, 1977.

62. Morris, T., Greer, HS, White, P. Psychological and Social Adjustment to Mastectomy. Cancer 40:2381-2387, 1977.

63. Andersen, BL, Hacker, NF. Treatment for Gynecologic Cancer: A Review of the Effects on Female Sexuality. Health Psych 2(2):203-221, 1983.

64. American Cancer Society: Cancer Facts and Figures, New York, 1985.

65. Wolcott, DL, Wellisch, DK, Fawzy, FI et al. Adaptation of Adult Bone Marrow Transplant Recipient Long Term Survivors. Transplantation 41(4):478-484, 1986.

A MODEL FOR PSYCHOTHERAPY WITH THE EARLY-STAGE CANCER PATIENT

Edward R. Kaufman, M.D.
Professor of Psychiatry & Human Behavior
Director, Psychiatric Education
University of California
Irvine Medical Center

Karen K. Redding, LCSW
Irvine Medical Center

CONTENTS:

A MODEL FOR PSYCHOTHERAPY WITH THE EARLY-STAGE CANCER PATIENT

Edward R. Kaufman, M.D.

Karen K. Redding, LCSW

ABSTRACT

Based on their own work over the past 10 years with cancer patients, the authors describe their integrated model of psychotherapy for early-stage, good-prognosis cancer patients. The therapy model includes psychotherapeutic and educational components, many of which can also be used at any point throughout the disease process as well as in the early stages. Previously unresolved conflicts become amenable to psychotherapy in many patients confronting a life-threatening illness. In patients whose cancer recurs, the model is intended to offer them and their families a means of coping with the disease.

INTRODUCTION

The psychosocial factors affecting cancer patients have been of interest to mental health professionals for the past 30 years. Earlier work primarily emphasized the patient with a poor prognosis and examined psychological risk factors. As a result of recent gains in the diagnosis and treatment of cancer, the patient currently diagnosed with cancer has a 49% chance of being alive five years after the diagnosis is made. This is a dramatic improvement over the 1930's when only one in 15 cancer patients survived five years (1).

These changes in survival are occurring across greater numbers of people across all age groups, as well as different tumor sites. Specifically, children with acute lymphocytic leukemia had a 4 in 100 five-year survival 20 years ago. Today, 75% of these children are alive after five years. In the past, the young adolescent with osteosarcoma generally died within two years following diagnosis. Today, as many as one-half are being cured whose cancer has not spread at time of diagnosis, and 70% of all patients are living 2 years following diagnosis. Adult women whith endometrial cancer have an 80% chance of recovering; 90% if the cancer is caught early. Improvement for testicular cancer is even more dramatic. Twenty years ago, barely 3 in 5 men survived the disease. Today, 90% can be cured in early stages. Thus, the psychological care of cancer patients with an excellent chance for survival is a progressively important clinical issue.

This chapter will focus on good-prognosis patients in the initial stage of cancer and on the methods best suited for psychosocial treatment. Underlying psychological issues will be examined, and a comprehensive system for psychotherapy will be presented. In these patients the cancer is at a level where the physician's goal is to eradicate or control it. Individuals in this stage who are hopeful about a cure generally have lower levels of anxiety than patients with a poorer prognosis, and seek meaningful communication with care givers and families. In some cases, these patients may be described as "aggressive optimists" (2). An aggressive optimist is one who has a very strong will to live, and is willing to exert all their energy towards their own fight for recovery. The average outlook for five-year survival of these good-prognosis patients is promising.

It has been our experience that for the most part, cancer patients, prior to the onset of their illness are essentially mentally healthy people who are confronting serious crisis in their lives. This crisis leads to a high incidence of acute anxiety and depression but for the most part, personality disorders are minimal. Derogatis et al (3) found the prevalence of personality disorders in cancer patients to be 3%.

AN INTEGRATED MODEL OF PSYCHOTHERAPY

The newly diagnosed cancer patient is an excellent candidate for crisis intervention (4). Psychological changes resulting from the illness may be viewed as an opportunity to resolve previously existing neurotic problems, ultimately enriching the quality of life (5). Education can play an important part in assisting the cancer patient in adapting to the situation. Gaining information about one's illness and its treatment may afford the patient a sense of control and mastery over the disease, thereby enhancing adaptive ability (6).

We have evolved an integrated system of psychotherapy with cancer patients that is based on prior work with other crisis-intervention patients. The therapy model may be divided into psychotherapeutic and educational components. The kinds of psychotherapy include individual, family, and group modalities. Individual therapy utilizes a crisis-intervention approach in which the therapist: (1) encourages the patient to ventilate feelings, (2) offers support and optimism, (3) clarifies feelings, (4) interprets thoughts in psychodynamic terms, (5) encourages the patient to act on his or her environment, (6) explores the current situation in the context of the past, (7) focuses on specific relevant psychodynamic issues, and (8) limits the duration of therapy (7). The therapeutic goal is not just to help the patient adjust to cancer but to utilize mobilized affects and issues to resolve previously existing conflict. The psychodynamic basis of the therapy for these patients is described in the next section.

Family therapy, an essential part of this therapeutic approach, incorporates a crisis-intervention model with an educational emphasis. The best technique for motivating the family to become involved in therapy is to point out the need all families have for help in communicating and coping when they must live with cancer (8). The spouse is helped to come to terms with the reality of the cancer, while providing support and nurturance, and may first have to ventilate his or her own fear, sadness, and anger. Relatives of the cancer patient may altruistically deny their own need for help while focusing on the illness and the patient's greater needs. This can be overcome by educating the relatives so that if they can learn to relax and cope with the cancer, the lowered anxiety level will, in turn, lower the stress on the cancer patient. Additional family and individual coping skills are provided by the American Cancer Society's, "I Can Cope" Program. This is an 8 week program, facilitated by an oncology nurse and/or social worker, that is provided without cost to patients and family members. Its goal is to teach and strengthen existing coping skills relevant to going through the cancer experience. Some of these

skills include: learning more about cancer and its treatment;
coping and understanding the side-effects of cancer treatments,
managing nutrition and diet; learning more about available
community resources; and improving existing communications
skills, especially as they relate to allowing expression of all
types of feelings, rather than only optimistic and positive ones.

In contrast to families who express hostility and criticism
to their members with psychiatric difficulties, the cancer
patient's family is more prone to express pity and
over-protection. Work should be done with spouses and other
family members to replace a smothering and over-protective
attitude with mutually supportive coping strategies.

Reestablishment of the sexual relationship needs to be
explored and encouraged (9,10). Cancer patient concerns about
sexuality may be classified as: 1) organ-specific; 2)
treatment-specific, and 3) psychosocial. Organ-specific
sexuality problems have generally been associated with the sex
organs (e.g. breast and gynecologic cancers; cancer of the
prostate, penis, colon, bladder). Some of the initial concerns
that patients have following surgical intervention involving the
sexual organs may include: 1) sterility, 2) loss of libido, and
3) limitations on sexual activity.

Treatment-specific concerns involve the effects that
chemotherapy, radiotherapy, or hormonal therapy may have on a
person's sexual functioning. These may involve:

- temporary or permanent sterility/infertility
- general fatigue

- nausea, vomiting
- loss of body hair
- weight gain or loss
- endocrine dysfunction, leading to premature menopausal symptoms
- radiation cystitis
- sense of touch either becoming dulled or sharpened to point of pain
- difficulty with sexual desire, arousal, or experience of orgasm

Other pharmaceutical agents, whether used alone for symptom management, or in conjunction with anti-cancer drugs, may have an adverse effect on sexual functioning. Such drugs include antihypertensives, antidepressants, anticholinergics, and pain medications (3).

Psychosocial concerns address a patient's identity as a sexual being. Common issues are:

1) self-esteem
2) vulnerability
3) mutilation
4) mortality
5) sexuality and sensuality

It is important to emphasize that sexuality involves more than physical intercourse. Sexuality can be defined as having several components (11): a person's view of himself/herself in terms of body image, attractiveness, worth, competency, and degree of satisfaction in experiencing pleasure (11); a variety of non genital behaviors including cuddling, stroking, kissing, touching and caressing (12) as well as masturbation, and sexual intercourse. The need for physical contact becomes much greater when a person experiences a debilitating illness. Yet both the patient and significant other have to surmount intital post cancer resistances to be able to exchange these needed intimacies.

Studies have shown that years of unacceptability, rejection and isolation cause more anxiety in cancer patients than do fears of recurrence, pain, and death (3). Most cancer patients experience sexual concerns and prefer to have the topic of sexual functioning initiated by their doctor or therapist. The topic can be introduced by asking questions related to organ-specific, treatment-specific, or psychosocial sexual concerns.

It is essential to work with the total family, particularly adolescent children. Cancer tends to pull adolescents back into the family with great intensity at a time when they are individuating and moving out on their own. Adolescents may also be stressed when they are misperceived as prematurely adult and pressured to assume family responsibilities beyond their wishes or capabilities. Couples and multifamily groups are particularly helpful with cancer patients, spouses and other family members as they permit the crisis to be shared with others, allowing for more cooperation in problem solving.

Group therapy is useful for cancer patients (14,15). Beneficial elements in these groups include: (1) altruism that diminishes self-absorption; (2) catharsis of "shameful", painful emotions; (3) group cohesiveness to deal with isolation and abandonment; and (4) the universality of shared experiences, feelings, and the fear of death (15). The educational component provides a system that the cancer patient can utilize to cope actively with the disease. This permits the psychotherapy to take place without rumination and preoccupation with cancer, while the feelings and issues tapped by the cancer can be used therapeutically. The psychotherapy of a cancer patient cannot occur in a vacuum that ignores a direct attack on the primary illness and relies exclusively on a psychodynamic approach.

The educational components of this therapeutic system include: (1) clarifying the state of the medical condition including diagnosis, and treatment alternatives; (2) teaching about the effects of the cancer and its treatments; (3) teaching methods for relief of anxiety by relaxation techniques, self-hypnosis, or biofeedback (16); (4) providing an individualized method of utilizing visual imaging to combat the cancer; (5) supporting compliance with medical regimens; (6) teaching about lifestyle, diet, and exercise; (7) teaching about the common reactions of patients, relatives, and friends to cancer; and (8) self-help groups.

Clarification of the medical condition and related treatments is important. Informed patients have less fear and anxiety, lower levels of stress, and more functional coping responses (17). Relaxation techniques help patients feel that they can exercise control over their bodies, as well as relieve pain and anxiety without extra medication (16). In addition, a lowered stress level may be associated with an enhanced cancer prognosis (16,18). This technique may help prepare the patient for visual imaging (16).

In our experience, patients often have difficulty in utilizing visual images of their bodies fighting off the cancer by reading the Simonton description of these images. Patients are better able to work with specific images devised with the therapist to meet individual needs. Although controversial, imaging techniques help patients feel more in control and less helpless.

Volunteer programs staffed by trained cancer patients provide empathy and teach common reactions shared by cancer patients. Self-help, volunteer programs provide a great deal of support, information, and role models for successful adaptation and recovery. Some such groups are (19):

1. I Can Cope- offered through the American Cancer Society (A.C.S.) addresses the educational and psychological needs of people with cancer.

2. Reach for Recovery (A.C.S.)- provides rehabilitation support for women who have had mastectomies.

3. United Ostomy Association- provide ostomy patients with mutual aid, moral support and education.

4. Leukemia Society of America- offers financial assistance and consultation services to cancer patients with leukemia and allied disorders.

5. Cancer Information Service administered by the National Cancer Institute (N.C.I.) is a toll-free telephone inquiry system

that supplies information about cancer to the general public. (General toll-free number is: 800-638-6694).

These psychotherapeutic and educational approaches are all helpful in management of the cancer patient. Whether they favorably alter the prognosis of the cancer remains to be proved. However, they definitely lower psychological distress and improve treatment satisfaction and compliance (14). The techniques of choice with each patient and family will depend on individual needs and the modalities available. No single educational or psychological technique has proved so successful that it should be imposed on every patient. An integrated approach selecting those techniques that are differentially helpful to a given individual is strongly suggested.

PSYCHODYNAMIC PSYCHOTHERAPEUTIC ISSUES IN CANCER PATIENTS

The psychodynamic aspects and psychological responses of cancer patients provide a foundation for the utilization of specific psychotherapeutic emphases. Feelings of loss, social isolation, alienation, mutiliation, and fear of rejection make up a large portion of the stress involved with having any catastrophic illness. perceived losses may involve control, professional identity, role, independence, sense of self, and change in body image. Loss of control over ones body and future are other important concerns of these patients. This uncertainty may lead to chronic anxiety or may facilitate the existencial leap into learning to live in the present.

As a general rule, the cancer patient suffers from more fear and anxiety than do patients with almost any other disease (6).

The critical issues characteristic of cancer are: (1) the helplessness or absence of personal control the patient has over treatment methods and success rates; (2) the physician's and patient's uncertainty regarding outcome; and (3) that the disease as well as its treatments can kill, cripple, disfigure, cause pain, and restrict functioning (2,6).

Cancer invariably elicits responses that should be addressed by the therapist and patient for successful treatment to occur. These include depression, anxiety, fear, guilt, denial, and conflicts over dependence and independence (6,20). The fears which are commonly seen in cancer patients should be addressed in therapy. These fears may be classified into those: (1) induced by the disease itself; (2) related to treatment; and (3) related to living in their external world with the reactions of others to their cancer.

Specifically these fears are:

FEARS INDUCED BY THE DISEASE ITSELF include:

    a) Loss of health

    b) Feelings of shame, punishment, or retribution

    c) Loss of control/disability

    d) Impending death

FEARS RELATED TO THE CANCER THERAPY focus on:

    a) Injury, mutilation

    b) Pain/suffering

    c) Change in physical appearance/sexuality

    d) Nausea/vomiting (a most uncomfortable aspect)

    e) Impairment of various body systems, including: skin

rashes; sores on mouth; sterility; heart damage; bladder
irritation; hair loss; depression of bone marrow with 1)
susceptibility to infection, 2) susceptibility to
bleeding tendency, 3) susceptibility to anemia; hot
flashes; fluid retention; numbness/tingling in fee/toes;
insomnia; fatigue

   f) Depression with loss of appetite, sleep, concentration
      and energy.

<u>FEARS RELATED TO LIVING WITH CANCER</u> include:

   a) Constant threat of recurrence

   b) Other's response; 1) avoidance; 2) pity; 3) ability to
      function without the patient

   c) Changes in relationships

   d) Being a burden

   e) Financial: insurance; ability to continue working

   f) Self-image

Fears of the reactions of others, particularly rejection and pity
often become greater than those of death itself. Thus these
patients should be encouraged to express fears about having
cancer and how their disease may affect goals, ambition and
self-concept. These fears may be expressed through crying which
needs to be supported and encouraged in order to help the patient
release tensions and come to terms with these feelings.

    The fears of rejection and pity emphasize the need for
family involvement which will be discussed later.

    The patient's psychological response to cancer is determined
by the premorbid personality, prior personal experience with

loss, and the availability of support systems (2,5). The nature and degree of the response can be predicted by assessing responses to major stressors of the past (4,6). According to Peck (20), anxiety (in 98% of the patients assessed), depression (in 74%), anger (in 49%), and guilt (in 36%) are the most common emotional responses to cancer.

Guilt fantasies focus on: (1) The cancer as deserved punishment for having magically caused the death or misfortune of others; (2) Sexual behavior as having led to the cancer; (3) Attribution of the cancer directly to anger or depression or to having permitted the level of stress to increase; (4) Not meditating, relaxing, or doing psychotherapy "well enough" so as to eradicate the potential for recurrence.

Denial is the cancer patient's most common defense mechanism (2,21) but it may provide only a partial filter for reality. Patients may know that they have a lethal disease yet maintain that it will not be lethal to them. Persons who deny aspects of their illness will reduce its impact, lower their stress level (22), and, perhaps, enhance their autoimmune response. A continual feeling of unreality may permeate the world of the cancer patient. As a general rule, denial is most harmful when it prevents the patient from receiving necessary treatment.

Some patients will maintain roles of responsibility and caretaking for others during their illness. Although this helps the patient avoid feelings of weakness and dependency, it may also prevent obtaining the support and nurturing that is needed (20). Existential issues are inevitably raised in patients struggling with cancer. A helpful aspect of treatmentis shifting the patient from a focus on outcome to an emphasis on process. Thus the patient is shifted from "why me?" to "where is this leading me?" In this shift the patient is helped to focus on increased openness, empathy, willingness to grow and insight (23).

Prior to surgery, patients with higher ego strength can be recognized by their ability to seek information, to use humor rather than fatalism, and to avoid blaming others (24).

Isolation of affect may help patients to speak of subjects as troublesome as the inevitability of death. However, it may also prevent the necessary expression of feelings that may serve to lessen the impact of the illness and lower stress levels. Rationalization is commonly employed by the cancer patient. Altruism is used by the patient who does not share feelings and concerns with others for fear they would be unduly burdened.

These patients should be encouraged to feel and react spontaneously to their experiences. They need to experience the process of grief rather than be plummeted into depression. Grief involves relief through letting go and obtaining support. Depression involves giving-up, feeling hopeless and becoming more socially isolated.

Identification with the physician and/or the psychotherapist is another defense mechanism. Identifying with the physician's active fight against the disease while attributing special healing powers to the physician assists in alleviating patient anxiety. It has also been found that a strong patient-doctor relationship can enhance medical compliance and deter a patient from seeking non-orthodox treatments. A psychosocial study conducted at the University of Arizona with patients choosing laetrile (unorthodox treatment) found that the biggest difference between patients choosing laetrile and those opting for experimental but sanctioned treatment was a difference in the patient-doctor relationship. Patients who sought laetrile did so because they were told there "was nothing left to be done". They felt abandoned by their physicians. Those opting for other experimental drugs, did so because, as a result of expressing their fight for life to their doctors, they were referred on to Phase I and II experimental protocols (25).

The nurturing aspects of the hospital enable many patients to postpone their depression throughout their hospital stay. Depression may not become manifest until as late as three to six months following discharge. During the hospital stay patients can first deal with concrete issues such as: symptom relief and management, learning about the disease and its treatment, and dealing with medical personnel. Later they can begin to deal with more existential issues such as: the nature of the cancer and treatment experience, the changes they have undergone, the shift from feeling normal, grief, uncertainty, and fears of death.

SPECIFIC COUNTERTRANSFERENCE ISSUES

Several unique countertransference problems arise in working with the cancer patient. These include a sense of omnipotence stimulated by fantasies of curing cancer, depression when and if cancer recurs, strong tendencies to be either overinvolved or too distant, and anxiety about caring for the patient who is attempting to cope with the possibility of dying.

The therapist's omnipotent feelings can usually be kept under control unless the cancer recurs. Then he/she may feel guilty about the incapacity to help the patient further, specifically in preventing the recurrence of cancer symptoms (26). Therapist depression in reaction to this disappointment can lead to withdrawal from the patient. "Therapists may even deny the existence of a recurrence to avoid the realization that the dream of cure by omnipotence has been shattered" (26). Therapist grief, on the other hand, may be very helpful in facilitating appropriate emotional grieving responses in patients and their families when there is a recurrence or less than expected response to cancer treatment regimens.

Therapists who are struggling with their own fear of death may distance themselves from the cancer patient, whose proximity to death is too threatening for them. Inadvertently, the distanced therapist may communicate pessimism to the patient, reinforcing feelings of isolation and despair. Unexplored personal issues in this area may also render the therapist too inhibited to help the patient deal with fears of death.

If therapists have not worked through their own feelings regarding friends and relatives who have died of cancer, these emotions can be readily tapped by the cancer patient (27). Thus, the therapist may experience reawakening of the grief attached to the death of a loved one or guilt about unresolved death wishes or the inability to save a loved one. The therapist may exhibit aloofness, rejection, or emotional withdrawal from potentially draining work with cancer patients. He/she may focus on intellectual interpretations as a defense against experiencing the cancer patients' powerful emotions. The patient may react negatively to, or identify with, the nonverbal message conveyed by the therapist's distance or his/her communicating a helpless, hopeless attitude toward cancer (27). More subtly, this same phenomenon may inhibit the therapist's empathy and capacity to experience spontaneously the patient's affect or material.

The parameters of therapist nurturing, giving and directiveness are much broader with these patients than any other group. This is because the powerful impact of their illness calls for more giving on the part of the therapist. The fine balance between being overly giving to a point where patient dependency is encouraged and therapist burnout enhanced (28) versus inappropriate neutrality and withholding is particularly delicate in these patients. All parameters of overt and covert giving and nurturing are used with these patients and their families but care must be taken to utilize these techniques for the patients growth and coping and not for the therapist's unresolved issues. Active involvement in medical issues, permissiveness about fees, increased frequency and length of sessions, including home and hospital visits, liberal use of interpretation or support, regular pep talks, physical contact, and therapist attendance at family functions are all permissible and indicated when patient and therapist needs are clearly separated and kept in context (27,29).

For successful psychotherapy to ensue, it is imperative that the therapist carefully explore his/her own countertransference issues. The therapist who has not resolved countertransference issues may be more at risk for burn-out or clinical depressions as a product of work with the cancer patient.

ADDITIONAL PSYCHOTHERAPEUTIC ISSUES

Several additonal themes that were not sufficiently emphasized in the previous literature include; developing a realistic attitude toward noncancer-related physical ailments, loss of a sense of omnipotence, assertion and competence, transference, fear of abandonment and blaming the patient for recurrences.

Developing a Realistic Attitude Toward Noncancer-Related Physical Ailments.

Patients may regard even an upper respiratory tract infection as a major catastrophe. They fear that the cancer has recurred or that they have been so weakened by it and chemotherapy or radiation treatment that they will never recover. On the other hand, patients should be encouraged to practice regular self-examination techniques as indicated.

The therapist should be supportive and reassuring at these times, as well as ensure that adequate medical evaluation and treatment take place.

Loss of a Sense of Omnipotence.

Cancer attacks the very core of omnipotent wishes. One patient maintained the fantasy that as long as he was "a good boy," e.g. worked hard, was obedient, ate well, exercised, and was a faithful husband, no ills would befall him. His cancer was a harsh confrontation that the fantasy did not offer him such wished-for protection. Psychotherapy facilitated the dissolution of this fantasy, permitting the patient to give up the myth that compliance guarantees nurturance and immunity from all ills. Such patients are also very vulnerable to self-criticism and condemnations when they've done all the recommended therapeutic techniques (e.g. relaxation, meditation, imaging) and their cancer recurs. This self punitive attitude should be countered by therapist support.

Assertion and Competence.

As these patients recover from the consequences of their cancer and its treatment, they begin to give up their helplessness and dependence and to return to their prior position in regard to assertion and competence. On the other hand, many of these patients retain a sense of humility which is very helpful for the rest of their years.

They often feel some regret and loss at giving up their nurtured, dependent state and returning to the competitive world. There also may be some experience of loss in how intensely one has experienced their feelings. Prior fears of success and the childhood roots of these fears are reawakened and rendered accessible in psychotherapy. Fears and inhibitions are rendered so trivial compared with the cancer that lifelong inhibiting patterns seem minor and conquerable. Having faced death, they are able to fight the struggles of day-to-day living.

Transference.

Cancer patients develop strong positive and negative transferences to different members of the treatment team as intense feelings toward the early good and bad parent are reawakened. One patient expressed appropriate fury at the surgeon who originally missed her cancer. Later, she developed an intense, dependent transference to the surgeon who successfully operated on her. The resolution of these underlying feelings, particularly to the "good surgeon," permitted her to resolve a lifelong pattern of splitting men into categories of all good or all bad. Positive transference to physicians may be quite helpful as they greatly enhance medical compliance (28). As these patients emerge from their post-cancer depression in psychotherapy, recover from their monor physical ailments, and do not experience a recurrence of cancer, they inevitably experience strong positive transference to their psychotherapist. This should be analyzed only if it interferes with psychotherapy, and it can be helpful if the patient needs to return to psychotherapy, particularly if the cancer should recur.

As the therapist is more giving, it is essential that he/she set appropriate limits and boundaries as necessary.

Fears of Abandonment, Rejection and Isolation.

Many cancer patients fear they will be rejected or abandoned as a result of the cancer. Persons with fears of abandonment may work them through as they deal with their fears of death as a result of cancer.

CONCLUSIONS

The efficacy of psychosocial factors in enhancing cancer prognosis is controversial. Cassileth and associates (27) noted that the following factors have been found in the literature to predict general longevity or survival: social ties and marital status, work and role satisfaction, use of psychotropic drugs, general life satisfaction, subjective view of adult health, hoplessness/helplessness, and adjustment to diagnosis. Their study found no significant relationship between the above seven factors and survival and time to recurrence. Most of the patients in their study had advanced cancers, past the stages in populations for whom we are suggesting psychodynamic crisis-intervention therapy. We suggest, however, that patient and family satisfaction would be positively augmented even in poorer-prognosis patients such as those studied by Cassileth if an integrated system of psychotherapy were utilized.

Other studies have demonstrated the effects of psychosocial factors on survival rates. Patients with a fighting spirit toward their breast cancer rather than helplessness and hopelessness have been shown (31) to have a higher five-year survival rate. Denial may act as a significant and dangerous distorter of reality or as an adaptive, healthy maneuver (32). Stavraky (33) suggested that cancer patients with the most favorable outcomes expressed their emotions, including hostility, in an open and direct fashion.

One controversial aspect of the system recommended by us is visual imaging. Although this technique's ability to enhance cancer prognosis favorably has not been demonstrated, it does help to counter the passivity of the disease and treatment process. In our experience, patients who use visual imaging feel a sense of mastery, assertiveness, and competence. One major problem with visual imaging is its use by fringe practitioners as a substitute for needed surgery, medication, or chemotherapy.

A review (34) of the literature investigating the success of intervention with cancer patients concluded that there were such methodologic inadequacies in the studies that the efficacy of psychosocial intervention remains equivocal (33). Definitive studies of the utility of a comprehensive therapeutic approach to the cancer patient and family are essential. The educational component of the method suggested by us is replicable. It is helpful and noncontroversial (with the exception of visual imaging) and may be cost-effective in the long run.

REFERENCES

1. American Cancer Society: 1988 Cancer Facts and Figures. New York, 1988.

2. Abrams, R.D. The patient with cancer: His changing pattern of communication. N Eng J Med 274:317-322, 1966.

3. Derogatis, L.; Morrow, G.; Fetting, J.; et al. The prevalence of psychiatric disorders among cancer patients. JAMA 249(6):1983.

4. Capone, M.A.; Westicks, K.S.; Chitwood, J.S.; et al. Crisis intervention: A functional model for hospitalized cancer patients. Am J Orthopsychiatry 49:598-607, 1979.

5. Trillin, A.S. Of dragons and garden peas. N Eng J Med 304:699-701, 1982.

6. Silberfarb, P.M.; Greer, S. Psychological concomitants of cancer: Clinical aspects. Am J Psychotherapy 36:470-478, 1982.

7. Marmor, J. Short-term dynamic psychotherapy. Am J Psychiatry 136:149-155, 1979.

8. Wellisch, D. Psychosocial problems of cancer, In: Haskell CM (ed): Cancer Treatment. Philadelphia, WB Saunders, pp. 1036-1045, 1980.

9. Pfeffenbaum, G.; Pasnau, R.; Jamison, K.; et al. A comprehensive program of psychosocial care for mastectomy patients. Int J Psychiatry Med 8:65-71, 1977.

10. Schain, W.S. Sexual problems of patients with cancer, In: Devita VT, Hellman S, Rosenberg SA (eds): Cancer: Principles and Practices of Oncology. Philadelphia, JB Lippincott,

pp. 278-290, 1982.

11. Redding, K.; Hotvedt, M.; Fordney, D.; et al. Guidelines for physicians in addressing sexuality concerns of patients with cancer. Arizona Med 107-110, Feb. 1982.

12. Kolodny, R.C.; Masters, W.H.; Johnson, V.E. Textbook of Sexual Medicine. Boston, Little Brown and Co., 1979.

13. Sutherland, A.M. The Physical Impact of Cancer. American Cancer Society. New York, 1960.

14. Jerse, M.A.; Whitman, H.H.; Gustafson, J.P. Cancer in adults, In: Roback HB (ed): Helping Patients and Their Families Cope with Medical Problems. San Francisco, Jossey-Bass, pp. 251-285, 1984.

15. Spiegel, D.; Bloom, J.R.; Yalom, I. Group support for patients with metastatic cancer: A randomized prospective outcome study. Arch Gen Psychiatry 38:527-533, 1981.

16. Fiore, N. Fighting cancer: One patient's outcome study. N Eng J Med 300:284-289, 1979.

17. Bloom, J.R.; Ross, R.D.; Burnell, G. The effect of social support on patient adjustment after breast surgery. Patient Counseling Health ED 1:50-59, 1978.

18. La Barba, R.C. Experimental and environmental factors in cancer. Psychosom Med 32:259-269, 1970.

19. Blumberg, B.; Flaherty, M. Services available to persons with cancer. JAMA 244: Oct. 10, 1980.

20. Peck, A. Emotional reactions to having cancer. Radium Ther Nuc Med 114:591-599, 1972.

21. Singer, B.A. Psychosocial trauma, defense strategies and

treatment consideration in cancer patients and their families. Am J Fam Ther 11:15-21, 1983.

22. Plumb, M.M.; Holland, J. Comparative studies of psychological functions in patients with advanced cases of self-reported depressive symptoms. J Psychosom Med 39:264-276.

23. Kushner. When Bad Things Happen to Good People. Schocken Books, NY, 1981.

24. Barber, J.; Redding, K.; Beutler, L.; et al. Psychosocial characteristics. J Psychosocial Oncology 2(34):93-109, 1984.

25. Novotny, E.S.; Hyland, J.M.; Coyne, L.; et al. Factors affecting adjustments to cancer. Bull Menninger Clin 48:318-328, 242-350, 1984.

26. Bleeker, J.A.C. Brief psychotherapy with lung cancer patients. Psychosom med 29:282-287, 1978.

27. Renneker, R.E. Countertransference reactions to cancer. Psychosom Med 19:409-418, 1957.

28. Redding, K. Coping strategies for the professional in working with oncology patients. Arizona Med 37(8):565-568, 1980.

29. Druss, R.G. Psychotherapy of patients with serious intercurrent medical illness. Bull Assoc Psychoanal Med 23:163-168, 1984.

30. Cassileth, B.R.; Lusk, E.J.; Miller, D.S.; et al. Psychosocial correlates of survival in advanced malignant disease. N Eng J Med 312:1551-1555, 1985.

31. Greer, S.; Morris, T.; Pettingale, K.W. Psychological

response to breast cancer: Effect on outcome. Lancet 2:785-787, 1979.

32. News and Comment. Cancer and the Mind: How are they connected? Sciences 200:1363-1365, 1978.

33. Stavraky, K.M. Psychological factors in the outcome of human cancer. J Psychosom Res 12:251-259, 1968.

34. Watson, M. Psychosocial intervention with cancer patients: A review. Psychol Med 13:839-846, 1983.

NEUROPSYCHIATRIC COMPLICATIONS OF CANCER AND ITS TREATMENT

Francisco Fernandez, M.D.[+]
Assistant Professor of Psychiatry

Valerie F. Holmes, M.D.[°]
Assistant Professor of Psychiatry

Joel K. Levy, Ph.D.[+]
Assistant Professor of Psychiatry

Mary Neidhart, R.N.[*]
Nurse Clinician

[+]Baylor College of Medicine
Psychiatric Consultation Service
St. Luke's Episcopal Hospital
Houston, Texas

[°]Section of Consultation/Liaison Psychiatry
Department of Psychiatry
State University of New York-Stony Brook
Stony Brook, New York

[*]AIDS Nurse Coordinator
Department of Internal Medicine
University of New Mexico
Albuquerque, New Mexico

All correspondence to: Francisco Fernandez, M.D., Chief, Psychiatry Consultation Service, St. Luke's Episcopal Hospital, 6720 Bertner Avenue, Room Y2439, Houston, Texas 77030

I.   OBJECTIVES

This chapter will address:

1.   the most common psychiatric problems in oncology;

2.   a systematic neuropsychiatric method for considering organic factors relevant to the differential diagnosis of abnormal affect, behavior and cognition;

3.   management of specific problems in cancer patients such as delirium, depression, anxiety, pain and treatment-related emesis; and,

4.   neuropsychiatric issues surrounding quality of life in oncology.

II.   DIAGNOSTIC CRITERIA

A lack of reliable diagnostic criteria for emotional disorders often leads to confusion for clinicians in psychiatric diagnosis and clinical decision making in oncology. As opposed to traditional conceptual models of illness in psychiatry, the medical model in contemporary medicine has three major components: 1) the identification of clinical syndromes, 2) the study of clinical-pathologic correlations, and 3) the discovery of the etiology. When applying the medical model to neuropsychopathology, the clinical syndromes would be disturbances in thought, emotion and behavior. A relatively recent interest in American psychiatry has been the application of the medical model in the delineation of psychiatric syndromes through the use of reliable and valid criteria. This series of developments has effectively paved the way for many investigations of clinical and pathologic correlations in psychiatric illnesses. The advancement of clinical assessments and neuropsychology have been critical to the development of a methodologically sound approach to the study of psychopathology.

The current edition of the Diagnostic and Statistical Manual of Mental Disorders (DSM-III) (1) has separated organic brain syndromes from idiopathic or functional disorders based on psychopathologic features. The approach taken by DSM-III is purely descriptive and the terms Organic Mental Disorders (OMDs), Affective Disorders and Schizophrenic Disorders are used to refer to a constellation of psychological or behavioral signs and symptoms without reference to etiology. For example, the DSM-III term OMD designates a particular brain syndrome in which the etiology is known or presumed. Separation of OMD according to the predominant area of psychopathologic features is done using specific criteria. This is expected to increase diagnostic reliability. After identifying a particular mental disorder a differential diagnosis must include associated medical disorders.

III.   A NEUROPSYCHIATRIC APPROACH IN EXAMINING CANCER PATIENTS

Although the criteria for the diagnosis of mental disorders have been standardized and tested for reliability and validity, they unfortunately do not specify the operations needed to arrive at the diagnosis. Most physicians rely on a brief mental status examination to grossly screen for brain function. Even when done in an orderly fashion, the traditional tests for a mental status examination fail to distinguish the more subtle cognitive impairments that are common in cancer patients. Neuropsychological batteries, although comprehensive, are time consuming and cumbersome and do not allow for a quick bedside diagnosis.

A simple test that has gained much popularity for screening medical and psychiatric patients is the Mini-Mental Status Examination (MMSE) developed by Folstein and colleagues (2). This test is comprised of eleven categories of questions requiring 30 responses and takes only 5 to 10 minutes to administer. Reliability and validity are quite high for differentiating dementia from functional conditions in all samples of patients and for monitoring the clinical improvement of treatable conditions. Its diagnostic accuracy, however, for the subtler impairments in cognition typical of cancer patients is poor. Folstein has recommended adding a visual analog scale to rate the level of consciousness and a tachistoscopic assessment to measure the capacity to attend and concentrate in combination with the MMSE in cancer patients (3). There are significant problems with this suggestion: the difficulty of teaching the use of the tachistoscope to cognitively impaired patients, the difficulty of using this instrument at the bedside of medically ill patients, and the time involved in completing such a complicated evaluation.

Furthermore, mental status exams of the verbal "bedside" type, when used alone, fall short of needed diagnostic sensitivity for at least two other specific reasons. Firstly, these tests rarely include measures of complex visuospatial function. Thus, they may not detect right hemisphere involvement (4,5). Secondly, these tests tend to measure mainly orientation and cortical language-associated functions of naming, repetition, verbal memory, praxis, and calculation. They usually do not include tasks involving sustained cognitive tracking, speed of cognitive processing, and delayed recall. These functions are often deemed "subcortical" functions (19), and are frequently impaired in cancer patients. The impairments may arise from the endocrine or metabolic disturbances and/or radiation or chemotherapeutic side effects.

Neurobehavioral assessment need not consume multiple hours and tax the patient's endurance. Mental status examinations that cover a broad range of cognitive functions that include some measurement of speed of cognitive processing exist [e.g., the Neurobehavioral Mental Status Examination (6)]. This screening allows for some detection of focal findings such as might appear with previously undiscovered intracranial metastases. When supplemented with other brief tasks of speed of cognitive processing [Controlled Oral Word

Association (7); Trail Making Test (8); Letter Cancellation (8); Stroop Color-Word Test (7); Finger Tapping Test (8)], which do not require cumbersome apparatus, evaluation of functions often subtly impaired as a result of the disease or its treatments can be effected.

IV. ORGANIC MENTAL DISORDERS IN ONCOLOGY

Screening oncology patients to rule out OMDs is of utmost importance. As many as 70% of outpatients and 90% of inpatients referred for "depression" at the U. T. M. D. Anderson Hospital and Tumor Institute are found to have OMDs (9). Given that cancer is a disease of older people who are concurrently at increased risk for benign senescent changes and OMDs, any psychiatric symptoms presenting for the first time in patients over 40 years of age merit careful scrutiny since functional psychiatric syndromes generally begin prior to that age.

A.   Delirium

Of all the OMDs, delirium is the most frequently encountered by physicians. It is estimated that as many as 25% of hospitalized medical/surgical patients have an undetected delirium (10). If geriatric patients are considered, the prevalence of delirium is closer to 40% (11). In a study of 100 cancer patients referred for depression, Adams demonstrated that 70% had an unsuspected organic disorder (12). Recent reports that cognitively impaired medical patients have higher fatality rates than cognitively intact patients are alarming (13). The detection of any OMD is clinically important because of the potential for reversibility (14) and the danger of letting delirium progress (15).

Delirium in cancer patients reflects diffuse cerebral cellular metabolic dysfunction (16). Often there is a prodromal phase in which the patients complain of difficulty thinking, restlessness, irritability, or insomnia associated in many cases with vivid nightmares. Identifying this prodromal phase should generate a search for a cause of the delirium and aid in preventing neuropsychiatric complications. A brief mental status examination focusing on arousal, attention, short term memory and orientation often reveals multiple deficits. Clinical variability of the signs and symptoms, especially diurnal variation (worse at night than during the day), is the hallmark of delirium. Abnormal involuntary movements such as tremor, multi-focal myoclonus, and asterixis are pathognomonic of delirium. A non-focal neurologic examination is generally the rule.

A discussion of the numerous causes of delirium is beyond the scope of this chapter. Certain common causes of delirium are life-threatening, may cause permanent brain damage, and require prompt diagnosis and treatment. These include Wernicke's encephalopathy, hypo- or hyperglycemia, hypoxemia, hemodynamic instability with cerebral hypoperfusion, infections, and metabolic dysfunctions including electrolyte disturbances. Additionally, leptomeningeal disease, cerebral metastases, meningitis or encephalitis, central nervous system paraneoplastic syndromes, neurotoxicities from chemotherapeutic agents, and radiotherapy should be included in the differential diagnosis of delirium in cancer patients.

The treatment of delirium has relied primarily on conservative management (17). Over the last fifteen years the safety and efficacy of high potency neuroleptics have gained them increasing popularity. Both oral and intramuscular haloperidol have been used without serious adverse effects (18-19). More recent reports have documented the safety of intravenous haloperidol either alone (20) or in combination with lorazepam for agitated delirious patients (21). Our experience with delirious cancer patients at the U. T. M. D. Anderson Hospital and Tumor Institute is that high doses of combination intravenous haloperidol with intravenous lorazepam are safe and effective. Attenuation of most symptoms can be achieved within 24 to 36 hours.

Swift attenuation of cognitive, affective and behavioral dysfunctions which increase the morbidity and mortality of delirium is the principle goal guiding rapid tranquilization. Although some physicians still consider high doses of intravenous haloperidol and lorazepam to be "dangerous", there is no evidence other than hypothetical to substantiate this claim. The ideal dose of any therapeutic regimen is the smallest dose which accomplishes maximal clinical effect; however, high initial doses of intravenous medications are indicated in cases where effective control of severely agitated delirium is essential to the patient's well-being.

B.   Dementia

Dementia generally refers to a group of disorders that are insidious and involve a destructive process of the cerebral mechanism (22). Diffuse and global deficits in higher cortical functioning are the prominent features of dementia. Unlike delirium, changes in arousal or attention are unusual until the terminal phases of the disorder. A list of the common causes of dementia can be found in Table 1. An important and useful distinction can be made between dementias associated with reversible organic illnesses (i.e., secondary dementias) and the dementias for which an organic cause cannot be demonstrated but is inferred (i.e., primary dementias). The contribution of chemotherapeutic agents in the subgroup of patients with drug-induced secondary dementias has not been systematically evaluated.

Exclusive of patients with the acquired immunodeficiency syndrome (AIDS), our study of the incidence of dementia in cancer patients indicates that 70.5% met criteria for an OMD of which 18% had a clinical dementia (9). Of these demented patients, 55% had specific reversible etiologies. Many patients with mild and benign senescent changes in cognitive functioning developed a clinical dementia following their treatment with either chemotherapy or radiation or both. In the latter subgroup of patients, most developed dementia after a prolonged and treatment-resistant delirium.

When dementia is suspected in cancer patients, a routine evaluation should include a CBC, arterial blood gases, serologic test for syphilis, serum chemistries, serum thyroxin and TSH, serum B-12 and folate levels, screening for toxicology and heavy metals, a formal coagulogram, urinalysis, chest x-ray, electrocardiogram, electroencephalogram, computerized tomography of the brain and a lumbar puncture (23). We have seen some patients whose evaluation is entirely negative and a paraneoplastic carcinomatous dementia has been considered the diagnosis by exclusion.

C.   Organic Personality Syndrome (OPS)

Personality changes are commonly associated with neoplastic disease. In many instances these changes are transient and are secondary to stress or distress caused by a life-threatening malignancy (24). However, personality changes may reflect an OPS such as described in DSM-III. These personality changes may be associated with metastatic disease, carcinomatous meningitis, partial seizure activity, metabolic imbalance, radiation encephalopathy or chemotherapy-related neurotoxicities (25-27). Destructive lesions of either the orbital areas or convexity of the frontal lobes have long been known to cause OPS (28). The patient with OPS secondary to a frontal lobe lesion is one who is either emotionally labile and impulsive or apathetic, pseudodepressed and indifferent. Our experience with the psychostimulants, specifically methylphenidate, is similar to that of others which indicates that the majority of OPS patients respond to these agents (29-33).

It is important to remember that the personality changes encountered with these lesions may also result from a variety of metabolic disturbances that are not of sufficient severity to produce a delirium. Uremia, hyper- and hypocalcemia, hypokalemia and hypoxemia, can produce varying personality changes that would meet DSM-III criteria for organic personality syndrome (34). Our experience with organic personality syndromes in cancer patients suggests that impending sepsis can also produce nonspecific changes in personality including alterations in initiative and energy, irritability and blunting of affect. Chemotherapy and/or radiotherapy-induced neurotoxicity can likewise produce similar effects (see Section VIII) specifically with agents such as interferon, dexamethasone, cisplatinum, methotrexate and cytosine arabinoside.

D.   Organic Affective Syndromes (OAS)

OAS are common in cancer patients secondary to treatment with ACTH, steroids, or any other hormones (35-37). Most of these disorders involve mania or hypomania followed by depression and delirium. When lithium is given prophylactically, steroid-related mania have been avoided (38). Although sometimes more difficult to treat, depression secondary to steroids has effectively responded to either psychostimulants alone or in combination with antidepressants (Dr. Frank Adams, personal communication). Paraneoplastic syndromes due to carcinoid tumors containing enkephalins and beta endorphins have been associated with both manic and depressive episodes (39). Manic psychoses from procarbazine (a mild MAO-I) and interferon have also been identified (see Section VIII). Direct brain insults particularly to the right hemisphere such as metastatic disease, subdural hemorrhage or surgical trauma with resultant partial complex seizures may induce mania. Likewise, left hemispheric lesions or trauma, steroids, vinca alkaloids, cisplatinum, L-asparaginase, analgesics, metabolic imbalances and isolation can all cause depressive symptoms.

E.   Other Organic Disorders

The remaining organic mental disorders (amnestic syndrome, organic delusional syndrome and organic hallucinosis) are less common. Amnestic syndromes are more typical in AIDS patients and can be an early complication of the disease. Herpes encephalitis with its predilection for the temporal lobes is a common cause of memory disorders in cancer patients (40). Vitamin deficiency and hemorrhages in the mamillary bodies giving rise to a Wernicke-Korsakoff-like syndrome have been associated with hematologic malignancies, particularly lymphoma (41). Transient episodes of amnesia in elderly patients receiving aggressive chemotherapy are most often due to temporary vascular insufficiency involving the inferior, mesial portion of the temporal lobes (42). Trauma secondary to surgical excision of metastases in the temporal lobes can also give a similar syndrome.

Organic delusional syndromes are sometimes present in cancer patients, but again, are more commonly found in AIDS patients secondary to the subacute encephalitis associated with Human Immunodeficiency Virus (HIV) infection. A similar syndrome can be found in patients with B-12 deficiency, probably due to impaired myelination (43).

Organic hallucinosis can occur as a result of various insults such as sepsis, neurotoxic drugs, analgesics, focal seizure activity, and partial blindness due to surgical enucleation of primary eye disease (44). Sensory deprivation has been reported to cause false perception in subjects and may be seen in patients who are either in a protective environment or in isolation.

V. DEPRESSION AND CANCER

Depression is commonly believed to the major psychiatric complication of cancer (45). Historically, writers as far back as Galen believed that melancholic states increased proneness to cancer (46). The literature is replete with impressionistic reports of depression predating the diagnosis of cancer that consider depression a possible etiology of the disease. This psychosomatic myth is compounded by a belief among physicians that cancer patients are understandably depressed and that it is therefore an expected consequence (i.e., "wouldn't you be depressed if you had cancer?"). This widespread yet erroneous notion ignores the neurobiological significance of behavioral and emotional changes in cancer patients (47). Furthermore, altered mental states may be trivialized by the traditional biopsychosocial model of psychiatry into psychological expressions of character pathology, life circumstance problems, coping and adjustment problems, "acting out" behavior, anxiety, and depression. When encountering patients who have symptoms across multiple psychiatric diagnostic categories, a thorough medical evaluation in every patient may obviate a psychiatric referral.

When the presence of an OMD has been ruled out, the diagnosis of depression should be considered. They psycho-oncology literature reports that major depressive episodes occur in as many as 50% of cancer patients (48). Without rigorous diagnostic criteria for the assessment of higher cortical functions, the diagnosis of depression in any medically ill population is suspect, as delirium and other OMDs can masquerade as depression (49,50).

Depression is a concept that easily generates confusion, even among psychiatrists. Unfortunately, depression is loosely used to describe a wide spectrum of behaviors and symptoms ranging from a mild and transient mood disturbance to a major affective disorder. Limiting depression to the definition found in the DSM-III (1) avoids misdiagnoses and medical mismanagement. In controlled studies using DSM-III criteria the prevalence of clinical depression in cancer patients is 6% (51-52). This rate is equivalent to that seen in the general population (53). These findings refute the argument that cancer patients in particular are depressed.

There are obvious difficulties in making the diagnosis of depression in cancer patients. For instance, it would be uncommon to find a patient who has not suffered from one or more of the somatic symptoms that overlap with the symptom complex of depression (54). Consequently some clinicians advocated reliance on cognitive or psychological symptoms of distress rather than on somatic signs and symptoms of depression. However, there is no evidence to suggest that these should be considered separately. In fact, a recent study suggests that the combination of both somatic and non-somatic symptoms appears more frequently among depressed cancer patients than among controls (52).

The treatment of depression in cancer patients is based largely on clinical experience and intuition. The available studies suggest that psychotropic drugs are either underused or used inappropriately in this population (55-57). This may be secondary to a popular and long standing bias against medical intervention for psychological symptoms or "psycho-pharmacologic Calvinism" (58).

At present, the choice of a tricyclic antidepressant for the treatment of depression is based on physician preference. All antidepressants have been reported to have an equivalent clinical efficacy in the treatment of depression. A particular choice can be made by knowing the different pharmacologic profiles of these agents and clinical information including a previous positive treatment response to a specific antidepressant, a first degree relative with a positive response to a particular antidepressant, or a positive response to a psychostimulant challenge test (59-62). Additionally, the patient's clinical presentation will determine whether one wishes a calming vs a stimulating effect (i.e., a serotonergic vs. a noradrenergic agent).

Standard clinical guidelines for antidepressant pharmacotherapy should be followed once treatment is initiated (63). It is the authors' experience that cancer patients appear to respond to antidepressants in a shorter time and at lower doses than physically healthy patients who are depressed. Treatment, therefore, should start with low doses and increases should be made as tolerated. After an adequate therapeutic effect has been reached over three to four weeks, the drug should be maintained for a minimum of six months at therapeutic doses. Should symptoms recur while tapering the medication, returning to a maintenance dose regimen (usually half of the initial therapeutic dose) and treating for another three to 12 months is indicated (64). Monoamine oxidase inhibitors (65) are generally not used as a first line agent in the treatment of cancer patients while undergoing antineoplastic therapy because of the fear of a hypertensive crisis or other drug interactions. Nevertheless, these fears should not interfere in the medical management of a depressed cancer patient given that the mortality associated with depression from suicide alone is as high as 15% (66). Likewise, fear of hematopoietic toxicities of agranulocytosis and neutropenia (67) should not interfere with medical treatment. We have treated many patients who are receiving concomitant marrow-depleting chemotherapy without any evidence for added toxicity.

The use of psychostimulants in cancer patients is rapidly growing (31,33). These agents are effective in quickly remitting the major signs and symptoms of depression without side effects. Our psychostimulant experience is highlighted by psychomotor activation, appetite stimulation, and qualitative improvement in higher cortical functions and in affect within hours. Treatment is typically initiated with 5-15 mg of methylphenidate (or its equivalent in either dextroamphetamine or pemoline) either by mouth, feeding tube, or suppository (prepared especially by our pharmacy) and adjusted as needed. A typical schedule would be 5-30 mg of methylphenidate administered at 7 a.m., 10 a.m., and 1 p.m. More than 30 mgs a day is rarely needed, but doses of up to 90 mgs of methylphenidate may sometimes be required. Even at these higher doses we have not encountered the side effects often anticipated (paranoia, hallucinations, suppression of appetite, sleep disturbance or cardiovascular complications).

We believe psychostimulant treatment to be the most effective treatment for various signs and symptoms of depression from various etiologies and it can be continued safely for several weeks or months after the patient becomes asymptomatic. Patients encountering anergia, fatigue and the so-called "chemotherapy blues" are commonly treated with psychostimulants for the duration of their chemotherapy. At times, this can be prolonged for up to a year without evidence of tolerance or drug abuse (32).

For depressed hospitalized patients, intravenous amitriptyline can be used without untoward effects (68). Treatment is initiated by infusing 10 mgs of the commercially available injectable amitriptyline in 100 ml of either normal saline or 5% dextrose solution over precisely 90 minutes at bedtime. Doses are then adjusted by 5-10 mg nightly until the patient shows improvement in target symptoms such as insomnia, tearfulness, and dysphoria. Many patients with abnormal ejection fractions, conduction defects such as left and right bundle branch blocks, doxorubicin toxicity, and pericardial windows have tolerated this procedure without cardiovascular side effects (e.g., rhythm and conduction disturbances or hypotension; 69). Nonspecific ST-T wave changes in the electrocardiogram have been found only in rare cases. We have found the effectiveness of this treatment to equal that of electroconvulsive therapy. While treating severely depressed outpatients, amitriptyline or imipramine can be used intramuscularly. In addition, tricyclic antidepressants or psychostimulants by rectal suppositories can be used in order to avoid hospitalizing these patients (70). Alternatively, a continuous infusion pump can be used at home for those patients with a ready access.

VI. ANXIETY DISORDERS

Anxiety is a universal accompaniment to any medical disorder including cancer. Cancer patients are prone to have reactive anxiety at differing times of crises: the initial discovery of the cancer, during diagnostic workups and reevaluations for restaging purposes and when a new treatment is started (71). Patients with a generalized anxiety disorder, panic disorder, obsessive/compulsive disorder or an atypical anxiety disorder preceding the diagnosis of cancer could experience a severe recurrence or exacerbation of their symptomatology requiring either an adjustment or reinstitution of their psychopharmacologic treatment.

Medical screening of anxious cancer patients is necessary. When anxiety is a prominent symptom, psychiatric evaluation should be generated only in addition to a complete medical workup. It is useful to remember that primary anxiety disorders are uncommon in patients after the age of 35. Therefore, the development of either obsessive/compulsive disorder, simple phobia, or panic disorder after the age of 35 requires the same initial complete medical evaluation.

Free-floating anxiety of insufficient severity to warrant the diagnosis of an anxiety disorder by DSM-III is a common feature of medical illness. When supportive measures and reassurance fail in abating anxiety, benzodiazepines (BZDs) remain the treatment of choice (72). All are equally effective anxiolytics and differ only by their elimination half-lives (73) and cost. Barbiturates, antihistamines, meprobamate, tricyclic antidepressants and neuroleptics should never be routinely used in cases of generalized anxiety since their safety and effectiveness do not compare with that of the BZDs.

BZDs fall into two groups: long- or short-acting agents. Those that are long-acting have longer half-lives because they are oxidized in the liver through multiple intermediate steps and have active metabolites (74). These intermediary metabolites have even longer half-lives than the parent compounds and are responsible for most of the drug-related side effects. It is useful to remember that the principal metabolite of diazepam, desmethyl-diazepam, has a half-life of 90-100 hours and thus takes longer to achieve a steady state (75). Once accomplished, compounds with long half-lives allow for once a day dosing.

The short- to-intermediate-acting BZDs are metabolized more simply, have a briefer duration of action requiring multi-dosing, and generally do not have active metabolites (76). Their lack of active metabolites make them safer for use in the elderly and in the cognitively impaired. Their short half-lives make them ideal for use in patients whose anxiety is limited to particular situations such as chemotherapy-related anxiety or while undergoing diagnostic or therapeutic procedures.

Given that elimination half-lives increase markedly with age, and that cancer patients have a higher likelihood of impaired clearance for varying reasons, our preference is to use short-acting BZDs such as lorazepam, oxazepam and alprazolam. Since lorazepam does not precipitate and form crystals at physiologic pH, it is the only BZD that should be given intramuscularly (77). It is our preferred parenteral BZD used in the treatment of anxiety, and in combination with haloperidol in managing both delirium (21) and treatment-related emesis (see Section IX). Alprazolam is our drug of choice in the following situations: adjustment disorders with single or mixed emotional features (usually anxiety and/or depression), "minor depression", mixed features of reactions to stress and distress. Although not approved for the treatment of depression, our experience, like that of others (78), is that it is an effective antidepressant devoid of the bothersome side effects commonly associated with tricyclic antidepressants.

Once the decision has been made to treat patients suffering from anxiety with BZDs, treatment for a brief period (i.e., two to three weeks) is recommended. Guidelines for long-term treatment are not firmly established but are similar to that for primary psychiatric disorders. We have noted virtually no risk for abuse.

VII. PAIN

Pain is a common symptom that occurs across various diagnostic categories in cancer patients. Effective analgesia is crucial for improving quality of life in cancer patients who suffer pain. Psychiatrists commonly encounter pain problems in cancer patients but, like other specialists, they frequently overlook the benefits of psychotropics in pain management. Adequate analgesia aids the recovery from associated symptoms such as insomnia, depressed mood, exhaustion and agitation. Narcotic analgesia is the preferred treatment for unrelieved organic pain associated with a malignancy. Therefore, psychiatrists should be familiar with potency and pharmacokinetics of typical narcotic analgesics (79). They should also be familiar with the current descriptive classification of pain syndromes and definitions, such as that of the International Association for the Study of Pain, to effectively diagnose and treat patients with cancer pain. This universal classification system has been the subject of a recent review (80). We will limit our discussion here to effective pharmacologic strategies in the treatment of these pain syndromes.

When choosing a narcotic analgesic it is always best to begin with a low potency narcotic and increase potency as necessary. Meperidine should be avoided whenever possible, since its active metabolite, normeperidine, is notorious for causing a variety of adverse central nervous system effects, including seizures (81). When pain becomes refractory to increasing doses of narcotic analgesics, it has become popular to add longer-acting agents such as methadone or controlled-release preparations of morphine. In the experience of the authors, regimens involving single oral narcotic analgesics are less neurotoxic than combinations of the short- and long-acting narcotics. We specifically avoid methadone because its analgesic effect is of short duration and does not correlate with its half-life or plasma concentration (82). Because methadone's half-life changes over time, there is generally a greater likelihood of cumulative toxicity. The use of long-acting or controlled-release preparations should be avoided, especially in the aged, the cognitively impaired or those who have multiple organ failure.

Our preferred parenteral narcotic analgesic is hydromorphone. This potent analgesic has few active metabolites, making it the most effective and, potentially, the least toxic of its class. It is comparable to heroin in solubility, kinetics and potency (83). Parenteral hydromorphone is five times more potent than parenteral morphine and four times more potent than oral hydromorphone. Doses are generally scheduled every three hours. On the other hand, in the outpatient situation, it is usually desirable to convert dosing to oral administration. Should unwanted side effects occur in converting hydromorphone from parenteral to oral preparations, then either conversion to a combination of cola syrup and injectable hydromorphone or oral morphine elixir (84) can be given with equal effectiveness and fewer side effects. The former is palatable and the experience to date is devoid of significant adverse effects, specifically nausea and vomiting. Doubling or tripling the regular dose at bedtime obviates the need to wake the patient during the night. Constipation remains the most serious side effect of any narcotic regimen and a bowel management program should be started concomitantly with the initiation of any narcotic analgesics.

Narcotic analgesics should not be combined. As a rule, combinations of these agents yield added toxicity rather than improved analgesia. One should not combine partial narcotic antagonists such as pentazocine, butorphanol, and nalbuphine with pure agonists, since the former agents will invariably precipitate a withdrawal reaction (83). Fear of dependency and abuse should not hinder clinical decision-making in the treatment of terminal or malignant pain since these fears are unfounded and only serve to generate and perpetuate poor clinical management.

The addition of specific psychopharmacologic agents as narcotic adjuvants should be reserved for pain refractory to optimal use of narcotic analgesics. Stimulants, neuroleptics, tricyclic antidepressants and anticonvulsants have been used for many years as analgesic adjuvants. Their choice should be individualized with an important goal of treatment being to obtain the most potent combination of drugs with the simplest regimen. At present there are no established criteria for choosing one psychotropic adjuvant over another. Physicians can follow simple guidelines based on the associated symptoms and character of the pain.

The success of tricyclic antidepressants as narcotic adjuvants rests largely on evidence that these agents act in reticular and limbic components of the central nervous system involved in pain transmission (85,86). Regardless of whether or not there is a clinical depression, tricyclic antidepressants can sometimes provide significant relief. Their effectiveness, however, has recently been called into question in a controlled study of the treatment of deafferentation pain associated with diabetic peripheral neuropathy (87). It may well be that the analgesic effect of tricyclic antidepressants is largely theoretical and these substances may have greater effectiveness in chronic pain than in organic pain of malignant or other origin. The routine use of tricyclic antidepressants, adopted from the model established in chronic pain clinics, should be avoided in cancer patients. Central antihistaminic and anticholinergic side effects (88) generally limit the use of these agents in cancer patients, many of whom are aged. In general, we recommend that the use of tricyclic antidepressants in cancer patients be restricted to situations in which depression coexists with a treatable pain syndrome, when insomnia is present despite adequate analgesia, when the use of benzodiazepines is contraindicated, or when in selected cases of deafferentation, causalgic pain is refractory to anticonvulsants alone (89).

The usefulness of neuroleptics (phenothiazines, thioxanthenes, and butyrophenones) to augment the effects of narcotic analgesia has long been known. Specifically, butyrophenones have been shown to potentiate the effects of morphine, both acutely and chronically (90). Additionally, some of these agents have been found to bind to opiate receptors (91) and thus further strengthen the observation of neuroleptanalgesia. Our preferred neuroleptic is haloperidol. Its potency and limited side effects, specifically the lack of anticholinergic and alpha adrenergic blocking properties (92), make it an ideal narcotic adjuvant in this population. Low doses of 1 to 2 mg four times daily can provide significant relief. Haloperidol's affinity for the mesolimbic dopamine pathways is theoretically of added benefit in diminishing the negative affective experience associated with pain.

The value of anticonvulsants in the management of deafferentation causalgic pain from various sources, including phantom breast, limb, bladder, and rectal pain, has recently been reviewed by Swerdlow (93). Carbamazepine, valproic acid, and clonazepam have all been found to be effective in reducing deafferentation-type pain. The clinical utility of anticonvulsants in the treatment of this severely debilitating pain syndrome is unsurpassed with up to 70% effectiveness sighted.

Stimulants potentiate the effects of narcotic analgesics, reduce narcotic requirements and counteract the adverse central nervous system effects of narcotics while restoring vital processes such as mood, affect, psychomotor activation, and other neurocognitive functions (31,68,94-95). Doses of 5 to 20 mgs orally of dextroamphetamine sulfate or its equivalent for methylphenidate can significantly improve the patients' quality of life. Again, arguments against these agents basically rely on questions about the addictive potential and tolerance of these agents with continued use. Abuse is a moot issue in the treatment of terminally ill patients in pain, and tolerance is rarely encountered.

VIII. NEUROTOXICITIES

Priestman has stated that cytotoxic chemotherapy is the art of differential poisoning, the aim being to destroy the tumor before the drugs kill the patient (96). Unfortunately, an often overlooked area is central nervous system (CNS) toxicity. CNS complications range between 5 and 86% for varying classes of drugs (97). Psychiatric disturbances are frequently poorly defined and little is known about their long-term sequelae. For the purposes of this discussion, cancer chemotherapeutic agents associated with neuropsychiatric toxicity will be described under the major groups of antineoplastic agents exclusive of steroids and hormones. This will be followed by a brief discussion of bone marrow transplantation and cranial irradiation.

Alkylating agents interfere with protein synthesis by causing DNA miscoding. They are lipophilic and thus cross the blood-brain barrier (98). These agents include five major classes and can be seen in Table 2. They are nitrogen mustards, ethylenimine derivatives, alkyl sulfonates, nitrosoureas and triazenes. Alkylating agents are powerful CNS stimulants with prominent cholinergic properties. They have been reported to cause toxic encephalopathies, depression, hallucinations, and other diffuse cognitive and affective effects (37,99-103). Sullivan also found that patients who experienced early toxicity with mechlorethamine and lived another 60 days or more tended to have delayed new neurotoxicities (101). Autopsy findings after nitrogen mustard treatment have included neuronal degeneration and demyelination, gliosis in both white and gray matter of the frontal, parietal, hippocampal and subependymal areas and coagulation necrosis (37,101).

The **antimetabolites** interfere with specific enzyme activity or cause the synthesis of a molecule that cannot function normally. Folic acid analogs, pyrimidine analogs and purine analogs are the major agents in this class (see Table 2; 100). Some of these agents cross the blood-brain barrier poorly and thus need to be used intrathecally as in the case of methotrexate. Well known acute and delayed CNS effects may occur which are not reversible and can be lethal. Methotrexate specifically can cause a multifocal leukoencephalopathy, the incidence of which increases with concomitant radiation and the use of intravenous methotrexate. Similar findings occur with cytosine arabinoside (37,99-101,105-110). While the mechanism of methotrexate-induced brain damage is not clear, it has been suggested that the CNS may act as a reservoir exposing nervous tissue to cytotoxic concentrations of methotrexate for prolonged periods, especially if the blood-brain barrier has been compromised by cranial irradiation. Even though its usual action is on dividing cells, methotrexate toxicity may be mediated by direct neuronal injury. Individual pharmacokinetics may also be widely variable (37,99,110). General antimetabolic effects on other CNS enzyme systems (biogenic amines, dopamine, serotonin, B-12-dependent enzyme processes) may contribute as well.

Electroencephalographic (EEG) examinations of patients with chemotherapy-induced neurotoxicity show diffuse slowing. Kaplan found that EEG at the time of diagnosis may be predictive of future neurotoxicity from prophylactic CNS treatment (99). Computerized axial tomography (CT) of the brain may or may not show white matter changes. Magnetic resonance imaging (MRI), however, can detect early white matter changes. There is a characteristic lesion with leukoencephalopathy seen vividly with MRI as increased signal density of the cerebral white matter in a periventricular distribution. This is similar to that seen with subcortical ischemia or demyelinating disease. The white matter changes are due to increased unbound water from treatment-induced damage. MRI, then, may have a role in influencing the course of leukoencephalopathy by allowing treatment modifications to be made before the leukoencephalopathy progresses further (100,111).

Neuropathology has complemented the MRI findings. Extensive myelin loss in deep cerebral white matter with progressive replacement of the white matter with a gliotic layer has been documented (37,100,105,111). Also, myelin basic protein, usually not present in normal cerebrospinal fluid, is elevated with leukoencephalopathy. Elevated levels have been seen with acute cerebral infarct and in demyelinating disease. Increasing levels may indicate progressive disease and may be an additional means of monitoring neurotoxic effects (105,107).

Frytak comments on the possibility of wide-ranging clinical consequences of leukoencephalopathy because white matter contains important "cross-talk" pathways for integrated neurological functions: short and long commissural systems, ipsilateral association pathways, main motor, sensory, visual and language fiber tracts (111). Mineralizing microangiopathy, on the other hand, primarily involves gray matter. Calcified mucopolysaccharides are deposited in and around small vessels. The putamen of the lenticular nucleus is always involved with or without involvement of deeper cortical regions (99). Agents in this class have cause symptoms of somnolence, mood lability, anxiety, delirium, Parkinson's syndrome, and dementia.

The **vinca alkaloids**, vincristine, vinblastine and vindesine, act by inhibiting cellular microtubule formation, blocking mitosis and cell replication (99). These agents differ in antitumor spectra and are used to treat different malignancies. They are known to cause peripheral and cranial nerve neuropathies as well as autonomic effects. Lipophilicity and neurotoxicity are highest with vincristine and lowest with vinblastine. Increased toxicity is often reported when vincristine is used in combination chemotherapy (99,112). Vincristine specifically has been shown to cause psychiatric toxicity ranging from irritability and dysphoric moods to depression, seizure and coma. Vinca alkaloids may exert their effects by inhibiting dopamine beta hydroxylase, the terminal enzyme in the conversion of dopamine to norepinephrine (113). Their relationship to other indole derivatives known to affect mood and behavior (LSD, reserpine, serotonin) may be of theoretical interest to those practicing in psycho-oncology (98).

Maytansine and the epipodophyllotoxins have similarities with the vinca alkaloids. They have minimal access to the CNS unless the blood-brain barrier is impaired (32,94).

Antibiotic agents penetrate the CNS poorly, but the anthracyclines do have neurotoxicity potential as seen primarily in animal models (see Table 2) (37,99).

L-asparaginase and SAGA are **enzymes** that rapidly inhibit synthesis of protein, DNA and RNA in tumor cells. As large proteins they are thought not to cross the blood-brain barrier. Nevertheless, there is a high incidence of CNS effects predominantly in adults (115). Lethargy, delirium, memory impairment and depression have been reported (99). Toxicity may be related to decreased protein synthesis in the brain, to elevated levels of aspartic acid, ammonia and glutamate due to asparagine breakdown by L-asparaginase, or to drug-induced hepatotoxicity with resulting metabolic encephalopathy. EEG examination has shown triphasic delta waves similar to those seen with hepatic encephalopathy (37,102).

Cisplatin is the first heavy metal used as an antineoplastic agent. It crosses the blood-brain barrier minimally and cerebral events are thought to be associated with significant metabolic alterations due to renal tubular dysfunction. Peripheral neuropathies involving vibratory and proprioceptive disturbances have been reported and microscopic examination has shown peripheral demyelination (37).

Procarbazine, a hydrazine monoamine oxidase inhibitor, crosses the blood-brain barrier and produces various psychiatric toxicities. Drowsiness to profound stupor, peripheral neuropathy, confusion, hallucinations, psychosis and disulfiram-like reaction to alcohol have been reported. Although pyridoxine has reversed primary sensory neuropathy induced by hydrazines, it has not been shown effective treating procarbazine-induced encephalopathy or peripheral neuropathy (37).

Among the remaining **miscellaneous agents,** the issue of CNS toxicity has not been thoroughly investigated. Hydroxyurea does occasionally cause drowsiness and hallucinations (37). Adrenocortical suppressants induce somnolence (37). Encephalopathies are reported with thymidine, and spirogermanium. Interferon, a biologic response modifier, has been shown to exert antitumor effects in a variety of neoplasia (116). It, however, also has been associated with a variety of neurobehavioral side effects (119) from behavioral changes measured psychometrically (114,116,117), to electrophysiologic alterations suggestive of encephalopathy (118), and psychosis (119). Peripheral neuropathies are seen with methyl-GAG and amacrine. Misonidazole is a potent electronaffinic hypoxic cell radiosensitizer that is markedly lipophilic and is found in high concentrations in the CNS. It is related to metronidazole (Flagyl) and has caused confusion and seizures. This neurotoxicity may be additive with vincristine therapy (99).

Steroids, as previously discussed under Organic Mental Disorders, have been known to cause psychosis, lability of mood and depression in cancer patients. Subtler subclinical changes may go unrecognized and untreated. Although the neuroleptics can be used effectively for steroid-induced mood lability, lithium carbonate should be considered prophylactically if patients are experiencing manifold mood changes.

Cyclosporine is a potent immunosuppressant used to prevent graft rejection following bone marrow transplantation (BMT) and to allay graft-versus-host disease (120). Patchell found CNS complications in 70% of BMT patients, primarily from infection and cerebrovascular dysfunction. Over one-third of these patients had metabolic encephalopathies due to respiratory, renal, hepatic or electrolyte disturbances, 34% of which were reversible. CNS manifestations usually occurred two months or more after BMT (109).

Neurological complications of cranial irradiation (XRT) are well known. Early reactions include ataxia, somnolence, anorexia dysarthria, dysphasia and irritability. Symptoms generally occurred between days 24 to 56 after XRT was begun and lasted 10 to 38 days. Effects were thought to be secondary to transient XRT-induced disturbance of myelination and autopsy has shown patchy demyelination in irradiated areas. Cerebral, cerebellar and basal ganglia calcifications have been found with XRT-induced blood-brain barrier alterations (100,121). Delayed reactions include late necrosis, seizures, headache, personality change, impaired level of consciousness and somnolence syndrome (121). The latter is a very frequent delayed reaction to cranial XRT. There is a rapid onset of lethargy, irritability and low-grade fever. During this time the EEG shows background slowing. Somatic symptoms of nausea, vomiting and diarrhea are common. The syndrome usually abates spontaneously in one to four weeks (99). Patients who experience the somnolence syndrome are at increased risk for developing late CNS dysfunction including learning disabilities and seizures (100).

Microscopic examination following cranial XRT discloses demyelination along with a macrophage reaction and perivascular inflammation. A virtually diagnostic change is fibrinoid necrosis of the blood vessel wall accompanied by extravasated fibrinoid material and recent parenchymal hemorrhage. Generally, 5000 rads fractionated over five weeks is safe for the brain, but higher doses are often used. For nervous tissue, smaller individual fraction sizes and increased number of treatments seem to help avoid late sequelae (121).

Long-term effects of whole-brain XRT with or without chemotherapy in children include adverse effects on intelligence and endocrine function. In Bamford's 1976 study of 30 children with brain tumors, 20% who underwent surgery plus XRT were profoundly disabled and 43% were educationally subnormal. Other studies strongly implicate XRT as a cause of intellectual deterioration reporting a decline in full scale IQ scores by 25 points or more. Scully states that 25% of children receiving prophylactic cranial XRT will have learning disabilities. Even children with normal IQs had learning disabilities and required special classes. Continued IQ deterioration has been seen longitudinally with math scores and performance skills affected more so than reading and verbal scores. Young children had more serious intellectual deficits with ages one to three years having a 60% change of being mentally defective with IQs of less than 69. Adverse effects on intellect may also not be evident for two to five years following XRT to the brain (122).

Endocrine effects include hypothalamic dysfunction, primary pituitary hormone deficiency, primary hypothyroidism and permanent adverse effects on growth hormone release (121,122). Other long-term sequelae include leukoencephalopathy, necrosis of the amygdala and hippocampus, hearing loss, oncogenesis, acceleration of atherosclerosis, cerebral atrophy, and intracranial occlusive vaculopathy leading to a stroke-like syndrome (100,121,122). As yet, there is no treatment for radiation necrosis and the effects on intelligence cannot be easily remedied (122,123).

High linear energy transfer (LET) radiation uses particles rather than electromagnetic radiation used in x-rays. These particles deposit energy more densely in tissues. Fast neutron particles have good antitumor efficacy, but cause diffuse damage to normal brain including progressive dementia and obtundation, myelitis and brain necrosis. Proton beams used in treatment of acromegaly cause transient diplopia, headache, anterior pituitary insufficiency, and carry a high risk of long-term injury such as cranial nerve palsy, chiasmatic injury, vertigo and seizures. Negative *pi* mesons affect deep structures and spare the overlying tissues. These particles cause more myelitis than x-rays and are potent neurotoxic agents (121).

Although the effects of chemotherapeutic and other antineoplastic agents on the central nervous system appear to be more prevalent than commonly believed, little attention has been given to a comprehensive neuropsychiatric evaluation of these cognitive, affective and behavioral issues. One must be careful to differentiate between physiologic treatment-related changes and reactive phenomena which are commonly attributed to patients undergoing cancer treatment. Diagnostic criteria must be carefully applied in evaluating cancer patients receiving psychoactive agents. Careful observation along with the development of better clinical assessments and use of the advances in the neurosciences will help to better delineate the occurrence of psychiatric toxicity and its pathophysiology.

IX. NAUSEA AND VOMITING

While aggressive therapeutic approaches to the treatment of cancer have resulted in increased cures and improved palliation and survival for many patients, there has likewise been an increase in the number of treatment-related side effects. Nausea and vomiting are chief among these secondary toxicities and are occasionally due to complications of disease, such as leptomeningeal infiltration. Standard antiemetic agents have generally proven ineffective in controlling nausea and vomiting when newer anti-cancer drugs or multiple drug regimens with varying emetogenicity are employed. Aside from the obvious physical discomfort, chemotherapy-induced vomiting can be dose-limiting and may precipitate problems from fluid loss and electrolyte imbalance. Changes in quality of life due to gastrointestinal toxicity may lead patients to question the value of therapy. It is important for psychiatrists working with cancer patients to have knowledge of the vomiting cycle itself and use of effective antiemetic agents that may insure improved patient comfort, satisfaction, and compliance to a potentially beneficial treatment regimen.

The exact mechanisms of chemotherapy-induced nausea and vomiting have not yet been defined. However, postulations are made based on animal research of the vomiting cycle. The first hint of localization of the Vomiting Center (VC) came in 1949 when Borison and Wang were able to continuously produce vomiting by electrical stimulation of an area in the lateral reticular formation of the medulla (124). Ablation of this designated

VC in dogs rendered them refractory to known emetic challenges. While electrical stimulation of the VC results in abrupt emesis, there is no evidence that the VC per se is clinically able to cause vomiting. Rather it is thought that other sensory centers act through the VC. The VC itself regulates and coordinates other medullary structures, i.e., salivation, respiratory and vasomotor functions, to produce the vomiting act.

Studies have shown that vomiting can be drug induced by stimulation of another medullary structure. Appropriately called the Chemoreceptor Trigger Zone (CTZ), this area has been localized to the floor of the fourth ventricle in the region of the area postrema and is accessible to both blood and cerebrospinal fluids (124). Many drugs stimulate this center, although precise mechanisms of action are unclear. It has been postulated that either the drugs themselves or metabolic byproducts cross the blood-brain barrier to stimulate the CTZ either by directly binding to specific receptor sites or by simulating the action of various neurotransmitters. Nausea and vomiting secondary to radiation have also been attributed to stimulation of this center (125).

Peripheral receptors located throughout the body in the alimentary canal, the uterus, kidneys, heart and semi-circular canals are another component to the vomiting process. Overdistention of an organ supplied with sensory receptors or direct stimulation by irritating substances will induce vomiting via afferent impulses to the VC.

Psychic phenomena may also initiate vomiting via the cerebral cortex. Unpleasant thoughts, sights, sounds or sensations may be a precipitating factor for vomiting. The VC is thought to be a major source of stimulation in patients suffering from anticipatory nausea and vomiting. Inability to obliterate the VC lies in the fact that it is positioned in close proximity to the center for respiratory control and does in fact share some neural components with the center.

Pharmacologic intervention in the vomiting cycle is also limited as it is unknown if chemotherapy-induced nausea and vomiting result from single or multiple site stimulation or the methods of stimulation themselves. The role of neurotransmitters and receptor binding is relatively unexplored. Research of antiemetic agents and their use in controlling chemotherapy-induced nausea and vomiting is a fairly recent phenomena. Prior to 1976, only 6 antiemetic trials had been reported. Well over 100 clinical trials have been published in the past 10 years. Until a decade ago, phenothiazines were the standard antiemetic treatments. Through a series of controlled clinical trials, Moertal was able to consistently demonstrate the superiority of prochlorperazine over placebo for 5-fluorouracil-induced vomiting (124). But in standard doses, the phenothiazines have been shown to be of marginal value. Antiemetic activity is believed to be related to blockade of dopamine receptors in the CTZ (124).

A second generation of antiemetic agents with varying modes of activity came into use over the past 10 years. Clinical trials have demonstrated antiemetic activity of antihistamines, steroids, neuroleptics, tranquilizers, and cannabinoids. A general overview of some agents will be given. The reader can seek further detailed information elsewhere.

Butyrophenones are a group of non-phenothiazine neuroleptics of which haloperidol and droperidol have antiemetic activity at the CTZ and vestibular sites (124). Haloperidol was shown to have efficacy in patients proven refractory to prochlorperazine, for post-operative vomiting, and for vomiting secondary to gastrointestinal disorders (124,126-128). Trials using both droperidol or haloperidol in combination with other agents report that combined therapy was more effective than either single agent (124).

Benzquinamide is a benzoquinolizine derivative with mild antihistaminic, anticholinergic and sedative properties. Clinical antiemetic trials report varying degrees of success. Moertal found benzquinamide to be less effective than prochlorperazine against 5-fluorouracil-induced vomiting while others report efficacy in controlling nausea and vomiting secondary to doxorubicin (124). Neidhart et al also found it to be occasionally effective in patients refractory to haloperidol or prochlorperazine (124).

Lorazepam is a benzodiazepine that has proven anxiolytic benefit. It is most often used in doses sufficient to induce drowsiness or sleep. Therapeutic benefit is derived from the sedative and amnestic properties (129). A major area of benefit seems to be the control of anticipatory nausea and vomiting. Additive antiemetic effect has been shown in combination with other agents (130).

Metoclopramide is a procainamide derivative with central and peripheral antiemetic activity. Reportedly, in addition to blocking CTZ dopamine receptors, it also affects gastrointestinal motility and promotes gastric emptying through cholinergic receptors. Antiemetic efficacy appears widely varied and dose-related. Low dose oral trials of metoclopramide produced conflicting reports but higher, frequent parenteral dosing regimens have proven antiemetic effect against cisplatin-induced nausea and vomiting (121). Metoclopramide is frequently used in combinational antiemetic therapies. Reported toxicities include diarrhea and CNS symptom including extrapyramidal reactions.

Corticosteroids have been used singly or in combination for antiemetic benefit. Rich postulated that antiemetic effect may be secondary to prostaglandin inhibition and found methylprednisolone to have antiemetic effect for various chemotherapeutic regimes (132). Mason et al reported high doses of methylprednisolone in combination with low dose chlorpromazine or droperidol effectively limit the acute gastrointestinal toxicity of cisplatin (133).

Numerous clinical trials have been conducted to evaluate antiemetic effect of THC and the synthetic cannabinoids (124). Varying degrees of antiemetic effect have been reported. However, the cannabinoids are usually not preferred by patients because of associated side effects including sedation, dysphoria and tachycardia.

Clinical trials have afforded numerous insights into treatment strategies. Combination antiemetic therapies have now become standard practice. Amended schedules of dosing and routes of administration have provided better coverage for anticipatory and late onset nausea and vomiting. It has been proven that failure to respond to one treatment regimen did not preclude a response to another regimen. Manageability of nausea and vomiting is essential and quite feasible in providing optimal care for the cancer patient receiving chemotherapy.

X. QUALITY OF LIFE

In 1948, Karnofsky developed a 10-point rating scale to measure subjective parameters and objective evidence of tumor shrinkage (96). Over the years other scales were developed to assess physical function, but these were also incomplete measurements of the overall functional quality of life (134).

During the 1960's and 1970's the focus of western policies shifted from purely materialistic goals (restoring welfare after World War II) to goals associated with psychological and social needs (135). Thus, not only were the cure and survival of patients important, but also their well-being especially in the areas of rehabilitation, chronic disease and cancer (135). Efforts to measure quality of life began with the 1960 report of

President Eisenhower's Commission on National Goals and have continued to the present (136).

As the management of cancer has become a more aggressive multidisciplinary approach, treatment-related morbidity has gained wider attention (137). Surgical interventions may be painful and mutilating. Radiotherapy has such side effects as fatigue, skin injury and emotional discomfort. Chemotherapy has frequently been considered the most burdensome treatment modality because it is given over extended periods of time and has many toxicities including alopecia, nausea, vomiting, fatigue and emotional problems (135).

Patients often rely on bodily sensations as an index of treatment success or disease recurrence. These are imprecise measures, at best, as positive treatment effects may not be immediate and adverse side effects may be severe and prolonged. This is especially the case in adjuvant chemotherapy for possible micrometastatic disease following primary radiation therapy or surgical removal (96,138). For patients receiving only palliative treatment with no expectation of a cure, the major objective is preservation of or improvement in quality of life. In those instances the issue of risks versus benefits often becomes paramount (139,140).

An often reported difficulty with quality of life studies has been the lack of a specific definition for quality of life even though the concept is widely accepted (134,135,137,138, 141). A recommended working definition generally includes the following categories: (a) physical, material and psychological well-being; (b) relationships with other people; (c) social, community and civic activities; (d) personal development and fulfillment; and, (e) recreation (136-138,142-145). Several authors emphasize that quality of life is not static, but rather a dynamic process with changing values, changing patterns of function and changing levels of satisfaction over time (134,142,143). Many suggest that quality of life can only be accurately measured by the individual and that well-meaning caregivers intrude on the patient's judgment with preconceived ideas of what is best for the patient (135,143,144, 146). Perhaps Gough put it most succinctly using a 10-cm linear analogue scale and a single, valid and reliable question: "How would you rate your quality of life today?" (139).

For those times when more detailed information is needed, Schipper (1985) has suggested seven requirements for a formal quality of life questionnaire: (a) cancer specific;

(b) functional orientation (e.g., activities of daily living); (c) self-administered; (d) questions generally applicable, easy and consistent interpretation, limited number; (e) repeatable; (f) sensitive; (g) valid, and reliable (134).

de Haes has commented that quality of life research tends to focus far more on the negative aspects of well-being rather than differentiate between the cognitive and affective components (135). A number of recent studies do not support the assumption that the quality of life of cancer patients in general is poorer than the quality of life of other groups (135,139,141,147). Cancer, even when cured, does not seem to carry social and psychological problems beyond those that occur with nonmalignant disease. Morris (148) found that in the week prior to their death, approximately 20% of terminally ill cancer patients continued to have functional, emotional, symptomatic and social reserves (148). Padilla found that information on coping was not as helpful as commonly thought, but that patients' ability to control aspects of their treatment was more important (149,152).

Traumatic events can lead to a relatively higher level of perceived quality of life in the victim and priorities may be reordered when compromise of physical status or shortened survival time occurs (137,150). It is important that care-givers encourage active patient participation whenever possible in the diagnosis and treatment of neoplastic disease and not underestimate human resilience in compensating for major infirmity (147,151).

SUMMARY

The prevalence of common psychiatric disorders in cancer patients has been reviewed stressing a neuropsychological approach to psychopathologic findings. Psychiatric symptoms and syndromes in oncology should not be considered as either/or (i.e., medical or psychiatric) phenomena. Medical illnesses such as cancer produce psychopathologic findings in a variety of ways and the appearance of psychiatric illness in this population requires a complete medical evaluation prior to a psychiatric consultation. Effective standard pharmacologic strategies for psychiatric disorders such as anxiety, depression, organic mental disorders, nausea and vomiting, and pain have been reviewed. Neurotoxicities of various antineoplastic treatments and quality of life issues have been discussed. More research and more teaching in the field of cancer pharmacology are needed in order to identify those situations in which psychopharmacologic interventions might be useful.

The psychiatric and neuropsychologic problems of long-term cancer survivors present a new arena of concern for which substantial research is urgently needed.

TABLE 1:   COMMON CAUSES OF DEMENTIA IN CANCER PATIENTS

Systemic Illnesses

> Pulmonary insufficiency
> Cardiac arrhythmia
> Anemia
> Hepatic or renal insufficiency
> Electrolyte imbalance
> Infection

Endocrinopathies

> Thyroid disturbance
> Hypoglycemia
> Cushing's/steroid treatment

Intracranial Conditions

> Neoplasm, primary or metastatic
> Hydrocephalus
> Seizure
> Anoxia

Collagen Vascular/Vascular Disorders

Deficiency States

> B-12, folate deficiency
> Malnutrition/malabsorption

Drugs

> Antineoplastic agents (see Table 2)
> Alcohol
> Anticholinergic agents

Cranial Irradiation

TABLE 2. NEUROTOXICITIES OF CHEMOTHERAPEUTIC AGENTS

CLASS	TYPE OF AGENT	NONPROPRIETARY NAMES	NEUROTOXICITY	
			Immediate	Delayed
Alkylating Agents	Nitrogen Mustards	Mechlorethamine (Mustargen)	Severe H/A	Depression
			Hallucinations	Personality change
			(with Procarbazine):	
			Disorientation	Confusion
			Confusion, H/A	Personality
			Lethargy	change
			Hallucinations	
			(with Cyclophosphamide):	
			Seizure	H/A
			Lethargy	Blurred vision
			Hallucinations	Hydrocephalus
			Vertigo, H/A	Aphasia
			Tremor	Focal sensory loss
			Paraplegia	
			Disorientation	
			(with Carmustine/other agents):	
			Severe H/A	Somnolence
			Disorientation	Blackouts
			Lethargy	Dementia
			Confusion	
			Tremor	
			(high dose IV or IA):	
			Peripheral neuropathy	
			Cerebral necrosis, edema,	
			Hemiplegia, seizures,	
			Hearing loss, vestibulopathy	
			Coma, death	

Table 2 (cont)

CLASS	TYPE OF AGENT	NONPROPRIETARY NAMES	NEUROTOXICITY
		Cyclophosphamide (Cytoxan)	Dizziness, mild intoxication Blurred vision SIADH (with WB-XRT + Busulfan): Multifocal necrosis of pons & cerebral peduncle
		Chlorambucil (Leukeran)	(with massive overdose): Seizures, "jerking movements" Irritability, ataxia, coma
	Ethylenimine Derivatives	Hexamethylmelamine	Peripheral neuropathy Encephalopathy (usually revers- ible): confusion, anxiety, hallucinations, depression, ataxia, tremor, dysphasia, Parkinsonism, somnolence, insomnia, respiratory dyskinesia, seizures
		Triethylenethio- phosphoramide (Thiotepa)	IT: Lower motor neuron disorder Ascending myelopathy -> respiratory paralysis & death Leukoencephalopathy (with IT MTX & ARA-C): Subacute myelopathy (Intracisternal: monkeys): Opisthotonus, extensor rigidity Neurologic death

Table 2 (cont)

CLASS	TYPE OF AGENT	NONPROPRIETARY NAMES	NEUROTOXICITY
	Alkyl Sulfonate	Busulfan (Myleran)	(with WB-XRT & Cyclophosphamide): Multifocal necrosis of pons & cerebral peduncle
	Nitrosoureas	Carmustine (BCNU)	Transient or delayed encephalopathy: confusion, disorientation Focal seizures Transient ischemic attacks Dizziness, loss of equilibrium Ataxia Necrotizing arteriolitis ? Synergistic with WB-XRT-> insidious dementia cerebral atrophy
		Semustine (Methyl CCNU)	(with post. fossa XRT): Spastic quadriparesis
	Triazenes	Dacarbazine (DTIC)	Acute encephalopathy Dementia Seizure, hemiparesis Cerebral hemorrhage
		Triazinate	Somnolence
Antimetabolites	Folic Acid Analog	Methotrexate (MTX)	IA: Coma, death

Table 2 (cont)

CLASS	TYPE OF AGENT	NONPROPRIETARY NAMES	NEUROTOXICITY
			<u>IT</u>: <u>Acute</u> Sterile men- ingitis, arachnoid- itis Transient or permanent paraplegia/ myelopathy ?seizures <u>High dose IV</u>: Mineralizing micro- angiopathy, stroke-like syndrome, leukoencephalopath <u>IT + WB-XRT</u>: Learning disability Behavioral abnormality Somnolence syndrome Leukoencephalopathy ?Optic atrophy <u>Intraventricular</u>: Reversible dementia & hemiparesis <u>Intratumor</u>: Cerebral edema with surrounding necrosis (without clinical sx) <u>IT + IV WB-XRT</u>: Seizures Hyperkinesis, ataxia Paraplegia Dementia Subnormal perceptual motor skills Intracranial calcifications	<u>Delayed</u> Leukoenceph- alopathy, often fatal Dementia Cortical atroph ?Myelopathy ?Cerebellar degen. Pontine abn. Tremors Seizures

Table 2 (cont)

CLASS	TYPE OF AGENT	NONPROPRIETARY NAMES	NEUROTOXICITY
	Pyrimidine Analogs	Fluorouracil (5-FU)	Acute cerebellar syndrome: dysmetria, ataxia of trunk or extremities, unsteady gait, slurred speech, coarse nystagmus, dizziness
			(with Allopurinol): Encephalopathy, seizures, hemiparesis aphasia, hemisensory deficit ataxia, brain stem dysfunction
			(with high doses): Lethargy, encephalopathy, coma
		Ftorafur	Extrapyramidal syndrome Parkinsonism Blurred vision, diplopia
			Encephalopathy: lethargy, confusion Seizure Forgetfulness Vertigo, dizziness, ataxia H/A, nervousness
		Cytarabine (Cytosine arabinoside, ARA-C)	IT: Acute arachnoiditis Myelopathy syndromes Peripheral neuropathy ?Predispose to necrotizing leukoencephalopathy

Table 2 (cont)

CLASS	TYPE OF AGENT	NONPROPRIETARY NAMES	NEUROTOXICITY
		5-Azacytidine (5-AC)	Progressive lethargy, confusion, irritability, somnolence Possible coma Neuromuscular toxicity: generalized muscle weakness, tenderness
		N-phosphonoacetyl-L-aspartate (PALA)	Acute or delayed encephalopathy and/or seizures poorly con-trolled with anticonvulsants
		6-Azauracil	Low dose: Drowsiness, lethargy Dizziness High dose: Hyperreflexia, Tremor, diplopia, dysarthria Expressive aphasia
		FMAU	Confusion, disorientation Somnolence Severe irreversible extrapyram-idal reactions
	Purine Analogs	Vidarabine (Adenine arabinoside, ARA-A)	Fatal CNS reactions preceded by tremors, myoclonus, dysarthria and coma
		Deoxcoformycin	Severe ocular toxicity Lethal encephalopathy

Table 2 (cont)

CLASS	TYPE OF AGENT	NONPROPRIETARY NAMES	NEUROTOXICITY
		Fludarabine	High dose: Delayed altered mental status, cortical blindness Progressive multifocal leukoencephalopathy Progressive demyelination (usually lethal) Generalized seizures Spastic or flaccid paralysis Quadriparesis Coma
Natural Products	Vinca Alkaloids	Vincristine (Oncovin, VCR)	Peripheral neuropathy Cranial nerve neuropathy Autonomic neuropathy Encephalopathy: confusion, delirium, agitation, hallucinations Depression Seizures, tremors Ataxia, athetosis Catalepsy, coma
		Vinblastine (Velban, VBL)	Similar to Vincristine
		Vindesine (DVA)	Similar to Vincristine Weakness more severe than sensory dysfunction Mental status changes usually reversible

Table 2 (cont)

CLASS	TYPE OF AGENT	NONPROPRIETARY NAMES	NEUROTOXICITY
	Epipodophyllo-toxins	Etoposide (VP-16)	Peripheral neuropathy Muscle atrophy, difficulty ambulating IA: Mild/moderate neuro-toxicity
		Teniposide (VM-26)	Similar to Etoposide
		Maytansine	Neuropathy similar to VCR Profound lethargy
Antibiotics		Doxorubicin	IA + Quelamycin: Massive brain edema & coma in 6 patients 3 deaths (Monkeys): Fatal necrotizing angiopathy (Rats): Neuronal necrosis in peripheral ganglia Posterior limb & fore-limb ataxia
		Bleomycin	Peripheral neuropathy Cerebral vascular accidents
		Mitomycin	(with MTX or CTX + 5-FU): Reversible disturbances of consciousness & cognition Possible acute encephalopathy

Table 2 (cont)

CLASS	TYPE OF AGENT	NONPROPRIETARY NAMES	NEUROTOXICITY
		Dactinomycin	(Animals: intracranial or direct injection into CSF): Seizure, tremor myoclonic jerks, encephalopathy, myelopathy with widespread demyelination and spongy necrosis
	Enzymes	L-asparaginase	Acute & delayed encephalopathy: Lethargy, confusion, somnolence, subtle memory or personality change
			Delirium with hallucinations
			Focal cerebral dysfunction & seizures, usually reversible; may progress to coma & death
			Depression
			Hemorrhagic & thrombotic stroke (drug-induced clotting abn.)
			(with VCR): Markedly increased toxicity if given with or before VCR; not if after
		SAGA	Similar to L-asparaginase
Miscel-laneous	Platinum Coordination	Cisplatin (CDDP)	Acute encephalopathy, reversible
			Ototoxicity - deafness may be permanent
			Vestibular toxicity - rare
			Seizures
			Peripheral neuropathy - vibration & proprioception
			Tetany due to decreased Mg++ & Ca++

Table 2 (cont)

CLASS	TYPE OF AGENT	NONPROPRIETARY NAMES	NEUROTOXICITY
			IA: Severe focal or general encephalopathy Ophthalmologic toxicity: papilledema, retrobulbar neuritis with blindness transient cortical blindnes
	Methyl Hydrazine Derivative	Procarbazine	Encephalopathy: altered level of consciousness, drowsiness to profound stupor, prolonged somnolence, confusion, hallucinations, agitation Depression, mania Psychosis Peripheral neuropathy, muscle weakness Acute cerebellar syndrome/ataxia Disulfiram-like syndrome
	Substituted Urea	Hydroxyurea	Rare H/A, dizziness, drowsiness, hallucinations
	Adrenocortical Suppressant	Mitotane	Somnolence, lethargy Vertigo, dizziness H/A, blurred vision Peripheral neuropathy - rare
		Thymidine (TdR)	Encephalopathy: somnolence, memory impairment, H/A visual illusions (with F-FU): Exacerbates cerebellar symptoms, reversible encephalopathy

Table 2 (cont)

CLASS	TYPE OF AGENT	NONPROPRIETARY NAMES	NEUROTOXICITY
		Methyl GAG (Methyl G)	Severe acute sensorimotor neuropathy, lower extremity weakness numbness & pain, decreased strength & sensation, peripheral paresthesias Profound malaise, lightheadedness, vertigo Confusion Tinnitus
		Amsacrine (mAMSA)	Peripheral neuropathy, stocking-glove paresthesia Grand mal seizures
		Spirogermanium	Acute encephalopathy: disorientation Isolated or delayed lateral gaze nystagmus, vertigo, ataxia, intention tremor, visual disturbance, paresthesias
		Misonidazole	Acute encephalopathy: Confusion, Obtundation Peripheral neuropathy Seizures Ototoxicity
		Interferon	Fatigue, neurasthenia, indifference, slowed cognition Affective disturbance Diffuse encephalopathy, primarily frontal lobe dysfunction with mild personality change, irritability, lability

Table 2 (cont)

CLASS	TYPE OF AGENT	NONPROPRIETARY NAMES	NEUROTOXICITY
		Cyclosporine	Seizures, tetany (? due to drug-induced decreased Mg++_ Tremors, ataxia Depression

Legend for Table 2
H/A = headache,   IV = intravenous,   IA = intra-arterial
WB-XRT = whole brain radiotherapy,   IT = intrathecal
CNS = central nervous system,   CSF = cerebral spinal fluid

REFERENCES

1. American Psychiatric Association, Committee on Nomenclature and Statistics: Diagnostic and Statistical Manual of Mental Disorders (3rd ed). Washington, D.C., American Psychiatric Association, 1980

2. Folstein MF, Folstein SE, McHugh PR: "Mini-Mental State", a practical method for grading the cognitive state of patients for the clinician. *J Psychiatr Res* 12:189-198, 1975

3. Folstein MF, Fetting JH, Lobo A, et al: Cognitive assessment of cancer patients. *Cancer* 53:2443-2449, 1984

4. Wettstein, RM: The Mini-Mental State in mild cognitive dysfunction (letter). *Am J Psychiat* 143:128, 1986

5. Dick JPR, Guiloff RJ, Stewart A, et al: Mini-mental state examination in neurological patients. *J Neurol Neurosurg Psychiat* 47:496-499, 1984

6. Mueller J: The mental status examination. In Goldman, HH (Ed.) Review of general psychiatry, Los Altos, CA: Large Medical Publications, 1984

7. Berg R, Franzen M, Wedding D: Screening for brain impairment: a manual for mental health practice. New York: Springer, 1987

8. Lezak MD: Neuropsychological assessment (2nd ed.). New York: Oxford University Press, 1983

9. Davis BD, Fernandez F, Adams F, et al: Diagnosis of dementia in cancer patients: results of 107 consecutive psychiatric consultations. *Psychosomatics* 28:175-189, 1987

10. Taylor MA, Sierles F, Abrams R: The neuropsychiatric evaluation, in Psychiatry Update, American Psychiatric Association Annual Review, vol. 4. Edited by Hales RE, Frances AJ. Washington, D.C., American Psychiatric Press, Inc., 1985

11. Lipowski ZJ (ed.): Delirium: Acute Brain Failure in Man. Springfield, IL, Charles C. Thomas, 1980

12. Adams F, Adams T: Cancer and quality of life: a cerebral affair, In The Biology and Treatment of Colorectal Cancer Metastasis. Edited by Mastromarino AJ. Massachusetts, Martinus Nijhoff, 1986

13. Rabins PV, Folstein MF: Delirium and dementia: diagnostic criteria and fatality rates. *Br J Psychiatry* 140:149-153, 1982

980

14. Cummings JL: Treatable dementias. Adv Neurol 39:165-183, 1982
15. Bedford PD: General medical aspects of confusional states in elderly people. *Br Med J* 2:185-188, 1959
16. Adams F: Neuropsychiatric evaluation and treatment of delirium in the critically ill cancer patient. *Cancer Bull* 36:156-160, 1984
17. Massie MJ, Holland J, Glass E: Delirium in terminally ill cancer patients. *Am J Psychiatry* 140:1048-1050, 1983
18. Donlon PT, Hopkin J, Tupin JP: Overview: efficacy and safety of the rapid neuroleptization method with injectable haloperidol. *Am J Psychiatry* 136:273-278, 1979
19. Tupin JP: Focal neuroleptization: an approach to optimal dosing for initial and continuing therapy. *J Clin Psychopharmacol* 5:15S-21S, 1985
20. Tesar GE, Murray GB, Cassem NH: Use of high dose intravenous haloperidol in the treatment of agitated cardiac patients. *J Clin Psychopharmacol* 5:344-347, 1985
21. Adams F, Fernandez F, Andersson BS: Emergency pharmacotherapy of delirium in the critically ill cancer patient. *Psychosomatics* 27:33-37, 1986
22. Cummings JL, Benson DF (eds): Dementia: A Clinical Approach. Woburn, MA, Butterworth Publishers, 1983
23. Wells CE, Duncan GW (eds): Neurology for Psychiatrists. Philadelphia, F.A. Davis Company, 1980
24. Weisman AD (ed): Coping with Cancer. New York, McGraw-Hill, 1979
25. Silberfarb PM, Bates GM: Psychiatric complications of multiple myeloma. *Am J Psychiatry* 140:788-789, 1983
26. Goldberg RJ: Psychiatric symptoms in cancer patients: is the cause organic or psychologic? *Postgrad Med* 74:263-273, 1983
27. Silberfarb PM: Chemotherapy and cognitive defects in cancer patients. *Annu Rev Med* 34:35-46, 1983
28. Blumer D, Benson DF (eds): Personality changes with frontal and temporal lobe lesions. In Psychiatric Aspects of Neurological Disease. New York, Grune & Stratton, 1975

29. Lipper S, Tuchman MN: Treatment of chronic post-traumatic organic brain syndrome with dextroamphetamine: first report case. *J Nerv Ment Dis* 162:366-371, 1976

30. Weinstein GS, Wells CE: Case studies in neuropsychiatry: post-traumatic psychiatric dysfunction - diagnosis and treatment. *J Clin Psychiatry* 42:120-122, 1979

31. Fernandez F, Adams F: Methylphenidate treatment of patients with head and neck cancer. *Head & Neck Surgery* 8:296-300, 1986

32. Fernandez F, Adams F, Holmes VF, et al: Methylphenidate for depressive disorders in cancer patients. *Psychosomatics* 28:455-461, 1987

33. Woods SW, Tesar GE, Murray GB, et al: Psychostimulant treatment of depressive disorders secondary to medical illness. *J Clin Psychiat* 47:12-15, 1986

34. Jefferson JW, Marshall JR (eds): Neuropsychiatric Features of Medical Disorders. New York, Plenum Medical Book Company, 1979

35. Ling MHM, Perry PJ, Tsuang MT: Side effects of corticosteroid therapy. *Arch Gen Psychiatry* 37:737-743, 1981

36. Palmer BV, Walsh GA, McKinna JA, et al: Adjuvant chemotherapy for breast cancer: side effects and quality of life. *Br Med J* 281:1594-1597, 1980

37. Young DF: Neurological complications of cancer chemotherapy. In Neurological Complications of Therapy, edited by Silverstein A: New York, Futura Publishing Company, 1982

38. Falk WE, Mahnke MW, Poskanzer DC: Lithium prophylaxis of corticotropin induced psychosis. *JAMA* 241:1011-1012, 1979

39. Pullan PT, Clement-Jones V, Corder R: Ectopic production of methionine enkephalin and beta-endorphin. *Br Med J* 1:758-759:1980

40. Corkin S, Cohen NJ, Sullivan EV, et al: Analyses of global memory impairments of different etiologies. In, Memory Dysfunctions: An Integration of Animal and Human Research from Preclinical and Clinical Perspectives, edited by Olton DS, Gamzu E, Corkin S. New York, Annals of the New York Academy of Sciences Vol 444:10-40, 1985

41. DeReuck JL, Sieben GJ, Sieben-Praet MR, et al: Wernicke's encephalopathy in patients with tumors of the lymphoid hemopoietic systems. *Arch Neurol* 37:338-341, 1980

42. Shuping JR, Rollinson RD, Toole JF: Transient global amnesia. *Ann Neurol* 7:281-285, 1980

43. Holmes JM: Cerebral manifestations of vitamin B-12 deficiency. *Br Med J* 2:1394-1398, 1956

44. McEvoy JP: Organic brain syndromes. *Ann Intern Med* 95:212-220, 1981

45. Greenberg DB: Psychiatric consultation in oncology patients. In Psychiatric Medicine Update: Massachusetts General Hospital Reviews for Physicians, edited by Manschreck T, Murray GB. New York, Elsevier, 1984

46. Bieliakas LA: Depression, stress and cancer. In, Psychosocial Stress and Cancer, edited by Cooper CL. New York, John Wiley and Sons, Ltd., 1984.

47. Cassilieth BR, Luck EJ, Miller DS, et al: Psychosocial correlates of survival in malignant disease. *N Engl J Med* 312:1551-1555, 1985

48. Bukberg J, Penman D, Holland JL: Depression in hospitalized cancer patients. *Psychosom* Med 46:199-212, 1984

49. Adams F, Larson DL, Goepfert H: Does the diagnosis of depression in head and neck cancer mask organic brain disease? *Otolaryngol Head Neck Surg* 92:618-624, 1984

50. Barclay LL, Blass JP, Lee RE: Cerebral metastases mimicking depression in a "forgetful" attorney. *J Am Geriat Soc* 32:866-867, 1984

51. Derogatis LR, Morrow GR, Fetting J, et al: The prevalence of psychiatric disorders among cancer patients. *JAMA* 249:751-757, 1983

52. Lansky SB, List Ma, Herrmann CA, et al: Absence of major depressive disorder in female cancer patients. *J Clin Oncol* 3:1553-1560, 1985

53. Robins LN, Helzer JE, Weissman M, et al: Lifetime prevalence of specific psychiatric disorders in three sites. *Arch Gen Psychiatry* 41:949-958, 1984

54. Popkin MK, Callies AL and Colon EA: A framework for the study of medical depression. *Psychosomatics* 28:27-33, 1987.

55. Goldberg IK, Kitscher AH, Schoenberg B, et al: Psychopharmacologic and analgesic agents employed in the terminal care of 100 cancer patients. In, Psychopharmacologic Agents for the Terminally Ill and Bereaved, edited by Goldberg IK, Malitz S, Kutscher A. New York, University Press, 1973

56. Derogatis LR, Feldstein H, Morrow G: A survey of psychotropic drug prescriptions in an oncology population. *Cancer* 44:1919-1929, 1979

57. Goldberg RJ, Mor V: A survey of psychotropic use in terminal cancer patients. *Psychosomatics* 26:745-748, 1985

58. Klerman GL: Psychotropic hedonism versus psychopharmacological Calvinism. Hastings Center Rep 2:1-3, 1971

59. Gelenberg AJ, Klerman GL: Preclinical pharmacology of antidepressants. In, Principles of Psychopharmacology, Part 2, Tricyclics, edited by Clark WG, Del Giudice J. New York, Academic Press, 1978

60. Morris JB, Beck AT: The efficacy of antidepressant drugs: a review of research. *Arch Gen Psychiatry* 30:667-674, 1974

61. Van Kammen DP, Murphy DL: Prediction of imipramine antidepressant response by a one day d-amphetamine trial. *Am J Psychiatry* 135:1179, 1978

62. Richardson JW, Richelson E: Antidepressants: a clinical update for practitioners. Mayo Clin Proc 59:330-337, 1984

63. Gelenberg AJ: The rational use of psychotropic drugs: prescribing antidepressants. *Drug Ther* 9:95-112, 1979

64. Gelenberg AJ, Klerman GL: Maintenance drug therapy in long-term treatment of depression. In, Controversy in Psychiatry, edited by Brady JP, Brodie HKH. Philadelphia, W B Saunders Company, 1978

65. Sheehan DV, Claycomb JB: The use of MAO inhibitors in clinical practice. In, Psychiatric Medicine Update: Massachusetts General Hospital Reviews for Physicians, edited by Manschreck TC, Murray GB. New York, Elsevier Science Publishing Company, 1984

66. Robins E: Psychiatric Emergencies: Suicide. In, Comprehensive Textbook of Psychiatry/IV, edited by Kaplan H, Sadock BJ. Baltimore, Williams and Wilkins, 1985

67. Blackwell B: Adverse effects of antidepressant drugs. Part 1: Monoamine oxidase inhibitors and tricyclics. *Drugs* 21: 201-219, 1981

68. Fernandez F, Adams F, Levy JK, et al: Depression and cancer: an update. *Texas Medicine* 82:46-49, 1986

69. Adams F: Use of intravenous amitriptyline in cancer patients. Twelfth Annual Education and Scientific Program of the Society of Critical Care Medicine, New Orleans, LA, May 1983 (abstract)

70. Adams FA: Amitriptyline suppositories. *N Engl J Med* 306:906, 1982

71. Massie MJ, Holland JC: Psychiatry and Oncology. In, Psychiatry Update, Volume III. Washington, D.C., American Psychiatric Association Press, 1983

72. Massie MJ, Gorzynski JG: Managing anxiety in cancer patients. Your Patient and Cancer: 53-60, 1982

73. Greenblatt DJ, Abernethy DR, Diroll MI, et al: Pharmacokinetic properties of benzodiazepine hypnotics. *J Clin Psychopharm* 3:129-132, 1983

74. Ballanger JC: Psychopharmacology of the anxiety disorders. In, Symposium on Clinical Psychopharmacology II, The Psychiatric Clinics of North America. Philadelphia, W. B. Saunders Company, 1984

75. Rosenbaum JF: The drug treatment of anxiety. *N Engl J Med* 306:401-404, 1982

76. Shader RI, Greenblatt DJ: Clinical implications of benzodiazepine pharmacokinetics. *Am J Psychiatry* 134:652-656, 1977

77. Raft D: Psychopharmacologic treatments of anxiety. In, Clinical Psychopharmacology, edited by Derogatis LR. California, Addison-Wesley Publishing Company, 1986

78. Feighner JP, Aden GC, Fabre LF, et al: Comparison of alprazolam, imipramine and placebo in the treatment of depression. *JAMA* 249:3057-3064, 1983

79. Foley KM: The treatment of cancer pain. *N Engl J Med* 313:84-95, 1985

80. Bouckoms AJ: Recent developments in the classification of pain. *Psychosomatics* 26:637-645, 1985

81. Kaiko RF, Foley KM, Grabinski PY, et al: Central nervous system effects of meperidine in cancer patients. *Ann Neurol* 13:180-185, 1983

82. Berkowitz BA: The relationship of pharmacokinetics to pharmacological activity: morphine, methadone and naloxone. *Clin Pharmacokin* 1:219-230, 1976

83. Cassem NH: Pain. In, Scientific American Medicine. New York, Scientific American, Inc., 1983

84. Walsh TD: Oral morphine in chronic cancer pain. *Pain* 18:1-11, 1984

85. Kocher R: The use of psychotropic drugs in the treatment of cancer pain. In, Recent Results in Cancer Research: Pain in the Cancer Patient, edited by Zimmerman M, Drings P, Wagner G. Berlin Springer-Verlag, 1984

86. Akil H, Koebeskind JC: Monoaminergic mechanisms of stimulation produced analgesia. *Brain Res* 94:279-296, 1975

87. Mendel CM, Klein RF, Chappell DA, et al: A trial of amitriptyline and fluphenazine in the treatment of painful diabetic neuropathy. *JAMA* 255:637-639, 1986

88. Richelson E: Antimuscarinic and other receptor blocking properties of antidepressants. *Mayo Clin Proc* 58:40-46, 1983

89. Fernandez F, Adams F, Holmes VF, et al: Adjuvant pain treatment in cancer: a case for psychopharmacology. *Texas Medicine* 83:60-65, 1987

90. Head M, Lal H, Puri S, et al: Enhancement of morphine analgesia after acute and chronic haloperidol. *Life Sci* 24:2037-2044, 1979

91. Maltbie A: Analgesia and haloperidol a hypothesis. *J Clin Pharmacol* 32:323-326, 1979

92. Black JL, Richelson E, Richardson JW: Antipsychotic agents: a clinical update. *Mayo Clin Proc* 60:777-789, 1985

93. Swerdlow M: Review: anticonvulsant drugs and chronic pain. *Clin Neuropharmacol* 7:51-82, 1984

94. Forrest WH, Brown BW, Brown CR, et al: Dextroamphetamine with morphine in the treatment of the postoperative pain. *N Engl J Med* 296:712-715, 1973

95. Twycross RG, Lack SA: Co-analgesics. In, Symptom Control in Far Advanced Cancer: Pain Relief, edited by Twycross RG, Lack SA. London, Pittman Books, 1983

96. Priestman TJ: Quality of life after cytotoxic chemotherapy: discussion paper. *J Royal Soc Med* 77:492-495, 1984

97. Peterson LG, Perl M: Psychiatric presentations of cancer. *Psychosomatics* 6:601-604, 1982

98. Calabresi P, Parks RE: Antiproliferative agents and drugs used for immunosuppression, in The Pharmacological Basis of Therapeutics, edited by Gilman AG, Goodman LS, Rall TW, et al. New York, Macmillan, 1980

99. Kaplan RS, Wiernik PH: Neurotoxicity of antitumor agents, in Toxicity of Chemotherapy. Edited by Perry MC, Yarbro JW. New York, Grune & Stratton, Inc., 1984

100. Scully RE, Mark EJ, McNeely BU: Case records of the Massachusetts General Hospital. N Engl J Med 311:653-662, 1984

101. Sullivan KM, Storb R, Shulman HM, et al: Immediate and delayed neurotoxicity after mechlorethamine preparation for bone marrow transplantation. Ann Int Med 97:182-189, 1982

102. Schilsky RL, Yarbro JW: Pharmacology of antineoplastic drugs, in Toxicity of Chemotherapy. Edited by Perry MC, Yarbro JW. New York, Grune & Stratton, Inc., 1984

103. Perry MC, Yarbro JW: Complication of chemotherapy: an overview, in Toxicity of Chemotherapy. Edited by Perry MC, Yarbro JW. New York, Grune & Stratton, Inc., 1984

104. Fanucchi MP, Leyland-Jones B, Young CW, et al: Phase I trial of 1-(2'-Deoxy-2'-fluoro-1-B-D-arabinofuranosyl)-5- methyluracil (FMAU). Cancer Treat Rep 69:55-59, 1985

105. Warrell RP, Berman E: Phase I and II study of fludarabine phosphate in leukemia: therapeutic efficacy with delayed central nervous system toxicity. J Clin Oncol 4:74-79, 1986

106. Cohen IJ, Vogel R, Matz S, et al: Successful non-neurotoxic therapy (without radiation) of a multifocal primary brain lymphoma with a methotrexate, vincristine, and BCNU protocol (DEMOB). Cancer 57:6-11, 1986

107. Bates SE, Raphaelson MI, Price RA, et al: Ascending myelopathy after chemotherapy for central nervous system acute lymphoblastic leukemia: correlation with cerebrospinal fluid myelin basic protein. Med and Pediat Oncol 13:4-8, 1985

108. Allen J, Rosen G, Juergens H, et al: The inability of oral leucovorin to elevate CSF 5-methyl-tetrahydrofolate following high dose intravenous methotrexate therapy. *J Neurooncol* 1:39-44, 1983

109. Patchell RA, White CL, Clark AW, et al: Neurologic complications of bone marrow transplantation. *Neurology* 35:300-306, 1985

110. Ettinger LJ, Freeman AI, Creaven PJ: Intrathecal methotrexate over dose without neurotoxicity: case report and literature review. *Cancer* 41:1270-1273, 1978

111. Frytak S, Earnest F, O'Neill BP, et al: Magnetic resonance imaging for neurotoxicity in long-term survivors of cancer. *Mayo Clin Proc* 60:803-812, 1985

112. Scheithauer W, Ludwig H, Maida E: Acute encephalopathy associated with continuous vincristine sulfate combination therapy: case report. *Invest New Drugs* 3:315-318, 1985

113. Silberfarb PM, Holland JCB, Anbar D, et al: Psychological response of patients receiving two drug regimens for lung carcinoma. *Am J Psychiatry* 140:110-111, 1983

114. Adams F, Quesada JR, Guetterman JU: Neuropsychiatric manifestations of human leukocyte interferon therapy in patients with cancer. *JAMA* 252:938-941, 1984

115. Holland J, Fasanello S, Ohnuma T: Psychiatric symptoms associated with L-asparaginase administration. *J Psychiat Res* 10:105-113, 1974.

116. Silberfarb PM, Oxman TE: The effects of cancer therapies on the central nervous system. *Adv Pyshcosom Med* 18:13-25, 1988

117. Mattson K, Niiranen A, Laaksonen R, et al: Psychometric monitoring of interferon neurotoxicity. *Lancet* 1:275-276, 1984

118. Mattson K, Niiranen A, Iivanainen M, et al: Neurotoxicity of interferon. *Cancer Treat Rep* 67:958-961, 1983

119. Quesada JR, Talpaz M, Rios A, et al: Clinical toxicity of interferons in cancer patients: a review. *J Clin Oncol* 4:234-243, 1986

120. Thompson CB, Sullivan KM, June CH, et al: Association between cyclosporin neurotoxicity and hypomagnesaemia. *Lancet* 2:1116-1120, 1984

121. Berger PS: Neurological complications of radiotherapy, in Neurological Complications of Therapy. Edited by Silverstein A. New York, Futura Publishing Company, 1982

122. Duffner PK, Cohen ME, Thomas PRM, et al: The long-term effects of cranial irradiation on the central nervous system. *Cancer* 56:1841-1846, 1985

123. Posner JB: Neurological combinations of systemic cancer. *Med Clin North Am* 55:625-646, 1971

124. Laszlo J (ed): Antiemetics and cancer chemotherapy. Baltimore, Williams & Wilkins, 1983

125. Wang SC, Renzi AA, Chinn HI: Mechanism of emesis following x-irradiation. *Am J Physiol* 193:335-339, 1958

126. Neidhart JA, Gagen M, Young D, et al: Specific antiemetics for specific cancer chemotherapeutic agents: haloperidol versus benzquinamide. *Cancer* 47:1439, 1981

127. Christman RS, Weinstein RA, Larose JB: Low-dose haloperidol as antiemetic treatment in gastrointestinal disorders: a double blind study. *Curr Ther Res* 16:1171-1175, 1974

128. Barton MD, Libonate M, Cohen P: The use of haloperidol for treatment of postoperative nausea and vomiting: a double blind placebo controlled trial. *Anesthesiology* 42:508-512, 1975

129. Maher G: Intravenous lorazepam to prevent nausea and vomiting associated with cancer chemotherapy. *Lancet* 1:91, 1981

130. Gagen M, Gochnour D, Young D, et al: A randomized trial of metoclopramide and a combination of dexamethasone and lorazepam for prevention of chemotherapy-induced vomiting. *J Clin Oncol* 12:696-701, 1984

131. Grall R, Itri L, Pisko S, et al: Antiemetic efficacy of high dose metoclopramide randomized trials with placebo and prochlorperazine in patients with chemotherapy-induced nausea and vomiting. *N Engl J Med* 305:905-909, 1981

132. Rich W, Ardulhayoglu G, Di Sara P: Methylprednisolone as an antiemetic during cancer chemotherapy - a pilot study. *Gynecol Oncol* 9:192-198, 1980

133. Mason B, Dambra G, Grossman B, et al: Effective control of cisplatin-induced nausea using high-dose steroids and droperidol. *Cancer Treat Rep* 66:243-245, 1982

134. Schipper H, Levitt M: Measuring quality of life: risks and benefits. *Cancer Treat Rep* 69:1115-1123, 1982

135. de Haes JCJM, van Knippenberg FCE: The quality of life of cancer patients: a review of the literature. *Soc Sci Med* 20:809-817, 1985

136. Flanagan JC: Measurement of quality of life: current state of the art. *Arch Phys Med Rehabil* 63:56-59, 1982

137. Danoff B, Kramer S, Irwin P, et al: Assessment of the quality of life in long-term survivors after definitive radiotherapy. *Am J Clin Oncol* (CCT) 6:339-345, 1983

138. Calman KC: Guest editorial: quality of life in cancer patients. *Current Concepts in Oncology* 6:2-3, 1984

139. Gough IR, Furnival CM, Schilder L, et al: Assessment of the quality of life of patients with advanced cancer. *Eur J Cancer Clin Oncol* 19:1161-1165, 1983

140. Brinkley D: Quality of life in cancer trials. Br Med J 291:685-686, 1985

141. Selby P: Measurement of the quality of life after cancer treatment. *Br J Hosp* Med 33:266-271, 1985

142. Padilla GV, Presant C, Grant MM, et al: Quality of life index for patients for cancer. *Res Nurs Health* 6:117-126, 1983

143. Young KJ, Longman AJ: Quality of life and persons with melanoma: a pilot study. *Cancer Nurs* 6:219-225, 1983

144. Kagan AR, Kagan JD: The quality of which life? *Am J Clin Oncol* (CCT) 6:117-118, 1983

145. Schipper H, Clinch J, McMurray A, et al: Measuring the quality of life of cancer patients: the functional living index-cancer: development and validation. *J Clin Oncol* 2:472-483, 1984

146. Presant CA, Klahr C, Hogan L: Evaluating quality of life in oncology patients: pilot observations. *Oncol Nurs Forum* 8:26-30, 1981

147. Morris T, Greer HS, White P: Psychological and social adjustment to mastectomy. *Cancer* 40:2381-2387, 1977

148. Morris JN, Suissa S, Sherwood S, et al: Last days: a study of the quality of life of terminally ill cancer patients. *J Chron Dis* 39:47-62, 1986

149. Padilla GV, Grant MM: Psychosocial aspects of artificial feeding. *Cancer* 55:301-304, 1985

990

150. Andersen BL: Sexual functioning morbidity among cancer survivors: current status and future research directions. *Cancer* 55:1835-1842, 1985

151. Spitzer WO, Dobson AJ, Hall J, et al: Measuring the quality of life of cancer patients: a concise QL-index for use by physicians. *J Chron Dis* 34:585-597, 1981

152. Lewis FM: Experienced personal control and quality of life in late-stage cancer patients. *Nurs Res* 31:113-119, 1982

BENZODIAZEPINES

Martin Guerrero, M.D.*
David V. Sheehan, M.D.+

CONTENTS:

1) Pharmacokinetic Properties
   a) Considerations in the Elderly
   b) Considerations in the Medically Ill
   c) Considerations in Pregnancy

2) Benzodiazepine Drug Interactions

3) Guidelines for Treatment of Anxiety Disorders
   a) Introduction
   b) Clinical Considerations in Initiating and Maintaining Treatment
   c) Guidelines for Withdrawal of a Benzodiazepine

4) Alcohol Detoxification

5) Treatment of Insomnia

6) Benzodiazepines as Antidepressants

7) Benzodiazepine in the Treatment of Psychoses, Mania and Agitated States
   a) Benzodiazepines in Psychoses
   b) Benzodiazepines in Mania
   c) Benzodiazepines in Delirious States
   d) Benzodiazepines in Aggression

8) Conclusion

* Assistant Professor of Psychiatry
  Texas Tech University Health Sciences Center
    Regional Academic Health Center
  El Paso, Texas

+ Professor of Psychiatry
  University of South Florida College of Medicine
  Director of Research, USF Psychiatry Center
  Professor of Psychology
  University of South Florida College of Social
    and Behavioral Sciences

BENZODIAZEPINES

Martin Guerrero, M.D.

David V. Sheehan, M.D.

The first benzodiazepines (BZs) were synthesized in 1933, but not systematically studied until the 1950's and ultimately introduced into clinical practice in the 1960's (1). Human and animal brain fractions specific for BZs were isolated in 1977 (2). Since then two receptor subtypes have been identified with specific properties (3). One receptor theory proposes a three-state model with sub-synaptic gamma-aminobutyric acid (GABA) and barbiturate sites which couple with BZs at their site in opening a chloride-channel complex (4). It is also believed BZs enhance the inhibitory effects of GABA (in cerebral cortex) and glycine (in brainstem and spinal cord) to produce their clinical effects (1-4). These clinical effects include anxiolytic, sedative-hypnotic, muscle-relaxant, and anti-seizure properties along with more recently discovered psychotropic effects which have made these compounds increasingly more popular and valuable. The mid-1970's saw an increasing use of BZs with a concomitant rise in re-evaluations of their indications, prescribing patterns, and warnings of their abuse potentials (2). This chapter will review the current knowledge of BZ pharmacology, kinetics, and clinical uses in psychiatry. BZ use in epileptic disorders will not be discussed here.

PHARMACOKINETIC PROPERTIES

The BZs are highly-lipophilic and readily pass the blood-brain-barrier (BBB) after intravenous (I.V.) injection. Various authors (1-4) assert that in order of increasing dosage all BZs exhibit 1) anxiolytic, 2) sedative-hypnotic, and 3) anticonvulsant effects. Furthermore, it is assumed that clinically there are no major differences between all members in this class and that they are relatively interchangeable. However, there are wide differences in absorption rates, routes of metabolism, and half-lives between the parent BZ compounds and their metabolites. It is wise to appreciate these subtleties which can make one BZ more desirable for a particular patient given his/her age, presence of concurrent medical illnesses, or desired therapeutic effect (as an example, anxiolytic vs. hypnotic). Table 1 summarizes general characteristics of the available BZs in the U.S. Dosages listed are recommended for healthy young individuals.

There are numerous pharmacokinetic features important in determining clinical consequences. These include 1) drug absorption, 2) plasma protein binding, 3) volume of distribution, 4) metabolic transformations, 5) rate of excretion and 6) route of excretion. Ultimate clinical response depends on the free concentration of drug and length of time at the active central nervous system (CNS) site. These factors in turn can be altered by numerous disease and physiologic states which eventually change the clinical profile of the particular drug. The following sections will review these alterations in reference to two important clinical groups: the elderly and the medically ill. The third section reviews clinical considerations during pregnancy.

CONSIDERATIONS IN THE ELDERLY

It is estimated that by the year 2030, the elderly will comprise 17% of the U.S. population or number about 50 million people. With anxiety disorders common among this group, and their relatively higher prevalence of moderate to severe psychopathology, BZs are an important therapeutic aid (5). Aging, however, can alter various physiologic functions which can potentially modify clinical responses to drugs (2,5). These alterations include increased gastric pH (which decreases absorption of acidic drugs), decreased splanchnic blood flow, and decreased functional gastrointestinal mucosal surface area (which decreases absorption of drugs). The elderly also have an increased volume of drug distribution due to the relative increase in their ratio of body fat to lean body mass. This increases the storage capacity of lipid soluble drugs and increases their half-life and duration of therapeutic action. All BZs are lipophilic but diazepam, chlordiazepoxide, and nitrazepam are more so and, thus, have larger distribution volumes in the elderly (5).

BZs are primarily metabolized in the liver by one of two pathways: 1) Phase I - mixed function oxidase system (demethylation, hydroxylation) or 2) Phase II - conjugation with glucuronic acid or glycine (5). Phase I metabolism is potentially reduced with increasing age due to decreasing microsomal enzyme function and decreased hepatic blood flow (2,5,6). Although the Phase II pathway has been postulated to be less effected by aging (2,5,6), clinically this has not been fully validated. In addition, other factors may possibly be involved in the elderly such as: 1) increased BZ receptor sensitivity and number, 2) increased permeability of BBB to drugs and 3) altered drug receptor interactions (5,6).

CNS depression, sedation, and impaired cognitive function are BZ side effects most commonly cited in the elderly (2,5-7). It is generally believed that sedation increases with progressive drug accumulation secondary to augmented drug half-lives in the elderly. Increased half-life in turn may be a result of increased volume of distribution and decreased metabolic clearance. For example, the half-life of desmethyldiazepam (DMDZ), an active metabolite of several BZs, can triple from 50 to 150 hours in the elderly. Desalkylflurazepam (metabolite of flurazepam) has a half-life which ranges from 60 to 120 hours in healthy young adults. In the elderly this can increase to 80-300 hours (5). On the other hand, BZs undergoing Phase II metabolism such as oxazepam and lorazepam have no active metabolites and therefore are less likely to accumulate and are fairly rapidly eliminated from the body (2,5,8,9). For these reasons, "conjugated" benzodiazepines have been advocated by some authors as drugs of choice for the elderly (2,9). However, rapid clearance may not be preferable in certain circumstances. Longer half-life compounds are eliminated more slowly than shorter half-life drugs and intrinsically taper themselves more gradually when discontinued abruptly. This minimizes risks of rebound effects of initial symptoms such as insomnia or anxiety (2,5,8,9). When tapering the dose of conjugated BZ compounds with shorter half-lives, it is advised to maintain a fixed hourly dosing schedule and successively decrease the dose rather than lengthening the dosage interval. More controlled trials comparing oxidized vs. conjugated BZs in the elderly are required to delineate further clinical differences.

CONSIDERATIONS IN THE MEDICALLY ILL

As a class, the BZs are relatively safe and minimally toxic (8,9) in particular when compared to barbiturates which had been used extensively for the same indications BZs are now used. Their advantages over barbiturates include 1) less steep dose-effect curve, 2) lower incidence of dose-related unwanted effects, 3) less likelihood of producing physiologic dependence, 4) less toxicity in over-dosage when taken without other CNS depressants, and 5) less capacity to induce hepatic microsomal oxidizing enzymes (thus, decreasing possible interactions with other drugs) (1,2,5,6,10-13). Despite their wide margin of safety, concerns over CNS, cardiovascular and respiratory depression are still voiced. Siris and Rifkin (14) reviewed general psycho-pharmacological considerations in the medically ill patient. Although correction of any underlying medical illness is first desirable before starting pharmacotherapy, frequently medication is necessary sooner because the underlying disease process cannot be adequately diagnosed, is untreatable or irreversible. At other times, indicated medical treatment may take too long to reverse symptoms. Sometimes, the patient's psychiatric state may be dangerous, disruptive, and compromising of his medical treatment (10,14,15). This necessitates immediate intervention.

In general, BZs are usually safe in patients with cardiac and respiratory disease (10,14,15). In the coronary care unit they can be used as an adjunct in decreasing post-MI anxiety and reducing cardiac hyperactivity (theoretically by lowering plasma catecholamines) (16-20).

Caution is advised when using BZs intravenously in patients with pulmonary disease, particularly in the presence of partial or past respiratory depression (10). However, they have been used successfully to decrease anxiety in helping wean patients off respirators (in low doses and with close monitoring) (15).

BZs are to be used cautiously in a patient with central-sleep apnea syndrome where CNS depression may further blunt or altogether terminate the respiratory drive (21).

Much has been written about the role of BZs in the presence of significant liver disease or compromised hepatic function. Numerous sources advocate the use of Phase II conjugated BZs in this setting (9,14,22-24). The reason is that glucuronide conjugation in the liver is least affected by hepatic dysfunction. Roberts, et al (9) found that the elimination half-life of intravenously administered chlordiazepoxide increased three-fold in patients with cirrhosis compared with age matched controls. The metabolite N-desmethyl chlordiazepoxide (N-DMCPZ) appeared at approximately the same time in both groups, while in the cirrhotic group the peak values were lower. These same investigators also found that patients with acute viral hepatitis also had prolonged elimination half-lives and reduced plasma clearance of chlordiazepoxide compared with controls. Concentrations of N-DMCPZ peaked at lower levels and at a later time in the hepatitis group than in controls. Roberts, et al (9) failed to demonstrate similarly altered kinetics in other patients with liver disease using oxazepam. They ascribed this difference to the fact that oxazepam is metabolized by conjugation and that this pathway is least affected in the presence of hepatic disease. Hoyumpa (22) has reviewed studies which suggest that oxazepam and lorazepam kinetics are unaffected by aging or liver disease and that these agents may be preferable in the elderly and in patients with liver disease. Similar suggestions for the use of BZs in the presence of hepatic pathology will be discussed in the section on alcohol detoxification.

There are few guidelines for BZ use in patients with kidney disease. Various reviews advise caution in patients with chronic renal failure regardless of its etiology. Levy (25) recommends avoiding BZs with pharmacologically active metabolites like diazepam. He suggests cautiously using BZs with inactive metabolites such as camazepam, clonazepam, flunitrazepam, lorazepam, nimetazepam, nitrazepam, oxazepam and temazepam. Levy (25) and associates recommend reducing the dose of BZs in renal failure patients to two-thirds the amounts given to patients with normal kidney function. Bennett, et al (26) caution that BZs may cause excessive sedation in chronic hemodialysis patients. Citing data for chlordiazepoxide, diazepam and flurazepam, they (26) noted no need to adjust dosage in patients with glomerular filtration rates less than 10 milliliters per minute. Taclob and Needle (27) report on four patients on chronic maintenance hemodialysis who developed encephalopathy (confusion, asterixis, somnolence, and EEG slowing) within 4 days of receiving flurazepam (30 mg hs) and diazepam (5 mg bid to qid). Two other patients developed the same symptoms after receiving only flurazepam. All symptoms developed without concurrent cardiovascular, pulmonary or hepatic abnormalities and remitted within five days of discontinuing the BZs. Chronic hemodialysis seems to prolong the half-life of chlordiazepoxide but it is not known if other BZs are similarly affected. It seems advisable, therefore, to closely monitor the patient with compromised renal function who is receiving benzodiazepines, use smaller doses, and select agents without active metabolites.

CONSIDERATIONS IN PREGNANCY

Because many women during their child bearing years are taking a benzodiazepine, they and their physicians are naturally concerned about the possible impact of benzodiazepines on pregnancy and lactation. While it is easy for the uninvolved to state that benzodiazepines are never to be used during pregnancy, the realities of clinical practice are full of complications that often make this recommendation difficult to implement. For example, how do we manage the chronic agoraphobic mother of five children on alprazolam or clonazepam who calls up and announces that she just learned today that she is 2-1/2 months pregnant? If we discontinue the drug too rapidly we may precipitate a miscarriage, possibly a seizure. If she becomes totally disabled off the drug who will care for her five small children? Will the ensuing panic attacks, phobic anxiety and depression in themselves have any complications for the fetus?

There is a problem in evaluating the evidence that bears on this question. Approximately 3% of all pregnancies result in an abnormal newborn infant (28). Of these only about 3% are associated with known teratogenic exposure (28). Consequently, even for the normal woman free of medication there is still a small risk of a fetal abnormality. If a baby born to a mother taking benzodiazepines has an abnormality, how can we be sure that this is due to the drug and would not have occurred because she is one of the small 3%?

In addition, there are several sources of possible error in the studies reported that could influence their results. Many consumers of benzodiazepines are a little older and may have had previous pregnancies - placing them at greater risk of producing children with congenital abnormalities. Their symptoms may lead them to use more analgesics, drink more alcohol and caffeine and smoke more cigarettes, all of which produce complications during pregnancy.

It is possible, but not yet known if the anxiety disorders themselves are associated with considerable physiological disturbance including alterations in vascular tone and blood flow. If this is occurring several times a week, could it have physiologically ill effects on the fetus? Is it possible that the benzodiazepines decrease the likelihood of spontaneous abortion of an already malformed fetus that would abort under normal circumstances? This could lead to an apparent increase in congenital malformations at term among women taking benzodiazepines. All these factors can color the evidence suggesting an association between benzodiazepines and fetal abnormalities. Good studies addressing this question are needed and should attempt to control for these compounding effects.

Several studies suggest that first or second trimester use of diazepam is associated with a small, but increased risk of cleft lip and/or palate (29-32) while others do not observe this association (33). First trimester use of benzodiazepines has also been associated with a small risk of inguinal hernia, pyloric stenosis and congenital heart defects (34). Second trimester use has been associated with hemangiomas and cardiovascular defects (34). When a woman smokes cigarettes in addition to taking a benzodiazepine, the risk of a resulting malformation increases four fold compared to those who do not smoke or use benzodiazepines (34). There have been isolated cases of skeletal defects (spina bifida, absence of left forearm, syndactly and absence of both thumbs) reported following benzodiazepine use in pregnancy (35-38).

In the third trimester and post partum, two other complications have been associated with benzodiazepine use. If the mother is taking a therapeutic dose of benzodiazepine at birth, a withdrawal syndrome is precipitated in the baby. This syndrome usually begins 2-6 hours after birth. At best this may only result in irritability, tremulousness, increased tone and hyperflexia, but at worst could lead to a seizure. For this reason, it is always advisable to have the mother entirely off benzodiazepines or on as low a dose as absolutely possible in the last two months of pregnancy to minimize withdrawal symptoms in the neonate.

Benzodiazepines readily cross the placental barrier. Because of the immaturity of the fetal liver, they are more slowly cleared by the fetus, often leading to levels that exceed those in the mother's blood. It is not surprising to find some cases of central nervous system depression in some of these infants at birth with hypotonia, lethargy, sucking difficulties and respiratory depression. Similarly, diazepam given parenterally to the mother during labor may produce apneic episodes, hypotonia, hyperflexia, hypothermia, and poor sucking in the newborn. However, diazepam has been found otherwise safe in labor in several studies (38) and does not significantly compromise fetal pH or Apgar scores (39).

Because benzodiazepines are excreted into breast milk and are then cleared more slowly in the neonate, they may cause CNS depression. Such mothers should choose between the use of benzodiazepines or breast feeding in the post partum period, but should not do both.

BENZODIAZEPINE-DRUG INTERACTIONS

There are few serious BZ-drug interactions. Physicians should note, however, that as sedative drugs, BZs should be used cautiously with other CNS depressants such as antihistamines, barbiturates, and alcohol. Since BZs are widely prescribed in both primary care and psychiatry, knowledge of potential drug interactions is important because many patients are frequently taking multiple medications (particularly the elderly and medically ill). As noted earlier, phase I metabolized BZs (see Table 1) are biotransformed by N-demethylation or aliphatic hydroxylation in the hepatic microsomes. Drugs that inhibit these microsomal enzymes may cause a rise in the plasma BZ level thereby prolonging or potentiating its effects through decreased metabolism. Conversely, drugs which induce hepatic microsomal enzymes may increase metabolism of the BZ. The following columns indicate some of the drugs and activities affecting this enzyme system.

Drugs Inhibiting Microsomal Enzymes	Drugs and Activities Inducing Microsomal Enzymes
Alcohol	Rifampin
Cimetidine	Xanthines (Caffeine, Theophylline)
Disulfiram	Barbiturates
Estogens	Smoking
Isoniazid	

Blackwell and Schmidt (40) point out that these interactions can be more complex. For example, anxious individuals taking BZs may also drink alcohol or smoke secondary to anxiety. These practices may alter the pharmacokinetics and clinical effect of the BZ.

Cimetidine alone may cause sedation which may compound drowsiness induced by BZ. A recent study (41), however, found that although the administration of diazepam to patients already taking cimetidine caused the plasma levels of diazepam and desmethyldiazepam to rise, the free fractions (unbound and active) were unaltered. In addition, there were no alterations in the pharmacokinetics of either compound. These authors conclude that in at least this healthy young population the interaction of diazepam and cimetidine is clinically insignificant (41). More controlled clinical studies are required to explore these interactions.

As shown in the above columns, there are potential BZ interactions with other commonly used drugs. Caffeine, in addition to inducing microsomal enzymes (and thereby reducing BZ sedation), causes CNS stimulation. Isoniazid can prolong diazepam's half-life by 30% through microsomal enzyme inhibition. Rifampin (commonly used together with Isoniazid), on the other hand, can supersede the effect of Isoniazid and increase the clearance of diazepam (42). Disulfiram (500 mg day) has been reported (43) to reduce the clearance and prolong the half-life of both chlordiazepoxide and diazepam. Unfortunately, the clinical effect on the patient was not reported in this reference (43).

Blackwell and Schmidt (40) contend, however, that these interactions are still clinically "tenuous and ill-defined" and, given the large population at risk, the available documentation suggests that these reactions may rarely be clinically significant.

Oral contraceptives (estrogens) have been shown to decrease the clearance of I.V. administered diazepam and result in elevated serum concentrations of diazepam. It is suspected that a similar phenomenon occurs with orally administered diazepam. Patients taking both medications should be monitored for side-effects and a possible dose reduction of the BZ.

Alcohol deserves special mention because of its widespread use and synergistic effects with other CNS depressants. Much is known about alcohol's interaction with barbiturates (44) including its synergistic lethal effects, i.e. death occurring in individuals with blood levels of both drugs in the non-lethal range. This is presumed to be due to the alcohol's inhibition of hepatic microsomal enzymes which hydroxylate phenobarbital and pentobarbital. Barbital and thiopental, on the other hand, are not dependent on these enzymes and thus interact only additively with alcohol not synergistically. The same may hold true with BZs that are hepatically metabolized (phase I) or conjugated (phase II).

Use of alcohol for a few weeks initially increases hepatic microsomal enzyme activity and thereby may decrease the effects of barbiturates and benzodiazepines through increased metabolism. In time, continued alcohol exposure may reduce metabolizing capacity. This occurs through a combination of hepatic structural damage and altered physiology. In addition, the sedative effects of barbiturates and BZs may be decreased if cross tolerance to alcohol has occurred.

Potentially, there are also BZ to BZ complications such that withdrawal syndromes from one BZ may not be adequately treated with another BZ. One case study (45) reports of a 68 year old man who developed delirium after being slowly withdrawn from alprazolam (0.5 mg tid) over 5 days. The delirium, on two separate occasions, was unresponsive to the administration of diazepam (40 mg over 14 hours) and haloperidol (3 mg I.M.). The delirium was corrected with readministration of alprazolam. Apparently, diazepam may not adequately treat withdrawal from alprazolam. Therefore, a withdrawal syndrome from a benzodiazepine is best treated with the particular benzodiazepine being withdrawn rather than substitution and tapering of a different BZ.

Other reported drug interactions include:

Digoxin: Diazepam (40) may raise digoxin serum levels and, therefore, levels should be monitored. However, the clinical significance is unknown.

Phenytoin: There is much controversy over effects of concomitant BZ use. Clonazepam has been reported to increase phenytoin levels (7,46). There are references citing both increased or decreased serum phenytoin levels when diazepam is added (47).

Carbamazepine: Clonazepam used concurrently with carbamazepine may increase its own metabolism and decrease its own plasma concentration (46,47). Carbamazepine levels do not seem to be affected (47).

Leva-dopa: Diazepam and chlordiazepoxide have been associated with decrease in control of Parkinsonian symptoms when added to a leva-dopa drug regimen (43,46).

Tricyclic Antidepressants: One reference reports increased elimination half-life and steady-state plasma level of amitriptyline when used with diazepam (46). Another source (40) reports a reduced side effect profile of the amitriptyline - librium combination at low doses compared to either drug alone. In some cases, however, the combination has produced additive, sedative and anticholinergic effects, including confusion. BZs may also increase the lethal potential of amitriptyline without increasing its plasma level (40). Steady-state plasma levels of both imipramine and desipramine have been reported to be elevated by concomitant BZ administration. Again, the clincial impact of this observation has not been discerned.

Aluminum and magnesium hydroxides: These may decrease the rate (but not extent) of G.I. absorption of chlordiazepoxide or diazepam. Antacids may decrease both rate and extent of conversion of clorazepate to desmethyldiazepam since transformation is dependent on an acidic pH in the stomach.

As noted in this section, there are few prospective studies showing consistent drug interactions with significant clinical impacts. When using BZs with other drugs which can be monitored, it may be wise to review blood levels periodically to confirm that there have been no changes in serum concentrations. Obviously, these interactions are to a large extent dependent on the patient's metabolism and handling of the drugs' pharmacokinetic profiles.

In general, BZs can be used quite safely with most other agents. The alert physician, however, should suspect a possible drug interaction when there is a change from the expected clinical course. Clues to such an occurrence include: over-sedation, a change in the patient's mental status, the appearance of toxic symptoms characteristic of the other medications, or poor anxiolytic response at standard doses.

GUIDELINES FOR TREATMENT OF ANXIETY DISORDERS

INTRODUCTION

Anxiety can be a symptom, a mood or a syndrome. In the latter category, it can be subdivided into phobic and non-phobic states (48). The classification in the current Diagnostic and Statistical Manual-Revised (DSM-III-R) of the American Psychiatric Association (49) divides primary anxiety disorders into 1) phobic states (agoraphobia, social phobia, simple phobia), and 2) non-phobic or anxiety neuroses (panic disorder, generalized anxiety disorder), 3) obsessive compulsive disorder, and 4) primary re-experiencing of a trauma (post-traumatic stress disorder). Current research is increasingly confirming biologic and physiological correlates to some of the anxiety disorders (48,50-53) such as the one-half molar lactate infusions which can reproduce panic attacks in susceptible patients (53).

Biologic treatment strategies for anxiety disorders are successful. However, non-psychopharmacologic approaches, including supportive psychotherapy, hypnosis, systematic desensitization and behavior modification paradigms are sometimes effective for certain patients in whom anxiety is circumscribed, related to an external stimulus, learned or conditioned (48,52).

The list of pharmacologic agents available for treatment of these disorders is extensive and, historically, has included alcohol, barbiturates, and propanediols. More recently clinicians have employed antihistamines, beta-blockers, neuroleptics, and anti-depressants (50,54-57). BZs now represent the fourth generation of anxiolytics and are currently the most effective, widely accepted, and perhaps safest agents in use. As noted previously, all BZs seem to have the same anxiolytic potential, yet only eight are marketed in the U.S as anti-anxiety agents, as illustrated in Table 1.

Sepinwall and Cook (58) reviewed the behavioral effects of BZs in animal models of anxiety and found that BZs can reverse the punishment induced response-inhibition of a task. Neither neuroleptics, antidepressants, antihistamines, phenytoin, morphine, chloral hydrate, nor ethchlorvynol exerted anti-punishment effects in these animal models. Meprobamate and some barbiturates also have this anti-punishment property. Amphetamine, on the other hand, suppresses even further the response-inhibition produced by punishment.

Several studies suggest that BZs may be more useful in treating non-phobic forms of anxiety. In contrast, tricyclic antidepressants (TCAs), such as imipramine and chlorimipramine (available in the United States only in specific research protocols) and monoamine oxidase inhibitors (MAOIs), such as phenelzine have been effective in phobic anxiety states (50,54,56,59,60).

In approaching the anxious patient, guidelines include ruling out organic diseases (such as hyperthyroidism, pheochromocytoma, carcinoid syndrome, mitral valve prolapse) as possible sources of the anxiety. Such a systematic work-up has been detailed elsewhere (61). Major depression or any other primary psychiatric condition (such as schizophrenia or paranoid disorder) in which anxiety may be a concomitant or secondary manifestation must be excluded.

For panic disorder, TCAs, MAOIs, or alprazolam are effective medications. If agoraphobia or avoidant behavior predominates, the above pharmacologic agents, in vivo exposure, behavior therapy and sometimes psychotherapy are indicated. For generalized anxiety disorders, BZs are still one of the drug classes of choice and can be supplemented with supportive therapy and education. If stage fright, tremor, or tachycardia dominate the clinical presentation, a trial of beta-blockers in medically stable patients can be considered.

CLINICAL CONSIDERATIONS IN INITIATING AND MAINTAINING TREATMENT

Benzodiazepines are prescribed far too casually and in haste in the average physician's office. Time spent in carefully preparing the patient about how to increase and adjust the dose of the benzodiazepine and the problems he may encounter while using it and if he abruptly discontinues it, is well rewarded. The success in using benzodiazepines in clinical practice is largely dependent on the attention paid to the precise regulation and the timing of the doses and the careful monitoring of side-effects.

Table 2 is an example of a chart we give to patients when we prescribe alprazolam for them. We generally start with a half tablet three times a day of an average dose for the benzodiazepine. We recommend that they take the tablet after each meal. When taken after food, the dose is absorbed more slowly, the blood level does not peak so dramatically and the effect may be somewhat more protracted. This may serve to minimize some of the side-effects. The dose is then increased by a half tablet every two days, until the patient either begins to experience some of the typical side effects like sedation or to have satisfactory benefit. Usually these tend to occur simultaneously. The patient may continue to do well on this dose for one to two weeks at which time they frequently develop a little tolerance to the benefit and the side effects.

The physician's skill lies in striking a safe balance between the side effects and the benefits. If the dose reaches two tablets three times a day after each meal, further increases may be made at the same rate by spacing the doses either four hours apart or one at each meal and one at bedtime. For those patients who have difficulty sleeping it may be sensible to shift some of the doses to bedtime at an earlier point on this schedule. However, since most anxious patients are anxious during their waking hours and many of them sleep reasonably well, doses taken at bedtime are often lost on the patient and are not doing any particularly useful work. We recommend writing out the directions as shown in Table 2 or giving the patient a printed copy of it. Many anxious patients forget the instructions they are given and this can often lead to either therapeutic failure or unnecessary toxicity. It also clearly conveys to the patient that we do not know precisely what dose he will finally need to achieve long-term benefit and that this is an individual thing to be arrived at by careful titration of the dose over the first several weeks. After four to eight weeks on this second plateau of doses, the patient may again develop some tolerance to the side effects and benefits and a further small increase in the dose may be necessary to again deliver the full benefit.

In general, one can anticipate that the typical patient taking benzodiazepines may need to go through two or three plateaus of tolerance like this before they reach their final effective long-term dose. If we do not anticipate that this will happen, we may leave the patient suspended in a state of partial recovery at a low dose when all that would have been necessary is a further small increase of the dose to achieve a satisfactory therapeutic result. In general, the final effective therapeutic dose is the dose at which the patient has very small amount of the mild side effects typically associated with that drug. Many physicians might consider that this prescribing principle only exposes the patient to unnecessary side effects. However, long experience with chronic anxiety disorders shows that when the patient is experiencing just a little of the typical side effects associated with that drug that they are unlikely to get a recurrence of their underlying disorder. On the other hand, if they have absolutely no side effects whatever from the medication, many of the patients do not have their condition under complete control. Adjusting the dose upwards to strike the best balance between the side effects and the benefit should be the focus of the clinician's effort. This can make a difference between a mediocre and a superior result.

Our experience has been that in the majority of cases tolerance to these medications is not an endless upward spiral. There does not appear to be a finite limit to the number of plateaus of tolerance the patient goes through before they reach their final effective therapeutic dose. It is probably fair to say that with the many effective benzodiazepines now available to us that the adjustment of the dose is far more important than the choice of drugs once we have chosen to put the patient on a benzodiazepine. The importance of fine-tuning the dose adjustment to get the best possible effect for each patient cannot be over-emphasized. In Table 2 the doses are spaced approximately four to six hours apart, since this corresponds with the duration of therapeutic action of many of the benzodiazepines. It should be emphasized that the half-life of the benzodiazepines is not a good guide to its duration of therapeutic action. The half-life of a drug, therefore, should never be used as a guide to space the doses throughout the day. With certain benzodiazepines, like clonazepam, the duration of therapeutic action is somewhat longer, i.e., six to eight hours, and other benzodiazepines, like alprazolam, have a duration of therapeutic action of approximately four to six hours. This may call for only bid or tid dosing of clonazepam while alprazolam may need to be prescribed on a tid or qid schedule.

For more severe anxiety disorders like panic disorder, the average effective dose may be somewhat greater than generally recommended in the PDR. In our panic disorders study, for example, we have found that the average final effective antipanic dose of alprazolam was approximately 6 mg per day at the end of a 10 week period. Naturally, the patient can never be started out on this dose but will only reach this dose after several weeks of treatment. We have never found it necessary to increase the dose to more than 10 mg per day in the case of panic disorder. Patients needing higher doses than 10 mg per day usually respond better to another antipanic drug, i.e., a tricyclic or a MAO inhibitor, in the long run. There is a wide range of effective doses with alprazolam with some patients needing as little as 2 mg per day and some patients needing as much as 6-10 mg per day to achieve a satisfactory therapeutic effect. Patients requiring very high doses of benzodiazepines may experience only minimal side effects at these higher doses. There seems to be no significant relationship between the severity of the patient's panic disorder and the dose needed to control the condition. The dose requirement of each patient is very individual and reflects more the rate at which the particular patient metabolizes that drug rather than reflects the severity of his disorder.

If the patient has not achieved a satisfactory improvement within four weeks of proper adjustment of his benzodiazepine, then it is unlikely that that particular drug will ever be useful for that patient. Consideration should then be given to switching to a more powerful anxiolytic, like an antidepressant drug. The Food and Drug Administration have not recommended the use of benzodiazepines for longer than four months. Very few careful long-term studies of benzodiazepines used in chronically anxious patients have been carried out. Unfortunately, severe anxiety disorders are often very chronic illnesses and many of these patients will regrettably require long-term medication management if they are to remain free of symptoms and disability. We generally continue the patients on the medication for six to twelve months, especially in the case of panic disorder and agoraphobia. Our long-term study does not show that patients require any further increase in their dose over this period of time compared to the dose that was needed in the first three months of treatment. Indeed there was even a marginal drop in the dose required to maintain their improvement. The longer they were on the medication, the better they continued to do over the first 12 months of treatment. At the end of this time the dose should be tapered very slowly over several weeks rather than over several days. In spite of this slow tapering, a considerable number of patients do experience a relapse of their original disorder. The number of patients who suffer a recurrence within several months of stopping a benzodiazepine, we believe is far higher than previously reported and as many as 60% of these patients may require another trial of a benzodiazepine to bring their symptoms once again under control. Given the crippling nature of some severe anxiety disorders, like panic disorders and agoraphobia, we do not hesitate to recommend that these patients should restart their benzodiazepines sooner rather than later. A risk benefit analysis comparing the potential disadvantages and dangers of the drug against the complications and disability of the disorder leave little doubt that in the majority of cases restarting the medication is justified.

It is much easier to treat the relapses in the early stages. If the relapse is treated quickly the patient suffers fewer complications. With each successive relapse, the patients become more practical in the management of their symptoms and blame themselves less. Their concern about depending on a medicine to provide relief gives way over time to the realization that the benefits significantly outweigh disadvantages of the drug and that their relapse is not a reflection of inadequate will-power, strength of mind or psychological work.

GUIDELINES FOR WITHDRAWAL OF A BENZODIAZEPINE

Special attention needs to be paid to the way in which patients are withdrawn from benzodiazepines. All benzodiazepines are powerful anticonvulsant drugs. The average physician would never consider withdrawing a patient from phenytoin, phenobarbital or corticosteroid on a rapid withdrawal schedule. Similarly, clinicians should not take patients off benzodiazepines as rapidly as they have been accustomed to do in the past.

The slow withdrawal of the benzodiazepine protects the patient against unpleasant withdrawal symptoms, against the danger of withdrawal seizures and to some extent, against rebound reactivation of their underlying anxiety disorder. To use specific examples, we do not recommend that alprazolam or clonazepam be withdrawn at a rate faster than a half a milligram every week or that diazepam be withdrawn at a rate faster than 5 milligrams every half week or 10 milligrams per two weeks. Although in the past many clinicians used withdrawal schedules that were more rapid, there is a risk that in a large population of such patients sooner or later one of the patients will have a withdrawal seizure on such a rapid schedule. Besides, there is no significant advantage to withdrawing a patient rapidly from a benzodiazepine while there are considerable disadvantages. The last three or four doses may have to be withdrawn at a rate somewhat slower than recommended above.

We would further advise that the clinician make no exceptions to this rule of slow withdrawal. There are several situations in which a physician may be tempted to ignore this. For example, if a patient is admitted on a high dose of benzodiazepine for emergency surgery or surgery that is planned within several days, the physician may be tempted to taper the benzodiazepine very rapidly so that the patient is not on any benzodiazepine at the time of surgery. This may precipitate extremely disruptive withdrawal symptoms at best and even a seizure in the recovery room after surgery. We recommend that in the majority of cases patients be kept on their effective dose of benzodiazepine right up to the night before surgery. The morning of the surgery they are not given any benzodiazepine and as soon as they are medically stable after surgery (usually within 24 hours after the surgery) they are restarted on their effective anxiolytic dose. Anesthesiologists should have no difficulty adjusting the dose of other medications they might need to use so as to minimize additive central nervous system depression. We have not encountered any difficulty with this regimen, but have frequently seen problems when the patient was too rapidly withdrawn prior to surgery.

Withdrawal symptomatology is more of a problem with usage of high doses. At least ten to fifteen percent of patients on low doses will manifest withdrawal symptoms, usually of an autonomic nature (tachycardia, tremulousness, diaphoresis, difficulty sleeping, increased sensitivity to lights and sounds, and rarely psychotic-like manifestations) if the drug is withdrawn abruptly. These symptoms must be differentiated from bona fide relapses, which are not uncommon. Relapse symptoms more closely resemble the previous anxious symptoms and occur at their characteristic times and generally reappear at seven to twenty-one days. Withdrawal symptoms appear sooner with shorter half-life drugs (from several hours to three days) and up to four to ten days with long half-life drugs. Additionally, some patients are reported to experience milder withdrawal symptoms intermittently for three to six months. If after discontinuing medication the patient rapidly redevelops the anxiety symptoms and has not mastered other methods of coping, the drug can be re-started for another two to four weeks, and again tapered and stopped. In general, the milder the anxiety disorder, the shorter the length of treatment that is necessary.

In a recent case series (62), clonazepam was found to have both anti-panic and antiphobic properties in doses adjusted to a maximum of 3-6 mg per day. The authors contend that clonazepam can be given on a bid or single dose/day regimen since its half-life is 20-40 hours. Our experience with clonazepam is not consistent with this duration of therapeutic action, which our patients report to be from 6 to 8 hours after each dose. Clonazepam has also been used to treat severe anxiety and agitation in adolescents and adults in dosages of 6-12 mg/day. However, the authors advise that in patients with a history of alcohol or drug abuse, imipramine may be preferable over BZs for treating panic disorders.

ALCOHOL DETOXIFICATION

Alcohol, by affecting every organ system in the body, can produce multiple and varied syndromes and diseases. Twelve neurological syndromes (63,64) and various endocrine disturbances have been reported secondary to alcohol use. In addition there are numerous syndromes associated with acute intoxication (65-67). There are four withdrawal syndromes described: delirium tremens, alcohol withdrawal seizures, alcoholic hallucinosis, and the protracted alcohol withdrawal syndrome which can last from one month to one year.

Management of intoxicated states and abstinent periods of chronic alcoholism has been outlined elsewhere (65-68). Withdrawal syndromes present a more complicated scenario. Their treatment is aimed at both reducing symptoms, and more importantly, preventing progression into more serious and life-threatening events like delirium and seizures. For mild withdrawal states, non pharmacologic treatment strategies have been advocated (10,65). For moderate to severe withdrawal, medical intervention is mandatory.

Historically, drugs with cross tolerance to alcohol, such as chloral hydrate, paraldehyde, and the barbiturates, have been used in detoxification. However, BZs are now the most commonly used sedatives in the treatment of alcohol withdrawal syndromes because of their advantages of being safer, causing less sedation, and having less toxic side effects.

Alcohol withdrawal symptoms can appear within hours of the last drink, usually peak in 24 to 48 hours, and resolve in 5-7 days. Table 3 lists the characteristics of three important withdrawal complications.

Alcohol withdrawal seizures are not a form of idiopathic epilepsy and EEG's performed after the seizure episodes are usually normal. Of the patients developing seizures, about one-third will have a single seizure, while the remainder will have multiple, often closely spaced, seizures. Typically these are generalized tonic-clonic seizures without focal features. One to 3% of these patients will progress to status epilepticus. Etiologies other than alcohol withdrawal should be sought if seizures (1) continue for an extended period; (2) progress to status or; (3) have focality. It has been suggested that BZs may be less effective in preventing withdrawal seizures than paraldehyde or chloral hydrate.

Similarly, delirium must be suspected and continuously ruled-out with thorough mental status examinations. Some patients may either slip quietly into this state or may superficially appear to be coherent while agitated.

Various protocols exist for detoxification and the physician can familiarize himself with one or two BZs for this purpose. Table 4 gives recommended dosages for BZs currently approved for alcohol withdrawal.

There is no satisfactory/conclusive evidence to suggest that any one BZ is superior to another in managing withdrawal. Various authors (69,70), however, suggest the oxazepam and lorazepam (phase II metabolism) may be preferable in the alcoholic patient because these compounds have no active (and potentially accumulating) metabolites. Furthermore, their metabolism via the conjugative pathway (and eventual excretion) may be less affected by concomitant liver damage secondary to alcohol abuse. Again, well-controlled studies are lacking to confirm the significance of this clinically.

In some instances, much higher BZ doses are required to manage alcohol withdrawal. One case report (71) describes a 33 year old man who required 780 mg of oxazepam in the first 24 hours. Over the next four days of detoxification he received 2,335 mg diazepam I.V. (maximum dose in 24 hours was 875 mg) which was discontinued on the fifth day. Oxazepam was given concurrently whenever oral intake was possible and over 9 days his cumulative dose was 21,255 mg (maximum 3,500 mg/day). Despite these massive doses the patient developed severe agitation, hallucinations and disorientation secondary to alcohol withdrawal. There was no respiratory or cardiac depression and only mild sedation after any one dose of either BZ. Mental status normalized on the seventh day. Plasma levels of diazepam and oxazepam were 10 to 100 times greater than those usually required in detoxification. The elimination half-lives of both parent compounds and their metabolites (desmethyldiazepam and temazepam) appeared to be relatively normal despite the patient's prior history of hepatomegaly, ascites, and micronodular cirrhosis per biopsy. During abstinent periods, liver function tests had been normal. It is possible that chronic alcohol ingestion or even withdrawal states may render individuals relatively resistant to the effects of BZs or other CNS depressants possibly due to changes at the receptor level. Thus, close monitoring of the patient's response to BZs is advisable regardless of the patient's concurrent medical status.

TREATMENT OF INSOMNIA

Insomnia, the subjective complaint of poor sleep (with resultant compromise in daytime functioning) is the most common sleep disorder. Approximately 30% of adult Americans report problems sleeping. Insomnia occurs more frequently in women, the elderly, individuals of lower educational and socio-economic status, and patients with chronic or multiple medical disorders (72-74). Insomnia may be either a primary disorder or a symptom of another underlying condition -- medical or psychiatric. The work-up includes a thorough history and physical, and current psychiatric status. Obtaining a "sleep log" may be helpful. This documents bedtime, sleep onset latency, awake-time, number and duration of nighttime awakenings, daytime naps, use of drugs (alcohol, etc.) and medications, and uncommon activities (i.e., physical work-out before going to bed). The assessments and differential diagnoses of insomnia, including neurological, medical, and drug-induced etiologies have been outlined elsewhere (21,72-74). These sources also discuss non-pharmacologic managements, which include psychotherapy, behavioral techniques, chronophysiologic manipulation, and improving sleep habits.

Pharmacologic treatment in general is reserved for transient or situational insomnia (one to three day duration) or intermediate insomnia (two to three week duration), both of which typically occur in individuals with regularly normal sleep (75). These forms of insomnia occur expectedly in relation to psychosocial (bereavement, hospital admission, public speaking), or physical stress (jet lag, premenstrual syndrome, or acute injury) (72,75).

In these situations, hypnotics may be useful. These have included barbiturates, barbiturate-like compounds (methaqualone, glutethimide, methyprylon, and ethchlorvynol), chloral derivatives, sedative antidepressants, antihistamines, L-tryptophan, and other miscellaneous combinations found in numerous over-the-counter (OTC) preparations.

Benzodiazepines have proven to be safe and effective agents, and are regarded as the hypnotics of choice over barbiturates, chloral derivatives, and antihistamines. However, like other hypnotics, flurazepam and temazepam reduce the percentage of stage IV sleep time (76). Triazolam has been found to either suppress or not alter stages III and IV density.

BZs do not seem to suppress REM sleep or increase REM latency to the extent tricyclic antidepressants do. The full clinical implications of this feature are not yet known. REM-suppression may be desirable in treating certain disorders such as nocturnal enuresis (76).

Almost all BZs can be used as hypnotics, although only three are marketed as such: flurazepam, temazepan and triazolam (see Table 1). Rapid absorption and thus rapid onset of action are preferable characteristics for hypnotics. BZs rapidly absorbed like diazepam, clorazepate, and flurazepam, can be given just prior to bedtime. Other BZs which are more slowly absorbed may have to be given up to an hour before bedtime. Hangover effects and daytime drowsiness may be due to the long half-lives of either parent compounds or metabolites. Flurazepam is rapidly converted to hydroxyethyl flurazepam and flurazepam aldehyde, both pharmacologically active metabolites. The parent compound is rapidly eliminated to undetectable blood levels in eight to twelve hours after a single dose. A third metabolite, desalkylflurazepam, appears more slowly and has a half-life of 40 to 150 hours in healthy adults, which may be prolonged to 300 hours in the elderly (7).

Although not marketed as a hypnotic, oxazepam was found to improve sleep parameters (by polysomnography) as well as flurazepam (77). However, unlike the latter, oxazepam did not produce significant daytime drowsiness. Drowsiness in the flurazepam group correlated with the appearance of desalkylflurazepam which is more potent than oxazepam on a nanogram for nanogram basis. Thus, oxazepam may have a desirable hypnotic profile.

Temazepam, with an intermediate half-life of 10 to 20 hours (in some individuals, up to 30 hours), will have an intermediate rate of accumulation. As it is metabolized by conjugation, its metabolic pathway is less likely influenced by old age.

Triazolam has an ultrashort half-life of 1.5 to 5 hours, and any given dose is almost completely eliminated in 12 to 15 hours, thus making it essentially non-accumulating. Although it is metabolized by two oxidative reactions, one study (78) found no effect of age (from 20 to 76 years in healthy controls) on the elimination of triazolam, in contrast to other BZs with similar phase I metabolism. The clinical implications of triazolam's low accumulation profile and kinetics in the elderly compared to other BZs are yet to be studied in a controlled fashion. On theoretical grounds, however, triazolam would seem suitable for the elderly.

More research is needed formally evaluating the other BZs in their hypnotic efficacy. Furthermore, studies comparing BZs to antidepressants and L-tryptophan in sleep pattern improvement and distortion are required.

BENZODIAZEPINES AS ANTIDEPRESSANTS

There is much recent interest in the literature (79,80) in the so-called second generation anti-depressants which follow the well-studied tricyclic antidepressants, MAOIs, stimulants, and electroconvulsive therapy. These new antidepressants do not claim to be more effective than the existing tricyclics or MAOIs, but may either work more rapidly, have fewer anti-cholinergic effects, or have less cardiotoxic effects (81). Alprazolam is the only benzodiazepine in this group. However, its possible antidepressant properties remain in dispute. It should be emphasized that no BZ has been approved for the treatment of major depression and that current indications are restricted to anxiety associated with depression.

Alprazolam might be an unusual benzodiazepine. It has a triazolo ring attached to the BZ nucleus much like trazodone (an antidepressant) has the triazolo ring attached to a pyridine structure. There is speculation that the triazolo ring may confer some of the antidepressant properties (81). Alprazolam has antipanic and antiphobic effects in addition to anxiolytic effects. Classic BZs have not been found to be effective in major depressions as discussed in reviews by Schatzberg and Cole in 1978 (82) and 1981 (83). One open-label study (84), without a control group, noted that depressed patients treated with alprazolam demonstrated reduction in their depressive symptomatology (as defined by improvement in the Hamilton Depression Scale scores). Responders were predominantly anxious, agitated, or suffering from insomnia. Of the five patients in the retarded subtype of depression, four were non-responders.

Other studies have compared alprazolam to a classical tricyclic antidepressant, imipramine, and placebo in a double-blind fashion (85-88). Using the Hamilton Psychiatric Rating Scale for Depression (HAM-D), Physicians Global Impressions scales, Patient's Global Impressions scale, and various other scales, these researchers found improved scores in groups treated with both imipramine and alprazolam compared to placebo. Mean daily doses of each medication ranged from 2.7 mg to 3 mg for alprazolam, and 117 mg to 133 mg for imipramine. In each of these studies, patients taking alprazolam reported fewer side effects--the most common being drowsiness and sedation--while patients on imipramine reported more anticholinergic effects such as dry mouth, blurring of vision, and urinary retention. Additionally, all four studies suggested that alprazolam's onset of action is more rapid than imipramine, although both medications produced the same response by the end of the studies at four to six weeks. It is interesting to note, however, that these four studies specifically excluded depressed patients having "involutional" depression (85), "melancholia" (86), or "predominantly psychomotor retardation" (87,88). This may have skewed patient selection into the more "anxious/agitated" subtype of depression. Furthermore, patients taking alprazolam demonstrated greater improvements in symptoms designated as "somatic-vegetative" compared to those "psychic-cognitive".

Two studies (89,90) have compared alprazolam to amitriptyline in double-blind formats. Draper and Daly (89) found that both alprazolam and amitriptyline significantly improved depressed patients' scores on the HAM-D over a six-week period of therapy. Mean total daily doses were 2.15 mg for alprazolam and 85 mg for amitriptyline. On the Hamilton Rating Scale for anxiety (HARS), there was no difference between the two drugs in anxiolytic effect and there was a suggestion that amitriptyline was slightly better. Unfortunately, there was no control group (placebo) in the study, and the mean dosage of amitriptyline may have been sub-therapeutic. In addition, patients were selected if they manifested "neurotic/reactive depression, i.e., depression-anxious-agitated-insomnia (initial) type" (89).

Another study (90) similarly compared the antidepressant effects of alprazolam and amitriptyline. However, patients were selected to meet Research Diagnostic Criteria for depression and were required to have at least one neurophysiologic abnormality associated with endogenous depression: 1) a rapid eye movement (REM) sleep latency less than 65 minutes by polysomnography, or 2) non-suppression by the dexamethasone suppression test. In a double-blind format (without a placebo-control group), at the end of six weeks 87% of patients taking amitriptyline had remitted compared to alprazolam 44% (as determined by the HAM-D). Improvement with alprazolam, when it occurred, was more rapid and usually evident by the first week, whereas amitriptyline took two to three weeks. The authors assert that their patients were selected for increased severity of illness and included 35% of their sample as inpatients. Furthermore, the reduced REM latency increased the likelihood of selecting a more endogenously depressed population. This study does not necessarily rule out the possibility of alprazolam's antidepressant effect, but rather that it may be more suitable for non-endogenous, anxious/agitated, non-psychotic or insomniac-somatic types of depression with normal REM latencies. Van Valkenburg (91) has reviewed the phenomenology and natural history of this new category of "anxious depressions." Lenox et al (92) in a double-blind study of inpatients fitting RDC criteria for endogenous-type depression, found that alprazolam paralleled the improvement seen with imipramine and electro-convulsive therapy (ECT) over the first ten days. Alprazolam improvement appeared to plateau after this period, while the imipramine and ECT groups continued to improve. In dividing items from the HAM-D scale into cognitive factors (reality disturbance, mood depression, and agitation/anxiety) and vegetative factors (somatization, diurnal variation, sleep disturbance, weight loss), alprazolam performed as well as ECT and imipramine in the vegetative cluster while it minimally altered cognitive symptomatology. The carefully done studies on the antidepressant effects of alprazolam appear at first glance divided in their endorsement. Most clinicians who have considerable practical experience using alprazolam have already concluded that it is not a particularly good antidepressant in spite of what may have been written to the contrary. How are we to make sense of this apparent discrepancy?

The most likely explanation is that the difference is due to an artifact in the Hamilton Depression Scale that frequently leads to misinterpretation in depression treatment studies. There are two factors on the Hamilton Depression Scale - an anxiety factor and a depression factor. Up to 8 of the 21 items on the Hamilton Depression Scale can be said to be anxiety items, the remainder being depressive items. Many anxiolytic drugs particularly benzodiazepines naturally have an impact on the anxiety items on this scale.

The impact on these items can be great enough to produce a statistically significant drop in the total Hamilton Score and thereby give the impression that the treatment is an effective antidepressant when it is really only an effective anxiolytic. The observation is supported by a study by Sheehan, et al (60) on the impact of alprazolam, imipramine and phenelzine on the depressive symptoms in panic disorder. The imipramine and phenelzine (as would be expected) significantly improved the depressive scores compared to placebo on the Hamilton Depression Scale, the Beck 21 Item Depression Inventory and the Montgomery-Asberg Depression Scale. The alprazolam was not significantly better than placebo in lowering the Beck or Montgomery-Asberg scores, although it did lower the Hamilton Depression Score. The Beck 21 Item Inventory and the Montgomery-Asberg are relatively pure depression scales uncontaminated by anxiety items and, therefore, would not be expected to respond significantly to an anxiolytic. When the impact of the alprazolam on the anxiety factor on the Hamilton Scale was removed, the remaining effect on the depressive factor was not significantly better than placebo. We suspect, therefore, that in the early depression studies with alprazolam that the noted drop in Hamilton Score was interpreted to mean that alprazolam was an antidepressant, when a careful dissection of the impact of the drug on the depressive factor would have failed to encourage such a speculation.

BENZODIAZEPINES IN THE TREATMENT OF PSYCHOSES, MANIA, AND AGITATED STATES

BENZODIAZEPINES IN PSYCHOSES

Recently there has been renewed interest in developing new approaches to the treatment of the psychoses, particularly non-neuroleptic pharmacology. Side effects of neuroleptics are well known and include acute and delayed dystonic reactions (and other extrapyramidal reactions); anticholinergic, and anti-alpha-adrenergic blocking (hypotensive) effects; and long-term complications like tardive dyskinesia. For these reasons (and the not infrequent finding of neuroleptic-resistant patients), non-neuroleptic medications are sought.

BZs have been tested for antipsychotic properties. Diazepam has been studied in schizophrenic patients (93-95) with variable results. In dose ranges of 20-80 mg/day, Hollister et al (93) found that only 9 out of 25 patients showed some clinical improvement as rated with the Brief Psychiatric Rating Scale (BPRS). The improvement was less than that expected with antipsychotic medication. Further analysis revealed that "paranoid" patients with symptoms of "hallucinations" and "unusual thought content" appeared to get slightly worse. Symptoms showing most improvement were anxiety, depression and somatic complaints. Jimerson et al (94) studied five schizophrenic patients and one with schizoaffective disorder in a double blind trial with high dose diazepam. The one schizoaffective female showed decreases in "abusive, impulsive, self-destructive behavior and a lessening of grandiose and paranoid delusions" in doses of 250-300 mg/day. Symptoms recurred upon dosage reduction. One schizophrenic female showed only modest decreases in global psychotic ratings, but appeared "calmer, more-spontaneous and sociable, and less hostile". Increased agitation, isolation and bizarre behavior was observed upon drug withdrawal. Although the authors concluded that diazepam did not demonstrate major antipsychotic effects, it is interesting to note that the patients who showed improvement had histories of previous improvement on neuroleptics. Beckman and Haas (95) studied high dose diazepam (up to 400 mg/day) in 15 consecutive schizophrenics. Unfortunately, there was no control group or neuroleptic-treatment group for comparison. Seven out of nine schizophrenic patients demonstrated a complete remission (noted by a decrease in hallucinations, conceptual disorganization, unusual thought, and uncooperativeness). Two other patients had moderate responses as determined by score improvements in the BPRS and Global Clinical Impression (GCI). Five patients had to be withdrawn from the study prior to day 10 due to worsening of symptoms and development of unmanageable excitation and insomnia. These five patients had diagnoses of schizoaffective disorder or cycloid psychosis. The authors were struck by the lack of sedative effects under continued high-dose BZ therapy and the development of feelings of well-being and euphoria with loss of social and sexual inhibitions in some of the patients. Additionally, blood gas analyses performed on four patients before and during the study revealed no hypercapnia on these high doses of diazepam. These authors concluded that diazepam may be beneficial in schizophrenics with lower levels of central arousal (retarded, affectively flattened, withdrawn and with concrete and over-exclusive thought disorder) rather than patients with active symptomatology of schizophrenia.

Kellner et al (96) studied the effects of adding chlordiazepoxide to six schizophrenic patients already on maintenance neuroleptics, (thioridazine or trifluoperazine). In a double-blind "multiple crossover" design, chlordiazepoxide was more effective than placebo in reducing "anxiety, tension and somatic symptoms". In addition, schizophrenic symptoms such as hallucinations, delusions, and thought disturbances improved in two patients. Two patients showed no response differences to placebo or chlordiazepoxide and one patient appeared to have become more depressed with chlordiazepoxide. It is interesting to note that patients responding to chlordiazepoxide had HAM-R scores of 13 or higher. Improvement with chlordiazepoxide occurred usually within one day. Usual mean daily doses of chlordiazepoxide ranged from 200 to 300 mg except one patient who had a non-statistical improvement on 150 mg/day. The authors suggest that there may be two types of anxiety occurring in schizophrenia. One type being the same as experienced by normal or neurotic individuals and independent of the schizophrenic process. The second form of anxiety may share a similar biochemical process in the central nervous system as that causing hallucinations and delusions in schizophrenia. The former would respond better to benzodiazepines and the latter to neuroleptics. It appears from this study that chlordiazepoxide and perhaps other benzodiazepines may be most beneficial as an anxiolytic for schizophrenics who are anxious. The diazepam studies (93-95) also suggest that in some schizophrenic patients core psychotic symptoms may benefit, but again only at high doses. McEvoy and Lohr (97) noted the dramatic reversal of catatonic immobility with I.V. diazepam in two schizophrenic patients. One of the patients began reporting hallucinations and grandiose paranoid delusions once the catatonia was decreasing. Thus in this case, diazepam selectively relieved only the neuromuscular component of catatonic schizophrenia and unmasked the underlying thought disorder. GABA has been theorized to modulate the hypothesized dopamine hyperactivity in schizophrenia particularly in potentiating the anti-psychotic activity of dopamine receptor blockers (98). As mentioned in an earlier section, BZs augment GABA activity and this inhibitory neurotransmitter in turn may decrease functional dopamine activity.

It is apparent from the above reveiw that BZs have not been found to have significant, primary antipsychotic properties and understandably have not been approved for use as sole agents in psychotic disorders. Nonetheless, it is clear that as supplements with neuroleptics, they are quite safe and effective in controlling selected symptomatology in the psychotic patient. Further guidelines are discussed in the following section on acutely agitated states.

BENZODIAZEPINES IN MANIA

Similar interest has expanded the use of benzodiazepines as adjuncts in the treatment of manic-depressive psychosis and manic agitation. Two studies (99,100) have examined the use of lorazepam as a supplement to simultaneous initiation of lithium therapy in acutely agitated manic patients. Modell et al (99) reported that lorazepam helped control mood and behavioral agitation in four bipolar patients within one week despite low-normal serum lithium levels. They contend that lorazepam was effective, well tolerated and did not exacerbate or prolong the acute phase of illness. No patient experienced hypotension, respiratory depression, syncope or increased aggressive behavior. There were few complaints of dysphoria and occasional ataxia (particularly when doses were greater than 10 mg per day). Lorazepam was administered 2 to 4 mg orally, I.M. or I.V. every 2 hours on an as needed basis to achieve sedation that allowed patient compliance with the milieu. Lenox et al (100) (the same authors as the previous study) reported on another group of manic patients treated with lorazepam and lithium and noted the same results. Patients seemed to improve within 5 to 10 days with the addition of lorazepam in average doses of 20 mg/day. One patient received 30 mg/day.

The authors assert that lorazepam is preferable over neuroleptics in treating acutely manic patients (even with psychotic features) as lorazepam has less side effects (including fatal ones like neuroleptic malignant syndrome). They noted that according to the DSM-III, the Manic Episode shares much of the symptomatology of Generalized Anxiety Disorder. Therefore, a benzodiazepine may be efficacious in alleviating these shared symptoms (anxiety, insomnia, agitation, excitement) within the first week while awaiting lithium's longer-term therapeutic effects. Further investigations are required to explore the potentials of BZs as adjuncts to the management of manic agitation.

On the other hand, the BZ clonazepam is said to itself have antimanic effects. Chouinard (101) reviewed his previous studies comparing clonazepam to lithium in a double-blind crossover design. Scores on the Inpatient Multidimensional Psychiatric Scale (IMPS) improved for patients in both groups. However, clonazepam was significantly better than lithium in improving motor activity and logorrhea. Patients taking clonazepam required a significantly fewer number of prn doses of haloperidol to control behavior compared with the lithium group. The mean dosages of haloperidol were also significantly smaller in the clonazepam treated group. It was also noted that patients on clonazepam had less Parkinsonian symptoms than those on lithium. This coupled with the fact that the clonazepam group required less neuroleptics potentially could minimize the risk of tardive dyskinesia. More patients manifested tardive dyskinesia in the lithium group but this was not statistically significant. In this study, the average daily clonazepam dosage was 10 mg/day with the highest dosage 16 mg/day in one patient. However, doses up to 40 to 60 mg per day have been used. Clonazepam, however, is still advocated as a third-line drug in patients resistant to lithium or lithium-tryptophan combination. Victor et al (102) described case reports of one bipolar and two schizoaffective patients whose agitation and psychosis failed to respond with either lithium or neuroleptics (the latter in high daily doses). With the addition of clonazepam in 0.5 to 2 mg/day all patients became calmer, more sociable and had decrease in pressured speech and threatening behavior. One patient had a decrease in delusions while another continued to have them but was able to be discharged and followed as an outpatient. Again, it is difficult to make any conclusions as to true antipsychotic and antimanic effects of clonazepam, but it does appear to be a safe and efficient adjunct in controlling agitation in some bipolar and other psychotic individuals. Further studies are needed to explore its range of applicability as a sole agent, supplement, or synergist in the treatment of this disorder.

BENZODIAZEPINES IN DELIRIOUS STATES

Lorazepam is gaining further popularity as an adjunct in treating agitation associated with delirium. For further discussion in assessing and treating the delirious patients refer to the chapter by Fernandez in this book.

Adams et al (103) reviewed their recent experience with intravenous lorazepam-haloperidol combination in the treatment of delirium of critically ill cancer patients. The authors note that haloperidol is the drug of choice in this setting. Yet some patients in severe delirium are refractory to even extremely high doses intravenously. Further increases in the neuroleptic alone would unlikely be helpful and the authors suggest that adding lorazepam has proven beneficial even in resistant cases. Furthermore, they contend that this combination may be an aid to diagnosing the cause of delirium since different response patterns (particularly difficult sedation) can provide clues to unsuspected organic conditions. They also note an absence of extrapyramidal reactions with this regimen. The combined effect of dopamine blocking and GABA-nergic stimulation may allow rebalancing of the cholinergic system which is postulated to be involved in some delirious states. Further, it appears that the sedation produced by the lorazepam-haloperidol combination is qualitatively unique in that patients do not enter a drug-induced coma. Patients will occasionally manifest stage 2 sleep patterns and can be aroused during chronically high doses. It is known that intravenous haloperidol causes increased nor-adrenergic activity in rats thus reducing their cataleptic response. A similar mechanism in humans may cause a paradoxical amphetamine-like effect which could prevent over sedation.

The authors recommend starting with 3 mg haloperidol followed immediately with 0.5 to 2 mg lorazepam (both I.V.). Behavioral control is usually seen in one hour and often occurs within 20-30 minutes. If there is little or no response in twenty minutes, follow with 10 mg haloperidol and 2-10 mg lorazepam hourly until the patient is soundly sedated. Medication can then be discontinued and the patient observed. If the patient become restless in 3 hours then medications are resumed on a three-hour schedule for the next 12-18 hours after which lorazepam is discontinued and haloperidol dosage schedule progressively lengthened. The key to determining maintenance doses and length of treatment is based on the patient's clinical response rather than on a set formula. All patients in this group had, in addition to their advanced cancer, at least two other serious medical complications such as cardiac dysrhythmias, myocardial infarctions, respiratory failure, pleural effusions, renal failure, profound myelosuppression, or shock (septic or hemorrhagic). No patient developed respiratory, cardiac, or hemodynamic complications during treatment. Some patients demonstrated normalization of heart rates and blood pressures. Ten out of 16 patients on respirators had resolution of their tachypnea and 7 had significant improvement of arterial blood gases and tidal volume once sedated (103). Ayd (104) reviewed the use of intravenous haloperidol as the treatment of choice of delirium particularly in the critically ill patient and commented on the addition of lorazepam as improving response where neither drug was efficient alone. He suggests that the combination is safe (both drugs do not have active metabolites) and is possibly synergistic. It is important to note the efficacy of the combination in a wide spectrum of complicated medical and surgical disorders. It is likely that such innovative treatments will become more common and that such interventions by psychiatrists on a consultation basis will increase.

BENZODIAZEPINES IN ACUTELY AGITATED STATES

Recently there has also been a focus in the pharmacologic treatment of aggression and violence. Unfortunately, management of the chronically violent patient remains controversial as this involves a more complex diagnostic schema and family/social considerations. These patients must be evaluated for the presence of personality disorders, alcohol and drug abuse, intermittent explosive conditions (episodic dyscontrol), mental retardation, organic mental states and neurological disorders in addition to ruling out primary psychotic of affective disorders.

Conn and Lion (105) outlined general principles in the approach to the acutely violent individual. In the emergency setting, calming the patient is the primary objective and it should be stressed that pharmacologic intervention alone is not adequate. Attempts to verbally calm and soothe the patient should be an on-going part of the treatment. This is particularly important in cases in which violence stems from feelings of helplessness and vulnerability. Medication may worsen aggressiveness if it causes a patient to feel he is losing self-control. Paranoid individuals may react with increased aggressiveness and suspiciousness when overly sedated. It is advisable not to deceive a patient as to the medication type he is receiving in this setting. it is also important to properly diagnose any conditions immediately precipitating or exacerbating the agitation when possible. This could help determine the most appropriate pharmacological agent. Rapid or partial neuroleptization is the most commonly used technique to achieve this. However, neuroleptics have potentially dangerous side-effects when used in rapidly accumulating doses. BZs can serve as a suitable alternative (alone or as adjuncts), in controlling the acute agitation and aggression of both psychotic and non-psychotic conditions. Because of their sedative effects and cross tolerance, BZs may be preferable in treating agitation associated with alcohol withdrawal using the guidelines outlined earlier. If BZs are insufficient alone, other medications such as haloperidol may be required. Neuroleptics should be used cautiously as they can cause hypotension, over-sedation, and lower the seizure threshold of the withdrawing patient.

BZs are also considered the drug class of choice in treating the acute aggressive behavior of phencyclidine (PCP) intoxication. PCP produces anticholinergic effects which may be exacerbated by neuroleptics and not by BZs.

Medication should first be offered orally. If oral intake is not feasible or preferred, I.M. lorazepam is a suitable alternative. As mentioned earlier, it is the benzodiazepine of choice given I.M. because it is more evenly and readily absorbed compared to other BZs. Blood levels peak in approximately 90 minutes after either p.o. or I.M. administration. As mentioned previously, lorazepam can be combined with neuroleptics to calm the acutely agitated patient.

Salzman et al (106) retrospectively reviewed the parenteral use of lorazepam in conjunction with the neuroleptic haloperidol in acutely disruptive patients in 1984, compared to using a neuroleptic alone in 1982 at the same center. The combination appears to provide rapid onset of behavioral control usually with no side effects other than sedation. The authors observed that patients receiving the combination in 1984 were given approximately one-half the mean dosage of neuroleptic per treatment episode and significantly less total neuroleptic dosage over a six-month period compared to patients receiving only a neuroleptic in 1982. The authors contend that one explanation to account for the reduced mean and total neuroleptic dosage was the addition of lorazepam, which allowed increased neuroleptic efficacy. Haloperidol was chosen because of its lack of orthostatic hypotension and lorazepam was preferred over other benzodiazepines because of its more rapid and uniform intramuscular absorption and shorter elimination half-life. The ratio used was 5 mg haloperidol to 1 to 2 mg lorazepam.

In 1972, Guz et al (107) compared the effects of lorazepam-haloperidol combination to haloperidol and placebo in psychotic patients in a double-blind study. The lorazepam group tended to do better than the placebo group in individual symptoms of anxious mood, insomnia, agitation and in some cases delusions and hallucinations; however, the differences were not significant on a global assessment. The authors assert that the lorazepam group did achieve control over some symptoms within the first week which was significantly earlier than the placebo group. By the fourth week, differences were no longer significant. It is possible that lorazepam can help reduce some target symptoms faster when used with a neuroleptic rather than using a neuroleptic alone. It is likely this is a result of indirect (GABA-mediated or B-adrenergic) effects rather than intrinsic neuroleptic-like properties.

CONCLUSION

The benzodiazepines represent a highly safe and clinically versatile class of psychotropic agents. As discussed in this chapter, their applicability to a wide spectrum of psychiatric disorders as well as numerous, independent target symptoms, make the BZ's an important tool in the pharmacopoeia of the modern psychiatrist. Careful understanding of their varied pharmacokinetic properties allows them to be used judiciously and effectively with the elderly and patients with concomitant medical illnesses.

BZ's are especially indicated for the treatment of primary anxiety disorders, particularly generalized anxiety, panic disorder, and agoraphobia. For such chronic illnesses requiring long-term BZ therapy, critical understanding of withdrawal kinetics is essential in successful management.

BZ's are the drug class of choice in the treatment of acute alcohol withdrawal syndromes and transient situational insomnias. Increasingly, BZ's are finding utility as adjuncts in the management of agitation commonly found in the psychoses, manic-states, deliria, and acutely agitated states.

TABLE 1

I. BENZODIAZEPINES METABOLIZED BY HEPATIC OXIDATION (HYDROXYLATION AND DEMETHYLATION) PHASE II

CURRENT BENZODIAZEPINES MARKETED IN THE U.S.

Generic Name (Half-life in Hours)	Trade Name	Active Metabolites (Half Life in Hours)	Approved Uses	Usual Daily Dose In Healthy Individuals In Milligrams	Absorption Rate	Approximate Equivalent Dose In Milligrams
Alprazolam (12-15)	Xanax	α-Hydroxyalprazolam ++ 4-Hydroxyalprazolam ++	A	(0.75 - 4.0)	Intermediate	0.5
Chlordiazepoxide + (5-30)	Librium	Desmethylchlordiazepoxide (18)	A,W,P	(15 - 300)	Intermediate	10
Clorazepate * (30-60)	Tranxene	Desmethyldiazepam (30-200) Oxazepam (3-21)	A,W,Ps,P	(15 - 90)	Fast	7.5
Clonazepam (18-50)	Klonopin	7-Aminoclonazepam ++	S	(2 - 16)	Intermediate	2.0
Diazepam +++ (20-50)	Valium	Desmethyldiazepam (30-200) 3-hydroxydiazepam (5-20) Oxazepam (3-21)	A,An,M,P S,W	(2 - 40)	Fastest	5
Flurazepam *** (30-60) (Rapidly Converted)	Dalmane	Desalkylflurazepam (47-100) Hydroxyethylflurazepam (2-4) Flurazepam aldehyde (2-4)	H	(15 - 30)	Fast to Intermediate	15
Halazepam (14)	Paxipam	Desmethyldiazepam (30-200)	A	(60 - 160)	Intermediate to Slow	20
Midazolam +++ (2-4)	Versed	Hydroxymethylmidazolam ++	An	(**)	Fast	2.5
Prazepam *** (30-60) (Rapidly Converted)	Centrax	Desmethyldiazepam (30-200) Oxazepam (3-21)	A	(20 - 60)	Slowest	10
Triazolam (1.5 -5)	Halcion	None	H	(0.125 - 0.5)	Intermed	0.25

* Prodrug rapidly converted to metabolites by decarboxylation in G.I. tract. Faster in Acidic ph.

** Dosage highly individualized, based on patient's weight and clinical response

*** Minimal parent compound concentrations found in plasma after oral administration due to first pass metabolism in liver.

+ I.V. use approved

++ clinically insignificant

+++ I.V. and I.M routes approved

A - Anxiolytic	P - Pediatric doses available
An - Light Anesthesia	Ps - Adjunct in treating partial-complex seizures
H - Hypnotic	S - Seizure control
M - Muscle relaxant	W - Alcohol Withdrawal

TABLE 1

CURRENT BENZODIAZEPINES MARKETED IN THE U.S. (CONTINUED)

II. BENZODIAZEPINES METABOLIZED BY HEPATIC CONJUGATION (PHASE II)

Generic Name (Half-life in Hours)	Trade Name	Active Metabolites (Half Life in Hours)	Approved Uses	Usual Daily Dose in Healthy Individuals In Milligrams	Absorption Rate	Approximate Equivalent Dose In Milligrams
Lorazepam +++ (10-20)	Ativan	None	A	(1 - 10)	Intermediate	1.0
Oxazepam (3-21)	Serax	None	A,P,W	(10 - 120)	Slow	15
Temazepam (10-20)	Restoril	None	H	(15 - 30)	Intermediate	15

+++ I.V. and I.M routes approved

A - Anxiolytic
AN - Light Anesthesia
H - Hypnotic
M - Muscle relaxant
P - Pediatric doses available
Ps - Adjunct in treating partial-complex seizures
S - Seizure control
W - Alcohol withdrawal

TABLE 2

DIRECTIONS FOR TAKING BENZODIAZEPINES

	Breakfast	Lunch	Evening Meal	Bedtime	Day
(tablets)	1/2	1/2	1/2	0	1-2
	1	1/2	1/2	0	3-4
	1	1/2	1	0	5-6
	1	1	1	0	7-8
	1 1/2	1	1	0	9-10
	1 1/2	1	1 1/2	0	11-12
	1 1/2	1 1/2	1 1/2	0	13-14
	2	1 1/2	1 1/2	0	15-16
	2	1 1/2	2	0	17-18
	2	2	2	0	19-20
	2	2	2	1	21-22
	2	2	2	2	23-24

*   If no side effects (drowsiness) or benefit occurs with medication, increase dose to next level every two days.

*   When coming off the medicine, do not reduce dose for any reason at a rate faster the 1/2 tablet every four days.

*   There are no food or drug restrictions with Benzodiazepines as with MAO inhibitors.

*   Caution when driving and operating high speed equipment is necessary.

*   Avoid alcohol consumption.

Reproduced with permission. Copyright Sheehan DV. 1985

TABLE 3

ALCOHOL WITHDRAWAL COMPLICATIONS

Syndrome	Onset	Peak	Comments
Seizures	7-48 hours	24 hours	Less than 3% progress to status epilepticus. May be correlated with hypomagnesemia and respiratory alkalosis.
Delirium	24-72 hours	4-5 days	History of 5-15 years heavy drinking. Associated with hypokalemia and respiratory alkalosis. Death rate 1%.
Hallucinosis	within 48 hours to a few days	unknown peak but usually recover in 1-6 days	Hallucinations are usually auditory but can be visual and olfactory. Content usually threatening. Absence of tremor disorientation or agitation.

TABLE 4

BENZODIAZEPINES USED TO TREAT ALCOHOL WITHDRAWAL

Drug	Withdrawal Symptoms		Comments
	Mild to Moderate	Severe	
Chlordiazepoxide	25-50 mg po qid	100-150 mg po qid or 50 mg po q 2 hours as needed until sedated I.V. use: 50-100 mg I.V. slowly and repeated in 2-4 hours if needed	I.M. not recommended
Diazepam	10 mg tid or qid first 24 hours followed by 5 mg tid or qid as per clinical response	5-10 mg I.V. slowly every 3-4 hrs. until sedated then switch to oral route when feasible	I.M. not recommended
Oxazepam	15-30 mg tid or qid	30-40 mg tid or qid	Taper slowly to prevent sharp plasma level decline due to short half-life
Clorazepate	30 mg po initially followed by 30-60 mg in divided doses first 24 hrs. Day 2: 45-90 mg/day-divided doses. Day 3: 22.5-45 mg/day-divided doses. Day 4: 15-30 mg/day-divided doses. Day 5-to termination: 7.5-15 mg/day (As per manufacturer)		

REFERENCES

1. Herrington RN, Lader MH: Sedatives and Hypnotics, in Handbook of Biological Psychiatry, Part 5, Van Praag HM, Lader MH, Rafaelsen OJ, et al (Editors), New York, Marcel Dekker Inc., 1981.

2. Greenblatt DJ, Shader RI, Abernethy, DR: Current status of benzodiazepines (first of two parts). N Engl J Med 306:354-358, 1983.

3. Gee K, Yamamura H: Subtypes of benzodiazepine receptors: cerebellar vs noncerebellar and central vs peripheral. Roche Receptor 1:3-4, 1984.

4. Polc P, Bonetti EP, Schaffner R, et al: A three state model of the benzodiazepine receptor explains the interactions between the benzodiazepine antagonist Ro 15-1788, benzodiazepine tranquilizers, B-carbolines, and phenobarbitone. Arch Pharmacol 321:260-264, 1982.

5. Cutler NR, Narang PK: Implications of dosing tricyclic antidepressants and benzodiazepines in geriatrics. Psych Clinics N Amer 7:845-861, 1984.

6. Shader RI, Greenblatt DJ: Clinical implications of benzodiazepine pharmacokinetics. Am J Psychiatry 134:652-655, 1977.

7. Shader RI, Weinberger DR, Greenblatt DJ: Problems with drug interactions in treating brain disorders. Psych Clinics N Amer 1:51-69, 1978.

8. Greenblatt DJ, Shader RI: Pharmacokinetic understanding of antianxiety drug therapy. Southern Med J 71 (Supp. 2):2-8, 1978.

9. Roberts RK, Wilkinson GR, Branch RA, et al: Effect of age and parenchymal liver disease on the disposition and elimination of chlordiazepoxide (Librium). Gastroenterology 75:479-485, 1978.

10. Boyer W, Chernow B, Lake CR: Psychopharmacology in the intensive care unit. Psych Clinics N Amer 7:901-907, 1984.

11. Cohen S: The anxiolytic agents. Drug abuse and alcoholism newsletter. Vista Hill Foundation 12 (5):1-4, 1983.

12. Greenblatt DJ, Shader RI, Abernethy DR: Current status of benzodiazepines (second of two parts). N Engl J Med 306:410-414, 1983.

13. Greenblatt DJ, Divoll M, Abernethy DR, et al: Benzodiazepine Hypnotics: Kinetic and Therapeutic Options. Sleep 5:S18-S27, 1982.

14. Siris SG, Rifkin A: The problem of psychopharmacotherapy in the medically ill. Psych Clinics N Amer 4:379-390, 1981.

15. Cassem NH, Hackett TP: The Setting of Intensive Care, in Massachusetts General Hospital Handbook of General Hospital Psychiatry, Hackett TP, Cassem NH (Editors), (Second Edition), Littleton, Massachusetts, 1987.

16. Freeman AM: Anxiety and Anxiety with Depressive Symptoms in the Patient with Cardiac Disorders. Monograph 8836-68, The Upjohn Co., 1983.

17. Lasagna L: The role of benzodiazepines in nonpsychiatric medical practice. Am J Psychiatry 134:656-658, 1977.

18. Billings CK: Management of psychologic responses to myocardial infarction. Southern Med J 73:1367-1371, 1980.

19. Hackett TP: Depression following myocardial infarction. Psychosomatics 26 (11-Supp):23-28, 1985.

20. Stern TA, Caplan RA, Cassem NH: Use of benzodiazepines in a coronary care unit. Psychosomatics 28:19-23, 1987.

21. Kwentus J, Schulz C, Fairman P, et al: Sleep apnea: a review. Psychosomatics 26:713-724, 1985.

22. Hoyumpa AM: Disposition and elimination of minor tranquilizers in the aged and in patients with liver disease. Southern Med J 71:23-28, 1978.

23. Greenblatt DJ, Divoll M, Abernethy DR, et al: Clinical pharmacokinetics of the newer benzodiazepines. Clin Pharmacokinetics 8:233-252, 1983.

24. Pillans PI, Robins AH, Straughan JL: Drug therapy in patients with hepatic encephalopathy - suggested guidelines for sedation and treatment of delirium tremens. SA Med J 66:711, 1984.

25. Levy NB: Use of psychotropics in patients with kidney failure. Psychosomatics 26:699-709, 1985.

26. Bennett WM, Muther RS, Parker RA, et al: Drug therapy in renal failure: dosing guidelines for adults. Part 2 -sedatives, hypnotics, tranquilizers, cardiovascular, antihypertensive, and diuretic agents; miscellaneous agents. Ann Int Med 93:286-325, 1980.

27. Taclob L, Needle M: Drug induced encephalopathy in patients on maintenance haemodialysis. Lancet 704-705, 1976.

28. Coustan DR, Carpenter MV: The use of medication in pregnancy. Resident and Staff Physician 31:64-70, 1985.

29. Safra JF, Oakley GP: Association between cleft lip with or without cleft palate and neonatal exposure to diazepam. Lancet 2:478-80, 1975.

30. Saxen I: Epidemiology of cleft lip and palate. Br J Prev Soc Med 29:103-110, 1975.

31. Saxen I: Association between oral clefts and drugs taken during pregnancy. Int J Epidemiol 4:37-44, 1975.

32. Calabrese JR, Gulledge AD: Psychotropics during pregnancy and lactation: a review. Psychosomatics 26:413-425, 1985.

33. Ezeizel A: Diazepam, phenytoin and etiology of cleft lip and/or palate. Lancet 1:810, 1976.

34. Bracken MB, Holford TR: Exposure to prescribed drugs in pregnancy and association with congenital malformations. Obstet Gynecol 58:336-44, 1981.

35. Stuart EJ: Drug associated congenital abnormalities. Con Med-Assoc J 103:1394, 1970.

36. Ringrose CAD: The hazard of neurotrophic drugs in the fertile years. Can Med Assoc J 106:1058, 1972.

37. Fourth Annual Report of the New Zealand Committee on Adverse Drug Reactions. NZ Med J 70:118-122, 1969.

38. Briggs GG, Bodendorfer TW, et al: Drugs in Pregnancy and Lactation: A Reference Guide to Fetal and Neonatal Risk. Baltimore, Williams and Wilkins. 1983.

39. Berkowitz RL, Coustan DR, Mochizuki T (Editors): Handbook of Prescribing Medications during Pregnancy. Boston, Little Brown. 1981.

40. Blackwell B, Schmidt GL: Drug interactions in psychopharmacology. Psych Clinics N Amer 7:625-637, 1984.

41. Greenblatt DJ, Abernethy DR, Morse DS, et al: Clinical importance of the interaction of diazepam and cimetidine. N Engl J Med 310:1639-1643, 1984.

42. American Medical Association: AMA Drug Evaluations (Fifth Edition), Philadelphia, W. B. Saunders, 1983.

43. Hansten PD: Drug Interactions (Fifth Edition), Philadelphia, Lea and Febiger, 1985.

44. Weller RA, Preskorn SH: Psychotropic drugs and alcohol: pharmacokinetic and pharmacodynamic interactions. Psychosomatics 25:301-309, 1984.

45. Zipurski RB, Baker RW, Zimmer BJ: Alprazolam withdrawal delirium unresponsive to diazepam: case report. J Clin Psychiatry 46:344-345, 1985.

46. McEvoy GK (Editor): Benzodiazepines, in Drug Information 1985. Bethesda, American Society of Hospital Pharmacists, Inc., 1985.

47. Stockley I: Drug Interactions, Boston, Blackwell Scientific Publications, 1981.

48. Ballenger JC: Psychopharmacology of the anxiety disorders. Psych Clinics N Amer 7:757-771, 1984.

49. American Psychiatric Association: Diagnostic and Statistical Manual of Mental Disorders, Third Edition - Revised, Washington, DC, American Psychiatric Association, 1987.

50. Sheehan DV, Coleman JH, Greenblatt DJ, et al: Some biochemical correlates of panic attacks with agoraphobia and their response to a new treatment. J Clin Psychopharm 4:66-75, 1984.

51. Bunney WE: Current biologic strategies for anxiety. Psychiatric Ann 11:21-29, 1981.

52. Kandel, ER: From metapsychology to molecular biology: Explorations into the nature of anxiety. Am J Psychiatry 140:1277-1292, 1983.

53. Carr DB, Sheehan DV, Surman OS, et al: Neuroendocrine correlates of lactate-induced anxiety and their response to chronic alprazolam therapy. Am J Psychiatry 143:483-494, 1986.

54. Sheehan DV: Current perspectives in the treatment of panic and phobic disorders. Drug Therapy 12:49-60, Sept 1982.

55. Waletzky JP: Alternative agents in the treatment of anxiety. Psychiatric Ann 11:49-53, 1981.

56. Altesman RI, Cole JO: Psychopharmacologic treatment of anxiety. J Clin Psychiatry 44:12-18, 1983.

57. Sheehan DV, Gorman J: Medical control of panic attacks. Acute Care Med 29-33, May 1984.

58. Sepinwall J, Cook L: Behavioral Pharmacology of Antianxiety Drugs, in Handbook of Psychopharmacology Volume XIII, Iversen LI, Iversen SD, Snyder SH (Editors), New York, Plenum Press, 1978.

59. Sheehan DV, Ballenger JC, Jacobson G: Treatment of endogenous anxiety with phobic, hysterical and hypochondriacal symptoms. Arch General Psychiatry 37:51-59, 1980.

60. Sheehan DV, Claycomb JB, Surman OS, Gelles L: A double blind placebo controlled trial of alprazolam, imipramine and phenelzine in the treatment of panic disorder. Papers presented at American Psychiatric Assoc Annual Meeting. Los Angeles, 1984.

61. Raj AB, Sheehan DV: Medical evaluation of the anxious patient. Psych Ann 18:176-181, 1988.

62. Fontaine R: Clonazepam for panic disorders and agitation. Psychosomatics 26 (12-Supp):13-18, 1985.

63. Nakada T, Knight RT: Alcohol and the central nervous systems. Med Clinics N Amer 68:121-131, 1984.

64. Adams RD, Victor M: Principles of Neurology (Third Edition), New York, McGraw-Hill Book Co., 1985.

65. Holloway HC, Hales RE, Watanabe HK: Recognition and treatment of acute alcohol withdrawal syndromes. Psych Clinics N Amer 7:729-743, 1984.

66. Miller G: Principles of alcohol detoxification. Amer Fam Physician 30:145-148, 1984.

67. Halikas JA: Psychotropic medication used in the treatment of alcoholism. Hosp Community Psychiatry 34:1035-1039, 1983.

68. Schuckit MA: Alcoholism and other psychiatric disorders. Hosp Community Psychiatry 34:1022-1027, 1983.

69. Gallant DM: Psychiatric Aspects of Alcohol Intoxication, Withdrawal, and Organic Brain Syndromes, in Alcoholism in Clinical Psychiatry, Solomon J (Editor), New York, Plenum Medical Book Co., 1982.

70. Lieber CS: Medical Disorders of Alcoholism: Pathogenesis and Treatment, Philadelphia, W. B. Saunders Co., 1982.

71. Woo E, Greenblatt DJ: Massive benzodiazepine requirements during acute alcohol withdrawal. Am J Psychiatry 136:821-823, 1979.

72. Byerley B, Gillin C: Diagnosis and management of insomnia. Psych Clinics N Amer 7:773-789, 1984.

73. Williams RL, Karacan I: Recent developments in the diagnosis and treatment of sleep disorders. Hosp Community Psychiatry 36:951-957, 1985.

74. Reynolds CF, Kupfer DJ, Sewitch DE: Practical geriatrics: diagnosis and management of sleep disorders in the elderly. Hosp Community Psychiatry 35:779-781, 1984.

75. Mendelson WB: Pharmacological Treatment of Insomnia, in Annual Review Volume V, Washington, American Psychiatric Press, Inc., 1985.

76. Wang RI: New alternatives for improved results in insomnia therapy. Insomnia Therapy, The Upjohn Co., Nov 1984.

77. Bliwise D, Seidel W, Greenblatt DJ, et al: Nighttime and daytime efficacy of flurazepam and oxazepam in chronic insomnia. Am J Psychiatry 141:191-195, 1984.

78. Smith RB, Divoll M, Gillespie WR, et al: Effect of subject age and gender on the pharmacokinetics of oral triazolam and temazepam. J Clin Psychopharm 3:172-176, 1983.

79. Richelson E: The newer antidepressants: structures, pharmacokinetics, pharmacodynamics, and proposed mechanisms of action. Psychopharm Bull 20:213-223, 1984.

80. Feighner JP: The new generation of antidepressants. J Clin Psychiatry 44:49-55, 1983.

81. Hollister LE: Second generation antidepressants. Rational Drug Therapy 16:1-5, 1982.

82. Schatzberg AF, Cole JO: Benzodiazepines in depressive disorders. Arch Gen Psychiatry 35:1359-1365, 1978.

83. Schatzberg AF, Cole JO: Benzodiazepines in the treatment of depressive, borderline personality, and schizophrenic disorders. Br J Clin Pharmacology 11:17S-22S, 1981.

84. Feighner JP: Open label study of alprazolam in severely depressed inpatients. J Clin Psychiatry 44:332-334, 1983.

85. Fabre LF, McClendon DM: A double-blind study comparing the efficacy and safety of alprazolam with imipramine and placebo in primary depression. Curr Ther Res 27:474-482, 1980.

86. Rickels K, Cohen D, Csanalosi I, et al: Alprazolam and imipramine in depressed outpatients: a controlled study. Curr Ther Res 32:157-164, 1982.

87. Feighner JP, Aden GC, Fabre LF, et al: Comparison of alprazolam, imipramine, and placebo in the treatment of depression. JAMA 249:3057-3064, 1981.

88. Feighner JP, Meredith NR, Chammas S, et al: A double-blind comparison of alprazolam vs. imipramine and placebo in the treatment of major depressive disorder. Acta Psychiatr Scand 68:223-233, 1983.

89. Draper RJ, Daly I: Alprazolam and amitriptyline: a double blind comparison of anxiolytic and antidepressant activity. Irish Med J 76:453-456, 1983.

90. Rush AJ, Erman MK, Schlesser MA, et al: Alprazolam vs amitriptyline in depressions with reduced REM latencies. Arch Gen Psychiatry 42:1154-1159, 1985.

91. Van Valkenburg C, Akiskal HS, Purzantian V, et al: Anxious depressions-clinical, family history, and naturalistic outcome comparisons with panic and major depressive disorders. J Affective Disorders 6:67-82, 1984.

92. Lenox RH, Shipley JE, Peyser JM, et al: Double-blind comparison of alprazolam vs imipramine in the inpatient treatment of major depressive illness. Psychopharm Bull 20:79-82, 1984.

93. Hollister LE, Bennett JL, Kimbell I, et al: Diazepam in newly admitted schizophrenics. Dis Nerv Syst 24:746-750, 1963.

94. Jimerson DC, Van Kammen DP, Post RM, et al: Diazepam in schizophrenia: a preliminary double-blind trial. Am J Psychiatry 139:489-491, 1982.

95. Beckman H, Haas S: High dose diazepam in schizophrenia. Psychopharmacol 71:79-82, 1980.

96. Kellner R, Wilson RM, Muldawer MD, et al: Anxiety in schizophrenia. Arch Gen Psychiatry 32:1246-1254, 1975.

97. McEvoy JP, Lohr JB: Diazepam for catatonia. Am J Psychiatry 141:284-285, 1984.

98. Van Kammen DP: Gamma-aminobutyric acid (Gaba) and the dopamine hypothesis of schizophrenia. Am J Psychiatry 134:138-143, 1977.

99. Modell JG, Lenox RH, Weiner S: Inpatient clinical trial of lorazepam for the management of manic agitation. J Clin Psychopharmacol 5:109-113, 1985.

100. Lenox RH, Modell JG, Weiner S: Acute treatment of manic agitation with lorazepam. Psychosomatics 27 (1-Supp):28-31, 1986.

101. Chouinard G: Antimanic effects of clonazepam. Psychosomatics 26 (12-Supp):7-12, 1986.

102. Victor BS, Link NA, Binder RL, et al: Use of clonazepam in mania and schizoaffective disorders. Am J Psychiatry 141:1111-1112, 1984.

103. Adams F, Fernandez F, Andersson BS: Emergency pharmacotherapy of delirium in the critically ill cancer patient. Psychosomatics 27 (1-Supp):33-38, 1986.

104. Ayd FJ: Intravenous haloperidol-lorazepam therapy for delirium. Int Drug Ther Newsletter 19 (9):33-36, 1984.

105. Conn LM, Lion JR: Pharmacologic approaches to violence. Psych Clinics N Amer 7:879-886, 1984.

106. Salzman C, Green AI, Rodriguez-Villa F, et al: Benzodiazepines combined with neuroleptics for management of severe disruptive behavior. Psychosomatics 27 (Supp):17-21, 1986.

107. Guz I, Moraes R, Sartoretto JN: The therapeutic effects of lorazepam in psychotic patients treated with haloperidol: a double blind study. Curr Ther Res 14:767-774, 1972.

PSYCHOLOGICAL ASPECTS OF ORGAN TRANSPLANTATION

A. Frances Brennan, Ph.D.
Associate Professor, Psychiatry
University of Louisville
Department of Psychiatry

Dennis J. Buchholz, Ph.D.
Clinical Associate Professor, Psychiatry & Neurosurgery
University of Louisville
Department of Psychiatry

Wolfgang F. Kuhn, M.D.
Clinical Assistant Professor, Psychiatry
University of Louisville
Department of Psychiatry

CONTENTS:

PSYCHOLOGICAL ASPECTS OF ORGAN TRANSPLANTATION

A. Frances Brennan, Ph.D.

Dennis J. Buchholz, Ph.D.

Wolfgang F. Kuhn, M.D.

Organ transplantation is a heroic technique that has evolved from the realm of experimentation into a viable therapeutic option for various end-stage medical problems. Organ transplantation in humans became a therapeutic option in the early 1960's, with the development and perfection of the technique for kidney transplantation (1) and the introduction of liver transplantation (2) and heart transplantation (3). Today, these are still the three major solid organ transplants performed, although recent advances have resulted in successful pancreatic and heart-lung transplants. Bone marrow transplant also continues to be an increasingly viable therapeutic option (4).

The frequency of kidney transplantation has increased yearly since the early 1970s. By 1981 the National Kidney Registry had data on over 20,000 cases (4) and since then, the annual number of kidney transplants in the United States has risen from less than 5,000 a year to over 10,000 in 1986 (5).

Since the first heart transplant in 1967, over 2500 heart transplants have been performed worldwide (6). There was a decline n the frequency of heart transplants during the early 1970s because of the relatively low success rates for these procedures due to problems with immunosuppression. A reversal of this trend occurred around 1978 following the discovery of cyclosporine, an immunosuppressant drug which dramatically increased survival rates with fewer serious side effects. The Registry of the International Society for Heart

Transplantation reports an exponential increase in heart transplant from 1976 when 21 transplants were performed, to 1985 when 962 were performed. The number of heart transplants in the United States alone has increased from 62 in 1981 to over 1300 in 1986 (5). The number of centers performing heart transplants have accordingly increased from 11 in 1983 to 80 in 1985 (7) and 106 by 1988 (8).

Available statistics show that by 1984, approximately 1000 liver transplants had been performed worldwide (9). In contrast, almost 1000 liver transplants were performed in the United States alone in 1986, along with approximately 45 heart-lung transplants and 130 pancreas transplants (5).

Heart and liver transplants are currently undergoing the most rapid increase of all types of transplants, showing a 25-fold increase between 1981 and 1986 (10). In the most extreme case of transplantation to date, at this writing a three year old child who was the first recipient of five organs died after surviving about six months. This procedure, performed at the University of Pittsburgh Medical Center, involved transplantation of the liver, pancreas, large and small intestine, and part of the stomach.

TYPES OF TRANSPLANT

This chapter deals primarily with heart transplantation patients since this is the basis of our own clinical experience. However, there are important medical and psychological differences among the types of transplant patients that deserve comment. The most obvious difference between kidney and other types of transplant is the possibility of using a living related donor for kidney transplant. This has medical implications since draft rejection is much less likely to occur with a living related donor organ. It also has psychological implications because it raises a host of emotional issues regarding the willingness of a family member to donate a kidney and the effect on the relationship between the kidney donor and recipient. A second major difference between kidney and other types of transplant is the fact that in case of graft failure, the renal patient can resort to hemodialysis as an available alternative, either permanently or pending re-transplantation. For other organ transplant recipients, graft failure is tantamount to death unless immediate re-transplant can take place. This difference may have a profound effect on the level of anxiety these recipients feel about potential organ rejection.

Despite the differences among these groups of patients, there are important similarities in their psychological reactions to the various aspects of the transplant procedure (4). Most of the research on psychosocial factors in transplant has been performed on recipients of kidney and heart transplants. While little has been written about psychosocial issues in other types of transplant, whatever information is available to us will be included where applicable.

THE ROLE OF THE PSYCHOSOCIAL TEAM

The improvement in survival rates and the subsequent increase in the number of transplant patients has been accompanied by a shift in emphasis from the strictly technical aspects of the procedure to a broader range of considerations, including the psychological factors affecting survival and quality of life following transplant. Throughout the history of transplantation, it has been suggested that involvement of psychosocial disciplines was important for the well-being of the patient. In time, an even more expanded role has emerged for psychiatry, psychology, and social work at various points in the transplantation process.

It has been our experience working with a heart transplant unit that the psychosocial needs of transplant patients are best met by a multidisciplinary team composed of a psychiatrist, a psychologist, and a social worker, all of whom should be full time members of the transplant team. To be most useful to the patient, these team members must not only understand the medical issues involved in transplantation, but must be recognized as functioning members of the transplant team and must be in constant communication with other team members.

The three members of the psychosocial team are equally able to attend to many of the needs of the patient. However, the particular expertise of each is necessary in certain defined areas. The psychologist must oversee psychological assessment, the psychiatrist must attend to the mental manifestations of medical illness and psychopharmacological management, and the social worker is best equipped to evaluate the family/social system. When it is impossible for any of these to be full time transplant team members, they should be available on a consultation basis.

The primary function of the psychosocial team is to care for the patient's psychological needs throughout each stage of the transplant procedure, both before and after the actual transplant surgery. Prior to the transplant surgery, the psychosocial team provides emotional support during the initial diagnosis of end-stage disease and the subsequent grieving process. Psychosocial consultation is also necessary to assess the patient's psychological suitability for transplantation (11,12). The psychologist may play a specific role in providing formal psychological test results that will aid in this evaluation of the patient.

Following the patient's acceptance for transplant, the psychosocial team will find itself providing emotional support during the stressful pre- and post-transplant periods as well as more formal psychotherapy or counseling during times of crisis. The psychiatrist plays a specific role in the pre- and post-transplant periods in monitoring medically-based psychological reactions (such as steroid-induced reactions in the post-operative period) and treating psychological crises through psychopharmacological intervention. As the patients discharges approach, it is important that patients receive counseling with respect to their new family and community roles, including career and leisure time goals (12,13). The social worker may play a key role at this stage in working with the patient and family to clarify these roles and help them contact social agencies appropriate to their needs. Finally, the psychosocial team will inevitably find itself confronted with assisting dying patients with the psychological issues surrounding their approaching death. More specific functions of the psychosocial team will be discussed in light of the medical and psychosocial factors associated with each of the stages of transplantation.

STAGES OF TRANSPLANTATION

The psychological assessment and treatment of organ transplant patients must consider both medical and psychosocial factors surrounding the transplant surgery. Prior to transplant, the surgeon must give attention to the medical indications and contraindications for transplantation and medical factors influencing survival. Immediately following transplant surgery, patients must be monitored for post-surgical medical complications and steroid-induced mental changes. Longer term attention must be paid to the side effects of medication and the patient's compliance with the medical regimen. The psychosocial factors that should be attended to include psychiatric diagnoses, psychological reactions to the transplant procedure, and, following transplant, longer term vocational rehabilitation, sexual functioning, and the more global area called "quality of life".

The transplant procedure has been divided into "stages" by many authors who have observed different psychosocial stressors and psychological reactions at various points in the protocol (14,15,16,17,18). Although different authors have delineated slightly different stages, there is some consistency noted in the overall progression of stages among the types of transplant patients (4).

The medical and psychosocial factors associated with transplantation will be discussed according to the following stages: (1) transplant proposal, (2) evaluation, (3) waiting period, (4) perioperative period, (5) recovery, and (6) post discharge. The specific intervention issues that must be addressed by the psychosocial team during each stage will also be discussed.

STAGE I. TRANSPLANT PROPOSAL

The major goal during the transplant proposal stage is to inform the patient of the medical diagnosis and to suggest the possibility of transplant. The major psychological tasks for the patient during this stage are: (1) accepting the severity of the medical condition, (2) receiving and understanding sufficient information about the transplant to make an informed decision, and (3) deciding to accept or decline a transplant if it is offered.

MEDICAL FACTORS IN THE TRANSPLANT PROPOSAL STAGE

Medical Causes. The assessment of organ transplant patients begins with a consideration of the diseases that lead to the end stage status of these patients. End stage kidney disease results from a variety of causes and mechanisms, most frequently immunopathogenic problems but also including coagulation problems, infection, metabolic disturbance, vascular disorders, congenital abnormalities, obstruction to urine flow, neoplasia, and trauma. Although different diseases vary in the details and rate of progression, all eventually result in progressive decrease in glomerular filtration rate (19).

End stage heart disease most frequently stems from: (1) cardiomyopathy secondary to viral infection, infarction, alcohol abuse, or idiopathic causes; or (2) coronary artery disease (ischemic heart disease) (4). Heart-lung transplant is primarily required due to primary or secondary pulmonary hypertension in addition to end stage heart disease (6).

End stage liver disease is most often the result of alcohol or postnecrotic cirrhosis (90%). Other causes include congenital biliary atresia, acute liver failure from fulminating viral hepatitis or toxic hepatitis, and malignant liver disease. An added medical consideration in the case of liver transplant is the timing of the surgery. This depends on a delicate balance between increasing progressive signs of liver disease and operating before the disease reaches a terminal stage (20).

Bone marrow transplant appears to be an increasingly reasonable therapeutic option for severe aplastic anemia, immunodeficiency diseases, and malignancies including childhood acute lymphocytic leukemias. Increasingly, it is utilized during periods of remission rather than in acute relapse (4). Pancreatic transplant continues to be more experimental but is primarily considered as a treatment for advanced degenerative complications of diabetes (4).

The end stage medical condition of patients at the time of transplant proposal creates a particular set of stresses that impact psychological functioning at this point. For many patients with end stage disease, there has been chronic declining course, with the patient becoming gradually weaker and progressively more ill and experiencing increasing changes in lifestyle and family roles.

For example, patients with ischemic heart disease have often experienced an extended course of disability and perhaps several surgical revascularization procedures. Kidney patients faced with transplant have usually endured a period of chronic uremia and hemodialysis. The symptoms of uremia include nausea, dizziness, fatigue, weakness, apathy, drowsiness, decreased concentration, restlessness, irritability, depression, and cognitive problems, including slowed speech, impaired memory, and confusion (21). Furthermore, the process of dialysis often results in a constant "washed out" feeling and physical sensation of illness, as well as "dialysis dementia" and confusion (21,22). For patients with chronic onset, the transplant proposal promises relief from the stresses associated with this pre-transplant period.

On the other hand, for patients with acute cardiomyopathy or acute renal failure, the diagnosis and transplant proposal causes a major and sudden shift in self image, perception of immortality, life expectancy, and future plans. This creates a very different impact which may result in shock, disbelief, and anger.

Cost of the Transplant. In addition to information concerning the medical aspects of transplantation, part of the information to be communicated to patients includes the financial cost and the question of whether the transplant will be covered by third party payors. The cost of transplantation is relatively high, with conservative estimates of first year costs (including post-transplant immunosuppression drugs) averaging $35,000 for kidney transplant, $95,000 for heart transplant, and $130,000 for liver transplant (23). Beyond the first year cost, the post-operative medical regimen may require a continuing annual cost of over $5,000 for immunosuppressant treatment. The costs for hemodialysis and kidney transplantation have been covered by Medicare since 1972. Transplantation of liver is now covered by Medicare in selected cases, primarily for biliary atresia in children. Heart transplant has been covered by Medicare since 1987 but only in selected centers. Kidney transplant is covered by most state medicaid plans and other third party insurers (96%), while only about 50-85% of these cover heart and liver transplant. We have known cases of patients declining transplant in order to keep their families from being burdened with the cost of their illness.

PSYCHOSOCIAL FACTORS IN THE TRANSPLANT PROPOSAL STAGE

Initial Psychological Reactions. When a patient is first approached regarding the end stage nature of the illness and the need for an organ transplant, the typical reaction involves a mixture of disbelief, anger, and denial as well as renewed hope (4,14,15,16,17). The course of the disease up to the point of transplant proposal may in part determine whether a particular patient tends more toward disbelief and anger or more toward grateful acceptance and renewed hope (18). If the disease has been chronic, as in ischemic heart disease or chronic renal failure, the emotional reaction to the transplant proposal may emphasize the positive hopeful aspects of the procedure. When the disease has an acute onset, as with viral myocarditis, the sudden shock of the news may elicit primarily anger and disbelief.

The period of denial, anger, consternation, and agitation may take several days to resolve before patients and their families are able to accept the severity of the illness and decide to proceed with the transplant evaluation. We have seen two cases in which patients were too ill to respond to the proposal of heart transplant themselves. In these cases, the families responded with similar emotions and were unable to proceed with the decision for several days. If a patient has not worked through this period of mourning and acceptance before the point of transplant surgery, there can be tragic results. We know of one case where a donor heart quickly became available for a patient who was not psychologically ready to receive it. This patient refused the procedure at the last moment resulting in the loss of the valuable donor heart and causing much anger among the medical staff.

Informed Consent. The patient's decision to consider a drastic transplant procedure is complicated by a number of potential barriers to full informed consent. As with any situation requiring informed consent, the quality of the consent given is compromised when insufficient information is provided, either because certain information is unavailable or inadvertently omitted, or because information is given in a way that the patient cannot fully comprehend. Information which the potential transplant patient must consider includes the risk of death during surgery, the financial cost, changes in lifestyle associated with a rigorous medication regimen, the elimination of alcohol and tobacco use, and the experience of periodic biopsy and rejection episodes.

Perhaps more important in the case of end stage disease, however, are the psychological processes of the patient that distort the information given, resulting in compromised informed consent. Some patients present for transplant with severe cognitive or psychiatric problems that impair their ability to fully comprehend the information provided. In these cases, third party consent is often given by a family member. More common, perhaps, is the effect of psychological denial on informed consent. For patients faced with certain death, there is a strong tendency to deny the risks inherent in the only possible reprieve, the organ transplant. The patient may "hear" only non-threatening information and may need to be repeatedly reminded of possible complications (22). Finally, subtle coercion by family, friends, and even medical staff can distort the patient's ability to freely chose to accept or decline this procedure. One patient who initially verbalized acceptance of the transplant later became demanding, angry, and irritable, and refused to cooperate with the evaluation process. This behavior increased when she was accepted for transplant and continued until it became clear that the patient had responded to significant family pressure to undergo the transplant while she herself did not really want it. Once this had been addressed, the uncooperative behavior disappeared and the patient declined the transplant, dying soon after.

INTERVENTION ISSUES IN THE TRANSPLANT PROPOSAL STAGE

At the time of transplant proposal, there is a strong need for support for both the patient and the family during the initial shock reaction. Help in working through the denial and anger may facilitate the patient's acceptance of the medical condition and the need for drastic medical intervention. It should be noted that a moderate degree of denial can be an important aid to patients in dealing with the anxiety and depression of this period and should be respected, as long as it does not interfere with appropriate decision making.

The movement toward a decision for transplant should also be monitored to ensure that the normal grieving process following diagnosis has been sufficiently worked through for a reasonable assessment of the costs and benefits of the transplant procedure. When necessary, the patient may need to be repeatedly informed of potential complications in order to overcome the tendency toward denial. Assessment and clarification of family conflict or pressure toward a particular decision is also important. These interventions should improve the quality of informed consent, ensuring that it is uncompromised by denial, unrealistic expectations, or undue external pressures, and facilitate a decision to proceed with evaluation or decline the transplant.

We have found that about 6% of our candidates decline an offer of heart transplantation. Patients who decline the procedure will require support, as well as assistance for their families, in working through the psychological aspects of dying.

STAGE II. EVALUATION

The major goal of the evaluation stage is to determine the patient's medical and psychosocial suitability for the transplant procedure. We have found that the majority of our heart transplant candidates during this period attempt to portray themselves in a good psychological light, "emphasizing the goodness of their character and the badness of their heart". The primary psychological task for the patient during this period is to resolve ambivalence and make a final decision for or against transplant surgery if it is offered (18).

MEDICAL FACTORS IN THE EVALUATION STAGE

During this stage, medical examinations are performed to ascertain that certain medical indications for transplant are present and that certain serious medical contraindications are not. Medical indications for kidney transplant include age less than 60 and end stage renal failure with not other systemic or debilitating illnesses (24).

The primary medical indication for heart transplant is New York Heart Association Class IV cardiac status, which reflects little realistic hope for recovery or survival past six months. Ninety percent of these patients die if not transplanted within three months (4). Age is a significant predictor of survival following heart transplant (25), and age over 60 is often considered a medical contraindication. Once age is accounted for, gender and type of heart disease (cardiomyopathy vs. coronary heart disease) are not associated with survival and are not considered as medical indicators. High pulmonary pressures constitute a contraindication to heart transplant, unless heart-lung transplant is possible.

Medical indications for a liver transplant include age less than 45 to 50 years old with a non-malignant disease that has not progressed to the terminal stage (20,26). Alcoholic cirrhosis is considered a relative contraindication for transplant, since the patient is often malnourished, prone to deterioration from infection, and usually unable to control drinking or comply with the medical regimen following surgery. Hepatitis B is also a relative contraindication because its recurrence would damage the newly transplanted organ. Children with biliary atresia are considered especially good candidates for liver transplant.

PSYCHOSOCIAL FACTORS IN THE EVALUATION STAGE

Once a patient has accepted the notion of a fatal illness requiring drastic medical intervention, the decision is made to undergo evaluation for transplant. The evaluation includes an examination of the patient's medical and psychosocial status, and this period may be characterized by anxiety about acceptance mixed with ambivalent fear of acceptance (15,17,18). An additional stressful and guilt-provoking aspect of evaluation for kidney transplant patients is the evaluation of family members in the search for a potential living related organ donor.

Need for Selection. During the evaluation stage, the psychosocial team attempts to determine whether the patient meets the psychosocial selection criteria for transplantation. The need for selection criteria arises from: (1) the scarcity of donor organs and the press for their most beneficial "rationing" (27); and (2) the ethical injunction to avoid a procedure that will make a patient worse. Psychosocial selection criteria exist primarily to assist in selecting patients who will benefit from the transplant and to identify patients at psychological risk for poor medical or psychosocial outcome following transplant.

The increased success of organ transplant has created a classic supply and demand problem, since the estimated number of appropriate transplant patients each year is considerably greater than the number of donor organs available. Approximately 2,000 donated kidneys become available for the 6,000 to 8,000 patients waiting for renal transplantation in the United States each year (28). Only 400 to 1000 donor hearts become available each year for the potential 14,000 heart transplant candidates waiting at any one time in the United States (29). Similarly, for over 4000 liver transplant candidates, only approximately 2000 to 2500 donor organs are available (20).

The competition for donor organs has resulted in protracted discussion of appropriate criteria for prioritizing cases for available organs. Most authors agree that this determination should attempt to balance the seriousness of the illness with the potential for long-term survival "at a reasonable level of functioning" (27,29). In effect, this suggests that the process of choosing appropriate transplant candidates must be based on a combination of medical and psychosocial criteria.

However, several authors have criticized the use of psychosocial criteria such as social support, IQ, mental illness, criminal record, employment, indigency, or even alcohol and drug addiction for determining potential long-term survival "at a reasonable level of functioning" (24,27). There has been a gradual move toward liberalization of selection criteria, as more recent research finds that some of these criteria are not as relevant to survival or quality of life as once thought. There is a parallel tendency toward avoiding subjectivity in determining priority for these life saving procedures, putting the burden of proof as to the relevance of any particular criterion on the professional.

Mostly, psychosocial selection criteria for transplant have been generalized from related areas of surgery and derived from clinical intuition about the relationships between certain psychological traits and potential adjustment following transplant. Many transplant units still follow the selection standards originated at Stanford in the 1970's. These standards exclude patients with documented psychiatric disturbance, history of drug abuse or addiction, history of poor medical compliance, or severe family dysfunction (30,31). In our heart transplant program, we have utilized the following relative psychosocial contraindications: (1) active antisocial behavior, (2) mental deficiency with lack of compensatory social support system, (3) ongoing substance abuse, and (4) active major depression or psychosis. Substance abuse and depression do not preclude consideration for transplant if they respond to treatment. The judicious use of these psychosocial criteria has resulted in our not accepting approximately 15% of patients either partially or wholly for psychosocial reasons. Four general classes of psychosocial selection factors for transplant (or their converse, "psychosocial contraindications") have been reported in the literature: psychiatric disorder, poor social conditions, cognitive deficits, and compliance problems.

Psychiatric Disorder as a Contraindication. The presence of
severe psychiatric disorder, especially severe depression, has
typically been used to exclude patients from transplantation
(14,15,31,32,33,34). In addition to overt depressive symptomatology,
clinical impressions that the request for transplant was a "suicidal
equivalent" (32) or that dramatic noncompliance with medical regimen
was a "depressive equivalent" (15) have been mentioned as
contraindications in this regard. Depression is not seen as a
contraindication if it can be successfully treated prior to surgery.
Several authors have noted that only the most severe psychopathology
should be deemed an absolute contraindication to transplant (33,35).

It should be pointed out that a degree of psychological distress
is normal under the circumstances of being evaluated for organ
transplant. Estimates of psychiatric disorder in these populations
during the evaluation period range from about 17% to 64%, with
estimates for kidney transplant candidates somewhat lower than for
heart transplant patients (36). More specifically, recent evaluations
of heart transplant patients have emphasized high levels of anxiety
(39-51%), depression (9-18%), substance abuse disorders (17%), and
personality disorders (17-42%), as well as some organic mental
disorders (11%) (15,17,37,38,39). Although these disorders are
classified differently in the various studies, it is likely that the
high frequency of anxiety and depression are primarily of the
"adjustment disorder" type. We have found about one in four of
the diagnosable mental disorders seen in our heart transplant patients
during the evaluation period are most appropriately considered

disorders of adjustment to the stress of newly-diagnosed severe cardiac disease requiring transplantation (39). Psychiatric disturbance may be even more frequent in liver transplant patients than in heart or kidney transplant patients, with one study observing obvious psychiatric disturbance in all children and adults interviewed both prior to and following liver transplant surgery (40). Many of these pre-transplant disturbances were organic brain syndromes (OBS). However, in addition, these patients showed depression and anxiety and, particularly in children, developmental lag, helplessness, and dependency. The lack of additional studies of psychiatric disturbance in liver transplant patients causes us to view this conclusion with some caution.

Several authors have noted a significant level of continued ambivalence in heart patients undergoing transplant evaluation and suggest that this may affect outcome following transplant if not resolved prior to surgery (15,31,37). Finally, in addition to psychological disorder, early reports noted a significant proportion of marital and family strain in families presenting for transplant (41,42). Again, these symptoms are likely to be reactions to the current stressful situation.

There are very few studies that document the level of psychological distress prior to transplant using standard psychological tests. However, in one study of kidney transplant candidates, Minnesota Multiphasic Personality Inventory (MMPI) profiles were more elevated than those of a control group of medical patients (21). We have found that the MMPI profiles of heart transplant patients were somewhat elevated compared to standardized norms, as did one other study in the area (43).

Social Problems as a Contraindication. The second major class of contraindications includes social conditions that have been found to adversely affect post surgical outcome following other types of surgery: severe family dysfunction (31), marked job instability and antisocial behavior (14), and poor social support (30). Recently, this last factor has been found not to be as important as initially estimated (34).

Cognitive Problems as a Contraindication. The third major class of contraindications include those conditions that will inhibit the ability to give quality informed consent or to participate in adequate medical self-care following transplant. These include active psychosis or mental deficiency (15,31,35). We have considered mental deficiency to be a particularly prohibitive factor when there is not a family member or other support system available to oversee the technical aspects of the patient's medical self-care.

Compliance Problems as a Contraindication. The fourth class of contraindications includes those disorders or behaviors which may threaten ability to comply with the complicated medical regimen following surgery: drug or alcohol abuse or addiction (15,31,34,44), ambivalence regarding the surgery (15, 31,34,37), and history of documented noncompliance or "personality unsuited to compliance" (15,33). Potential for compliance is such as critical factor that it has even been suggested that severe psychopathology is not necessarily a contraindication unless it directly affects potential for compliance with the medical regimen. It appears to be the case that some personality disorders characterized by antisocial or aggressive behavior render patients particularly unsuited to adequate medical compliance (34). Because alcoholism is the leading cause of liver failure in the United States, the issue of noncompliance due to alcoholism is particularly salient in liver transplantation.

INTERVENTION ISSUES IN THE EVALUATION STAGE

The identification of relevant selection criteria and psychosocial contraindications for transplant patients is one of the earliest functions performed by psychosocial professionals in transplant units. The role of the psychosocial team in assessing, evaluating, and determining the appropriateness of patients for the transplant procedure has been emphasized since the early transplant operations.

Given that there is probably a higher than normal level of psychiatric distress among pre-transplant patients, it is important to determine which psychiatric disorders should be considered as contraindications to the transplant procedure. In other words, are there certain psychosocial characteristics of a patient that influence prognosis following transplantation? As previously mentioned, most of the psychosocial selection criteria have been developed without strong empirical research. As pressures grow to move away from choosing patients for transplant procedures based on arbitrary standards (24,27), it will become more important to scientifically demonstrate the predictive relationship between these social and psychological traits and post-transplant medical outcome and quality of life. The following section will present the evidence that is available about these predictive relationships.

Predicting Medical Outcome. The most common psychological

factors examined in attempts to predict medical outcome (including survival) include depression and anxiety. These have been shown by some to be related to organ rejection and non-survival following kidney transplant (45,46,47). We have not noted this phenomenon in our heart transplant patients and there is reason to believe that symptoms of depression and anxiety prior to cardiac transplantation do not adversely affect outcome (38). A more systematic study in this area also failed to provide empirical support for this contention (48). However, there is a great deal of research in related areas showing, for example, the relationship between depression and medical status post coronary bypass surgery (49). Thus, although definitive research has not been performed in this area, there is reason to believe that severe and chronic depression, untreated, would constitute a strong contraindication to transplant. "Reservations about psychiatric suitability" for heart transplant (based on depression, substance abuse, and personality disorder traits) was found to predict perioperative survival as well as psychiatric morbidity (50).

More recently, a few studies have attempted to use standardized psychological test instruments to predict medical outcome following heart transplant. One of these studies suggests that higher scores on the somatic subscale of the General Health Questionnaire prior to transplant are associated with non-survival one year following transplant (38). We have found in heart transplant patients that pre-transplant MMPI profiles reflecting personality traits of low frustration tolerance, impulsivity, and social alienation predict poorer medical outcome (including survival) six months following transplant. An important factor in this relationship appears to be the increased tendency of patients with those personality traits to be more noncompliant with the medical regimen.

The validity of using standardized psychological instruments such as the MMPI with medical patients has been repeatedly questioned (51). These instruments are normed on psychiatric samples and the presence of medical symptoms may spuriously elevate certain scales, particularly those measuring depression or hypochondriasis. In addition, medical patients tend to produce rather defensive, "socially desirable" profiles which emphasize physical complaints and deny emotional problems. The few studies that utilize psychological tests with transplant patients are not sufficient to resolve these questions and results obtained with these populations must currently be interpreted with caution. However, we feel that the results of validity studies such as those we are currently conducting to predict medical outcome and quality of life from MMPI profiles can be useful guide to using this test with these patients.

Predicting Compliance. Compliance has been found to be poorer in younger patients, females, single or divorced patients, and those with lower education. Adolescent females, especially those with depression and decreased family support, appear particularly at risk (33,52,53). It is generally agreed that extreme denial, lower tolerance for frustration, acting out of aggression, and poor family support are significant predictors of noncompliance in transplant patients. We found that MMPI profiles indicative of these traits were strongly related to noncompliance in heart transplant patients. Finally, it has been suggested that medical compliance during the waiting period for a donor organ may also provide a good predictor of post-transplant compliance (54).

Although not directly applicable to the transplant situation, several studies of renal dialysis patients may also shed light on factors associated with compliance in a similar population. These studies also found that lower frustration tolerance, acting out potential, inappropriate adjustment to the sick role (dependency), increased emotional reactions, and poor impulse control were related to noncompliance (55). One study (57) found that a high level of pervasive denial in renal dialysis patients was associated with noncompliance, while denial that does not distort cognitions was not associated with noncompliance.

Predicting Quality of Life. A number of psychosocial factors appear to be related to post-transplant quality of life. Poor family support, inadequate family communication, less favorable pre-transplant psychological status, and the presence of psychiatric diagnoses are all associated with poorer post-transplant quality of life and dissatisfaction with the results of cardiac transplantation (21,35,37,50,54). In addition, we have found that pre-transplant diagnoses of personality disorder are significantly associated with poorer quality of life following transplant, while pre-transplant diagnoses of anxiety, depression, or cognitive problems did not predict post-transplant quality of life (58).

Recently, there has been growing agreement on the relatively greater adverse effects of chronic personality disorder than pre-transplant anxiety or depression on post-transplant outcome. It appears that personality disorder may be a causative factor in post-transplant behavior management problems and poor quality of life

(36,38,58). In contrast, the relatively high levels of anxiety and depression often seen prior to transplant are more likely to be a reaction to the current medical situation and are thus considered more "normal". In fact, these are not as predictive of post-transplant complications (34,36). The strong relationship of personality disorder and substance abuse problems to medical outcome is illustrated by the case of a female heart transplant patient who was retrospectively determined to be characterologically quite antisocial as well as alcoholic. Her transplant was one of the first locally and caused her to be a very "special" person with much media attention. She showed a good medical course for about 6 weeks following the transplant. However, after this, she began to pilfer drugs, became manipulative toward staff, and lied about disregarding smoking and dietary restrictions. During eleven months of alcohol drinking and questionable adherence to immunosuppressant medication, she was re-hospitalized several times and finally died from factors related to tissue rejection shortly after admission to a psychiatric unit for alcoholism treatment.

Living Related Donors. Although the evaluation of potential living related kidney donors is beyond the scope of this chapter, the dynamics of the pre- and post-transplant relationship between the organ donor and recipient are briefly considered. There has been some suggestion in the literature that the recipient experiences more psychiatric distress following the transplant of a kidney from a living related donor than an anonymous cadaver donor (59,60). However, it appears that this depends to a large extent on the pre-transplant relationship between the donor and recipient. There are numerous anecdotal reports of poor adjustment (including kidney rejection) when the relationship with the donor is conflictual (48). In particular, it has been noted that the potential for conflict between a parent and child (perhaps especially an adolescent child) may be great due to activation of preexisting authority and rebellion issues.

The issue of living related organ donation obviously applies only to kidney transplant. However, in these cases, special attention may need to be paid to the emotional relationship between donor and donee. For a more detailed review of this issue, see the 1977 book entitled "Gift of Life" by Simmons, Klein, and Simmons (61).

The Patient's Decision. During the evaluation, there should be an assessment of the patient's ability to make an informed decision about the transplant procedure and give consent based on realistic criteria. In addition to limitations imposed by severe cognitive problems or psychosis, it has been noted that certain personality styles may hinder the decision-making process that must occur during this stage (18). Obsessive-compulsive candidates are likely to deal with anxiety through indecision and preoccupation with details. Narcissistic persons may have trouble accepting the "imperfection" implied by the necessity for transplant. Paranoid people may have difficulty with the evaluation period and its attendant invasive procedures which may be experienced as a threat. They may decline transplantation, since "surgery may be seen as an assault" (18).

The decision by the medical staff for or against transplant is also likely to be handled differently by persons with different personality traits. Dependent persons may get depressed if not accepted, while histrionic patients may become charming and impressive in their efforts to gain acceptance. Narcissistic individuals are likely to become demanding and feel that they are entitled to be accepted. The psychosocial team must also be prepared to help patients deal with their reactions to the medical decision.

Summary. In summary, the role of the psychosocial team during the evaluation period is to identify patients with severe psychiatric disorder, especially severe personality disorder and severe depression, as well as social and family dysfunction. Furthermore, evaluators should be alert to signs and traits associated with post-transplant noncompliance: low frustration tolerance, denial, potential for impulsive acting out, and poor social/family support.

The purpose of identifying poor prognosis patients during the evaluation period may be to exclude certain psychosocially inappropriate persons from transplant, or to anticipate psychosocial problems in certain patients and provide necessary active support and intervention to prevent these. For example, certain problems may be anticipated during different stages of the transplant procedure depending on the personality type (18). During the waiting period, passive dependent individuals are often frustrated and angry, while compulsive individuals become overcritical of the staff, alienating them at a time when they most need emotional support from them. During post-operative recovery, compulsive individuals may do well, as they channel their perfectionistic energies into complying with the medical regimen, while antisocial persons may have difficulty overcoming impulsivity and frustration to allow unimpeded compliance. During recovery, histrionic persons may have particular difficulties with body image and appearance distortion due to steroids, and dependent persons are likely to feel over-anxious at discharge. Anticipation of these difficulties should allow a more preventive and individualized approach to the counseling, support, or other intervention a particular patient will need at various stages of the transplant procedure.

STAGE III. WAITING FOR DONOR ORGAN

The major goal during the waiting period is to manage the deteriorating medical condition of the patient and achieve survival long enough to obtain a donor heart. The primary task for the patient is to cope with the increased stress and anxiety of the waiting period to arrive at transplant in a psychological condition conducive to the success of the surgery and post-operative course.

MEDICAL FACTORS IN THE WAITING STAGE

The waiting period is a stage of increased psychological stress and very few medical procedures, except for stabilizing treatment of the deteriorating medical condition. The shortage of donors and the increase in transplant centers has resulted in increasingly long waiting lists and has dramatically lengthened the time the average patient must wait for a donor heart (62). The tendency for less acutely ill patients to return home during this period is often stressful for the patient and family, and results in less contact between patient and medical personnel. During the evaluation period, the patient had been the center of attention from family and medical staff. The decreased activity during the waiting period and the prolonged wait at home can result in feelings of abandonment, misperceptions of the patient's priority on the waiting list, and a sense of competition with the other patients waiting for a donor organ.

The rapid medical deterioration of several of our patients during this period required the temporary use of ventricular assist devices (VADs). Information concerning the psychological effects of these devices is not available since these have been successfully used as a bridge to transplant in relatively few cases.

PSYCHOSOCIAL FACTORS IN THE WAITING STAGE

Much has been written about the unique stresses of the waiting period on transplant patients. In some ways it is the most difficult stage for the patient because of increasing anxiety and stress as the wait is prolonged, fear of death before a donor organ becomes available, and an increased state of dependence. It is a period characterized by vacillation between anxiety and fear of death on the one hand, and hope and euphoria on the other (17,18).

In addition to the usual increases in anxiety and depression during this period, there are reported instances of the development and exacerbation of severe psychopathology, or the development of an acute adjustment disorder "characterized by social withdrawal, indecisiveness, and morbid dependence" (p. 45) (34). This occurs most often during a prolonged period of waiting in which the elation of acceptance for transplant gives way to depression and anxiety (32,62). We have found that almost half of our transplant patients exhibit psychiatric symptoms of anxiety, depression, or behavioral management problems during the waiting period. One 56 year old patient, initially relieved over acceptance for heart transplant, experienced increasing irritability and anxiety as the waiting period lengthened, which erupted into outright distrust and anger when another waiting candidate was transplanted ahead of him. His anxiety made hospitalization intolerable and he twice left against medical advice. Finally, he died after emergency admission to another hospital. Another patient became increasingly demanding and controlling during the waiting period, denying anxiety and feigning medical symptoms to elevate his position on the transplant priority list. This patient refused to comply with his medical workup and he eventually began verbalizing his suspicion of a conspiracy to keep him from getting a donor heart.

A patient's felt and/or expressed wish for the death of a donor is a common phenomenon associated with the waiting period (18,32). Ruminations and fantasies about the death of potential donors from traffic accidents tend to increase during rainy weather or holiday weekends. The frequency of this phenomenon suggests that it is a normal part of the transplant process during the waiting period despite the fact that these thoughts often result in guilt feelings. Over half of our waiting heart transplant candidates have directly expressed a wish for a potential donor to die and many felt guilty about this thought. One patient, anxiously awaiting a donor organ, was preoccupied with incidents of car accidents which might produce donors. Upon hearing of a medical staff member's upcoming weekend trip, she stated to her: "I hope someone who is traveling home over the Thanksgiving weekend will die in an accident so I can get a heart". This statement was overtly "unrelated" to the staff member's trip and the patient was apparently unaware of any connection between her statement and the staff member's trip.

We have also observed that almost one in four of our patients expressed a concern that the new heart would impart some personality traits from the donor, such as gender-specific characteristics. This blurring of identity has been documented also among kidney transplant patients, where family members sometimes anticipated a transfer of certain characteristics, such as an "even-tempered personality", from the donor to the recipient (4).

Denial is a commonly used mechanism to deal with the stress of the waiting period. We join others in noting pronounced levels of denial concerning the heart, the donor, or the transplantation process in many of our waiting patients (39,63). A tendency for waiting patients to distance themselves from patients experiencing graft rejection has also been noted during this time (64).

A recent study of family reactions to the various stages of transplant notes that during the waiting period, the significant other of the patient becomes devoted to keeping the patient alive and comfortable (65). The family perspective for the future is that "life will return to normal". This phase is characterized by an "immersion" process in which the significant other frees the self from all other unnecessary commitments, takes on necessary roles of the patient, and symbiotically merges with the patient in terms of emotions and monitoring the patient's contact with the world.

INTERVENTION ISSUES IN THE WAITING STAGE

Assisting Patients. During the waiting period, interventions should focus primarily on supporting patients and their families, as well as monitoring patients for serious exacerbations of psychopathology. An acute adjustment disorder during the waiting period has been described which looks like organic brain syndrome (OBS) but is completely treatable by transplant and therefore must be distinguished from OBS (34). Helping the patient to understand how anxiety can increase physical symptoms is also helpful during this period.

Strong denial and other defenses against death, depression, and anger in transplant patients may cause resistance to looking at the implications of the illness and may thus prevent the "work of worrying" that could facilitate better post-transplant outcomes (66). However, it has been our experience and that of others that these defenses are an integral part of the coping process during this waiting period.

Therapy or counseling groups have proved helpful for some transplant patients and their families. Although there are not specific descriptions of transplant patients participating in these groups during the waiting period, it stands to reason that group support at this time could help by letting waiting patients obtain concrete medical information and share common experiences in an educational format (67). However, this needs to be approached with caution, since group experiences have sometimes been counterproductive to waiting patient's needs to maintain denial and to distance themselves from patients who may encounter medical problems.

During this period, family members who are "immersed" with the patient may be more interested in maintaining emotional stability than in realistically processing information about possible post-transplant complications and it appears that this preference should be respected as far as possible (65).

Staff Reactions. The waiting period can be utilized by staff for extended observation of patients' ability to manage themselves and comply, as behaviors under this stress may predict acting out behaviors at future stressful points in the transplant procedure (18). Although the patient has already been accepted for transplant and this evaluation is not necessarily part of the "selection" process, it may be useful in targeting high risk patients for special future intervention and support.

Most of the anxiety and depression that we have encountered in our waiting patients has responded to supportive psychotherapy and reassurance by the staff. However, a few patients have required antidepressant or anti-anxiety medication. In kidney transplant candidates who are on hemodialysis, the effects of the dialyzability of the particular drug must be considered. Drugs such as lithium, which are readily dialyzable, are not able to be maintained in sufficient levels to be effective. Medication of the heart transplant candidate without renal or liver insufficiency appears to be less complex, although certain antidepressant medications must be used cautiously with heart transplant patients during the pre-transplant period, as they may prolong intra-cardiac conduction times and possibly produce blocks.

During the waiting period, communication between medical staff and patient is critical, particularly because misperceptions about administrative matters such as priority on the transplant list can easily arise. Medical staff can also be particularly helpful in allaying guilt about such feelings as wishing for the death of a donor, be emphasizing that these are normal feelings (62). However, staff sometimes tend to avoid waiting patients during this stage, because they may feel helpless to assist the patient in any concrete way with the emotions of the period. They may have difficulty coping with the unanswerable questions about survival and they may be too personally affected by the fading optimism and sense of hopelessness which sometimes occurs during an extended wait. This can make the lack of communication and misunderstanding between staff and patient even worse (62).

STAGE IV. PERIOPERATIVE STAGE

The major goal during the perioperative period is survival from surgery, including management of immediate post-surgical medical complications. Psychosocially, this period has been noted to be "without a special adaptive task... as euphoria clouds other considerations" (pg. 110) (18). However, management of postoperative delirium or drug-induced psychosis may be required.

MEDICAL FACTORS IN THE PERIOPERATIVE STAGE

With one year survival hovering around 80% for all three of the major types of transplant (kidney, heart, and liver), there has been an increasing tendency to view these as viable therapeutic procedures. Furthermore, short term survival is not the pressing issue it was early in the history of transplantation. Survival statistics have greatly improved over the history of transplantation from the 1960s to the 1980s. Better techniques, increased experience, and better identification and management of tissue rejection and infection appear to be responsible for this improvement (68). In particular, the introduction of cyclosporine in the late 1970s had a dramatic effect on reducing rejection rates.

Statistics on kidney transplantation show that two year patient survival approximates 100% with living related donors and 84% with cadaver donors (69). However, some of these patients survive by returning to dialysis or being re-transplanted. Actual graft success is somewhat lower: 83 to 94% at one year for living related donors and 50 to 54% at one year for cadaver donors (69,70). These statistics tend to remain constant in the subsequent years following transplant because most acute rejection for kidney transplant occurs during the first year. Problems that arise in subsequent years are manageable by re-transplant or return to chronic hemodialysis. In general, the survival rate for kidney transplant patients appears much better than the primary alternative treatment, chronic hemodialysis.

Survival rates associated with heart transplant have increased dramatically since the introduction of cyclosporine around 1978 and with the improvement in transplant techniques during the past ten years. In 1968, only 22% of heart transplant patients survived one year while 23% survived less than one month (71). By 1986, approximately 79% of the patients survived one year and 77% survived five years (6). The use of cyclosporine continues to influence survival --one year survival is only about 66% in those current cases that are managed without cyclosporine, as opposed to 79% cited above (25). Survival rates associated with heart-lung transplant are approximately 54% at one year.

For liver transplants, one year survival ranges from approximately 68% to 80%. Prior to the introduction of cyclosporine, the one year survival rate using "conventional immunosuppression" (1963-1979) was only 32% (20).

PSYCHOSOCIAL FACTORS IN THE PERIOPERATIVE STAGE

The most common psychological reaction following transplant is euphoria at the "rebirth" aspects of the transplant and the second chance at life (38,60,72). For kidney transplant patients, the transplant comes as a welcome escape from the stresses and routines of chronic hemodialysis treatment. For liver and heart transplant patients, it is seen as a reprieve from certain death within a circumscribed time period.

Early in the history of heart transplant, there was a great deal of attention given to hypomanic reactions resulting from the steroid medications used for immunosuppression. A high incidence of postoperative psychosis (33%) was reported for the first nine heart transplants performed at Stanford in 1968. This was attributed in part to the steroid drug regimen (32). Less intense reactions were noted by others, including aberrant behavior associated with organic syndromes during the first month and when increased steroids were used to treat subsequent rejection episodes (42). One study showed that 7 of 83 heart transplant patients had "acute psychotic episodes, characterized by bizarre or inappropriate behavior, paranoid ideation and hallucinations" (pg. 686) (73). This was attributed to a combination of premorbid personality, situational stress, and corticosteroid medications.

Both euphoria and psychiatric distress immediately post-transplant have been attributed to steroid reactions (31,74,75). However, steroid-induced mental changes were more typical in the perioperative period before cyclosporine was used, when higher doses of steroids were necessary. More recently, better managed doses of immunosuppressant medication seem to result in fewer steroid reactions immediately after the operation. We found that about 18% of our heart transplant patients showed some impairment of orientation immediately following transplant, but none with obvious steroid-induced psychosis. Another recent study reported an organic mental disorder in 17 of 70 cardiac transplant patients, with 10 of these conforming to steroid-induced syndromes (50).

INTERVENTION ISSUES IN THE PERIOPERATIVE STAGE

Psychological issues are not of primary concern during this stage. However, patients should be monitored for signs of delirium, and appropriate measures should be taken as needed to aid in the management of steroids and the counteraction of steroid reactions. It has been noted that many steroid induced mental changes resolve themselves over time.

STAGE V. RECOVERY

A major focus of the recovery period is to teach the patient self care techniques related to medications, diet, weight, exercise, and infection control (13). The primary psychological task for the transplant recipient is to attain a normalized life in the face of stressful medical events such as biopsy, rejection management, and medication side effects.

MEDICAL FACTORS IN THE RECOVERY STAGE

As the euphoria of transplant begins to wear off, two inevitable medical processes begin to occur. One is the ongoing process of organ rejection which waxes and wanes but never totally subsides. The first biopsy is often a concrete reminder that cuts through the patient's euphoria and results in high levels of anxiety (15). Intervention to manage anxiety prior to scheduled biopsies is often indicated. Although patients are usually aware that rejection episodes of some magnitude are expected, the first substantial rejection episode often results in a significant reactive depression requiring intervention.

The second ongoing medical process is immunosuppression. Psychosocial side effects of the immunosuppression medication may include acute steroid psychosis as well as longer term medical complications such as increased risk of infection or carcinoma, and cosmetic side effects known as Cushing's Syndrome which is characterized by moon facies.

The increase in immunosuppressive medication which often accompanies rejection episodes can exacerbate steroid psychosis. One patient with a premorbid narcissistic personality disorder underwent treatment for rejection with increased steroids. He was apprehended trying to enter ICU to "heal" another transplant patient by "laying on hands" and likened himself to Jesus Christ in that both had been "sacrificed and returned from the dead". This abnormality resolved with haloperidol.

The more chronic medical and cosmetic side effects of immunosuppressive medication cause a considerable amount of concern among transplant patients and produce additional stress during the recovery period. Among the medical side effects are capillary fragility (bleeding), osteoporosis (fractures), glaucoma and cataracts, and increased risk of serious bacterial or viral infection or carcinoma. The major cosmetic side effects include Cushingoid symptoms ("moon facies") and acne. Although not a result of the immunosuppressant medication, children and adolescents with kidney transplant suffer additional cosmetic problems including orthopedic deformities, stunted growth, and delayed sexual maturation.

PSYCHOSOCIAL FACTORS IN THE RECOVERY STAGE

Recovery and long term convalescence have received the most attention in the literature concerning psychosocial adaptation to transplant. The recovery stage can be the beginning of the normalization process, at least when serious medical complications do not prevent this. For many patients, the psychological reactions caused by the medical condition begin to abate during this period and old coping styles can once again become effective. One patient with obsessive-compulsive personality traits was extremely irritable and demanding during the waiting period. This worsened with the length of the wait. Following transplant, he became very conscientious about his medical regimen and took pride in his cardiac rehabilitation accomplishments. He voiced much satisfaction over having more control and being able to actively contribute to his recovery. However, irritability and exacting demands continue to be problems when complications develop.

On the other hand, the recovery stage is also characterized by several unique stresses. The two major stressors associated with the post-transplantation period are fear of organ rejection and concern about side effects of immunosuppressant medication, including medical and cosmetic effects.

Fear of Graft Rejection. The chronic fear of graft rejection has a pervasive influence on all aspects of post-transplant life for both adults and children (21,52,53,60,76,77). The level of fear experienced may be directly related to the degree to which the patient has successfully psychologically incorporated the organ (72,78).

Patients go through three stages in the process of incorporating the transplanted organ. In the first, the "foreign body" stage, the organ feels alien, and the patient is preoccupied with its presence or can "feel" it inside, and may have fantasies or dreams about the organ falling out or being torn from the body. During this stage, the organ is truly not psychologically part of the person. One patient voiced concern over the possibility of his stitches coming loose and heart falling out. In the "partial incorporation" stage, the organ is experienced more as part of the body. Although it may still be referred to as a separate entity, during this stage the intense preoccupation with the organ as an alien object is lacking and the organ is only experienced as foreign when patients are reminded of the transplant. In the "total incorporation" stage, little thought is given to the organ as a separate part of the body and little time is spent in active concern about is viability or rejection possibility. By one year post-transplant, there appear to be few severe problems of psychological incorporation and over 80% of heart transplant patients report rarely or never thinking about the heart (79). However, a more subtle expression of awareness has been noted in that over half of kidney transplant patients report occasional comments/jokes about the kidney belonging to the family member who donated it (21).

Even when a patient has achieved a sense of total incorporation, certain medical complications or procedures such as symptoms associated with complications or rejection or the need for a routine biopsy can cause a regression to the stage of "foreign body" (72,78). This is consistent with our finding that about one-fourth to one-half of our heart transplant patients show depression, anxiety, or behavioral management problems at times of biopsy or graft rejection. There is a tendency for anxiety to be the most predominant symptom at biopsy and increases in depression are apparent with graft rejection (39). Despite overall good adjustment, one female patient showed periodic management problems and seriously increased irritability requiring medical management prior to scheduled biopsies.

These "regressive" phenomena are considered normal reactions in post-transplant development for several years, although it has been suggested that major problems with incorporation lasting beyond two years is aberrant (78). Much of the work on problems with psychological incorporation and fear of graft rejection has been done on kidney patients. However, it stands to reason that fear of graft rejection would be at least as severe and preoccupying for liver and heart transplant patients. For these patients, there is no interim alternative such as dialysis and immediate re-transplant would be the only possible life saving procedure in the event of serious organ rejection.

An additional problem associated with incomplete psychological incorporation concerns changed body image and abnormal identification with the organ donor (32,42,80). We have noted that almost one in three of our post-transplant patients exhibited pronounced curiosity about the characteristics of donors and the circumstances of their death. This type of phenomenon may not be as frequent in liver transplant patients, where only one child (of 14) and two adults (of 20) reported thoughts about the origin of the liver or its donor (40). A common concern involves gender differences, where patients have wondered about taking on the sexual characteristics of the donor, including feminization or renewed virility and sexuality (42). However, patients have anticipated acquiring many different types of traits through transplant, ranging from "generosity" to "foreign language ability" (72).

Immunosuppressant Medications. Immunosuppressant side effects are among the most salient problems for post-transplant patients. Only two of our operated patients experienced a steroid induced hypomanic reaction during the recovery period. However, other heart transplant centers have recently reported an 18% to 25% incidence of mental changes after cardiac transplantation, including acute delirium and psychosis. This usually occurred in the third to fifth week post-operatively, following the onset of increased immunosuppressive medication for rejection management (15,34,38). These reactions were not necessarily more common in those with previous psychiatric histories.

Although superficial and often time-limited, cosmetic problems due to immunosuppressant medications constitute very serious problems and often become the reason for non-compliance with the immunosuppressant regimen. Dissatisfaction with appearance appears to be a primary factor leading to poorer emotional and behavioral adjustment in children and adolescents, including problems with the medical regimen, problems with incorporation of the organ, and trouble coping with rejection (81). Emotional adjustment in adolescent kidney transplant patients was found to be significantly poorer when the effects of their disability and medication side effects were more "visible" (82).

Denial. Denial of feelings is a particularly common mechanism for coping in transplant patients. Denial concerning either the graft or the donor is particularly frequent in the recovery period, with up to 90% of heart transplant patients exhibiting this coping device during this period (63). It appears that denial plays an important protective and adaptive function, and is not to be automatically discouraged.

Family Concerns. Immediately following transplant when the patient begins to regain strength, significant others may be reinforced in their perception that life will return to normal and they may begin to move back toward independence from the patient. During this "passage" stage (65), the significant other may for the first time allow the full impact of the feelings held back prior to transplant. However, subsequent emergence of medical complications during this period causes a "crack" in the family's perception of life returning to normal and usually leads to an awareness of the need to "redesign the dream" for the future.

INTERVENTION ISSUES IN THE RECOVERY STAGE

Psychopharmacology. During the in-hospital recovery period, interventions may be needed to deal with psychiatric crises. Psychopharmacological treatment of transplant patients has been mentioned only briefly in the research literature. Cautions concerning the use of psychotropic drugs with transplant patients include: (1) the possibility that these will mask symptoms of a developing organic brain syndrome and (2) concern with residual renal insufficiency in kidney transplant patients (or additional renal insufficiency in other transplant patients) which may affect drug metabolism (4).

The use of neuroleptics, minor tranquilizers, and antidepressants has been recommended at usual doses as needed for most transplant patients. Concern has been raised about the use of some antidepressant medications with heart transplant patients due to potential adverse cardiac effects (54). However, it has recently been countered that "there are no contraindications to the use of antidepressants in heart transplant recipients" (pg. 143) because their hearts are usually well-functioning and, since they are denervated, vagal blockade and atrioventricular conduction effects are of no concern (83). We have also found that antidepressant medications used at regular doses can be safe and effective in treating depression in heart transplant patients.

The successful management of six renal transplant patients with affective psychosis by somatic therapy has been reported (84). The therapy included electroconvulsive treatment as well as the use of phenothiazines, tricyclic antidepressants, and lithium carbonate. These authors noted that these affective psychoses, which appeared to be related in part to the effects of steroid medications, could be rapidly and safely remitted with these therapies without reducing immunosuppressant dosages.

Psychotherapy. Both individual and group psychotherapy have been used to provide support for patients' emotional reactions and to assist in the management of behavioral problems, including noncompliance. Two types of individual psychotherapy for transplant patients have been discussed in the literature. The first involves more brief, time limited psychotherapy (counseling) that deals with current situational crises, does not attempt personality change, and may be carried out by medical staff rather than trained psychotherapists (85). The second, a more traditional approach, deals with personality dynamics as they relate to the medical transplant situation (86). The latter type may be suitable for patients experiencing more severe psychopathological reactions and/or having more serious preexisting psychopathology.

Brief Counseling. The major assumption underlying the use of brief psychotherapy is that many transplant patients do not need traditional psychotherapy or are not capable of benefitting from it. In support of this assumption, it appears that for kidney and heart transplant patients, post-transplant psychiatric problems are usually precipitated by medical crises or in response to medication side effects, and are not common or chronic in the absence of these complications (21,38,59,60,87). Thus, brief therapy which attempts to help patients through the mechanical aspects of their medical treatment, may be more relevant for most transplant patients than insight-oriented psychotherapy (72). This time-limited counseling often emphasizes the role of anxiety in exacerbating problematic symptoms (11) and may encourage catharsis in the over-anxious patient, along with support and structured advice. It can also provide structured help for problems with compliance (86) and can help patients to overcome intensive denial which may be hindering compliance. Brief counseling with family members during the recovery stage should allow for their emotional catharsis and assist them to deal with their growing awareness of potential medical complications and the probability that life will not return to "normal" (65).

Some types of brief psychotherapy which focus on relevant problems can be carried out by interested, friendly, and sensitive medical personnel without specific training in psychotherapy. This service plays an important role in a transplant unit where traditional psychotherapy is often not feasible (85). This type of treatment seems particularly appropriate for reactive depressions; it emphasizes a common sense approach to problem solving, support, and active intervention and may also include relaxation training, biofeedback, and/or psychopharmacology as appropriate.

Traditional Psychotherapy. Where a more traditional type of psychotherapy is indicated, a question arises concerning the patient's defenses against the medical condition. Specifically, should the individual be encouraged to confront the severity of his illness and concerns about death? Some writers emphasize that discussing possible impending death provides a common ground between therapist and patient and is a necessary early step in the psychotherapeutic process (88). However, others focus on the need for a moderate level of denial, which allows for some reactive depression and anxiety but prevents overwhelming levels of these (86). A moderate level of denial prevents the maladaptive effects of either highly intensive or insufficient denial. These have been described as follows: "Highly intensive denial results in a nearly total repudiation of the disease situation and the understanding of its treatment. In the case of insufficient denial, the patient tends to overly fear the disease and its treatment with the consequence of relapsing states of death anxieties and/or hopelessness" (pg. 257) (86). Either extreme results in problems with compliance or serious difficulties in the face of medical problems and complications. This view has been supported by recent findings of the prevalence and positive function of denial in heart transplant patients and the need for respecting this denial by avoiding probing or intrusive questions about feelings and reactions (34).

One case report illustrates the need for a combination of brief and traditional psychotherapy. Supportive interventions at different stages of transplant aided with mastery of immediate crises, while more in-depth psychotherapy helped integrate fantasies, anxieties, and personality structures with the trauma of the medical treatment (89). The case concerns the interaction of kidney failure and transplant with the already-existing pubertal conflicts of a 16 year old male adolescent. The body image problems often associated with transplant were intensified by the patient's delayed pubertal development, his enforced dependency on parents and hospital, and the physical changes induced by immunosuppressant medication. These factors resulted in high levels of anxiety in this adolescent for whom adaptation to the normal physical changes of puberty were not yet effectively consolidated. Pre-transplant emotional assessment did not predict these problems, although they are seen as a reaction to both the medical problems and the preexisting state.

Group Psychotherapy. Group psychotherapy for transplant patients promotes identification, acceptance, and cohesiveness as a result of sharing common medical conditions, but it may threaten the maintenance of denial that is so necessary to the coping of many patients (67,86). However, some specific benefits of a group experience for kidney transplant patients and their spouses have been observed. These include: (1) obtaining concrete medical information and sharing common experiences, which may calm anxieties that can develop in isolation; 92) symptomatic relief by safely ventilating negative emotions without directly confronting medical personnel; (3) modeling of independence for those who become "stuck" in the sick role, as well as concrete help in the social aspects of reintegrating into society and employment settings; and (4) feelings of hope from observing others successfully negotiate the post transplant course.

The educational nature of these groups is emphasized, with little focus on dynamic interpretation of patients' motivations or psychopathology. The recent explosion of the self help model for medical patients supports the effectiveness and acceptability of these educational meetings. The average medical patient has low motivation to talk with a psychiatrist and this type of group may be less threatening, while allowing for some reduction of denial concerning their illness. Information about the medical aspects of transplant can also decrease anxiety and depression.

Early reports with children undergoing dialysis or transplantation noted the spontaneous formation of a "mothers club" which provided a network of communication prior to the formal institution of a parents group (90). More recently, the benefit of self help groups have also been recognized for heart transplant patients and their family members (18,34).

A two-stage model has been proposed for groups of transplant patients where the first four meetings are primarily educational and are followed by 10 to 15 meetings during which more personal, psychological issues are discussed. For some patients, the first four meetings seem sufficient while for some, the second stage is necessary. Of course, there are patients who are too threatened by any exposure to benefit at all from meetings.

Consultation Functions. In addition to individual or group psychotherapy, the psychosocial team can fill several non-traditional functions on transplant units. These include informal inpatient visits, consultation with surgeons, and support for staff in their dealings with difficult patients (91). The primary medical staff should be involved in the "psychotherapeutic" activities and this function should not be "split off" for the mental health consultation liaison person. Many have proposed monthly service meetings for this purpose (86,91).

The psychosocial team assists medical staff to deal with the non-medical care of transplant patients by encouraging staff to ventilate their own feelings at depressed, angry, denying, manipulative, or acting-out patients as well as by helping them identify specific modalities to help the patients (91). It is particularly important for the psychosocial team to continue to remind the medical staff of the complex interactions between psychosocial and medical factors (34). Discussion of the patients' character structures and defenses and the symbolic meanings of certain dependent, regressive, or aggressive behaviors can often help to defuse overreactions or strong countertransferences on the part of the staff. In particular, the medical team should understand the meaning of the illness to the patient as well as the degree of threat and usual defensive styles utilized by the patient (4).

STAGE VI. POST DISCHARGE

The major task of the post-discharge period is the resumption of a normal life outside the hospital despite a significant chronic medical condition. This requires re-focusing on meaningful life activities and prior family roles, while also concentrating on maintaining physical health. Life normalization involves coping with the social (or media) attention attendant to the "transplant patient" role and overcoming the tendency to fall into sick role dependency behaviors.

For child and adolescent transplant recipients, family issues are particularly salient. Family issues to be dealt with include: (1) reintegration of the child and family; and (2) new dilemmas posed by the donor-patient relationship (often a parent-child relationship). Children who have spent a protracted period of time in the hospital may show a particular tendency to regress and successful reintegration with the family following discharge requires a reduction in the child's sick role behavior. Furthermore, the tendency toward continuing overprotectiveness by parents can impede successful adjustment and must be counteracted. For children or adolescents who have received a kidney from a parent, the dynamics involving parent-child "obligation" and "authority" issues may result in particularly serious conflict.

Becoming comfortable with long-term compliance to the medical regimen is a major issue for all transplant recipients. Finally, dealing with the deaths of other transplant patients increases stress significantly during this period (13).

MEDICAL FACTORS IN THE POST DISCHARGE STAGE

Medical Complications. The problem of moving from the sick role to a healthy role following discharge is exacerbated by continuing uncertain medical prognosis and especially the recurrence of specific medical problems. In particular, the need for re-hospitalization may raise acute anxiety and cause regression to the sick role. A number of our heart transplant patients experienced an increase in psychiatric symptoms at times of re-hospitalization for medical procedures.

Noncompliance. Compliance with the medical regimen following transplant is one of the most important variables affecting the long-term medical outcome of post transplant patients. The effects of noncompliance with medical regimen on survival and graft success are well-documented. One study of heart transplant patients showed that noncompliance in nine patients resulted in irreversible graft failure and death in eight, and reversible graft failure in the other one (33). Noncompliance was also reported to be a major factor in 7 of 27 deaths in 39 other patients. We have shown that of the heart transplant patients operated on during the first 24 months of our program, those who were designated as having poor medical outcome had a significantly higher rate of noncompliance than those with good medical outcome.

Although compliance is a critical determinant of medical outcome and survival, the degree to which patients comply depends extensively on psychosocial factors. There are numerous stressors associated with the medical regimen which cause patients to compromise the level of their compliance. The side effects of immunosuppression medication, especially cosmetic side effects, and the complexity of the regimen are among the primary impediments to adequate compliance. For child and adolescent kidney transplant patients, the cosmetic effects of the illness and immunosuppression medications are particularly salient, especially the Cushingoid symptoms, the lack of normal growth, and the lack of normal sexual maturation (52,53,76,81,92). There have been numerous reports of these patients discontinuing medications because of cosmetic side effects. In particular, a subset of female adolescent patients with relatively poorer psychological adjustment was found to be more noncompliant with the medical regimen (52,53). It was determined that their noncompliance was mostly due to cosmetic concern about the side effects of the immunosuppressant medication, but also included some adolescent rebellion and wish to deny the entire transplant process. We have not seen this among our mostly adult heart transplant patients, where most compromised compliance appears to stem from the complexity of the regimen and lack of tolerance for the frustrations associated with it.

PSYCHOSOCIAL FACTORS IN THE POST DISCHARGE STAGE

The long-term psychosocial adjustment of transplant patients can be summarized best under the term "quality of life." As long term survival becomes a more expected outcome of transplant, issues of quality of life become as important as length of life. Even where transplant is the only viable alternative to death, many consider that it is not a procedure for everyone and that issues of post-transplant quality of life should be an important consideration. Although physicians may be satisfied with "wound healing" after surgery, patients often evaluate success more in terms of their subjective feelings and their ability to carry out the routine tasks of everyday life (93).

Experience at the Stanford program showed that 97% of those who survived heart transplant for one year or more achieved NHYA Class I status and the majority returned to employment. All patients had Class IV status before transplant, with expected survival of less than 6 months. However, beyond medical status, there are still issues of quality of life, including potential psychiatric complications, family problems, sexual dysfunction, and financial and employment problems. the general term quality of life encompasses more than the mere absence of ill health or psychopathology, or even employment status. It includes the concept of long-term rehabilitation that enables the patient to opt for return to active employment or another activity of choice (94), as well as a more subjective evaluation by the individual as to the worthwhileness of existence (95). Recent endeavors to measure quality of life have taken a broad approach, including physical, occupational, social, family, and sexual satisfaction, rather than focusing on any one indicator of quality of life such as "return to work" (93,96).

Post-Transplant Psychiatric Disorder. Although the absence of psychiatric symptoms by itself is not a good indicator of quality of life, the presence of these can be a serious obstacle to good quality of life. Most authors find long-term psychological morbidity rates between 32% and 50% (36,38,60,97,98). We found that about 1 in 3 of our patients showed depression, anxiety or behavioral problems following discharge and that fully 1 in 5 experienced themselves as so different from others that this caused problems for them or hindered management. Some estimates of psychological problems in post-heart-transplant patients approach 100%, with one study reporting that all 28 patients who survived 3 months post-heart-transplant evidenced some psychological problems, including mood alterations, marital stress, family problems, and problems coping with chronic pain, changing body image, compliance, impotency, and decreased libido (16). In addition to depression and anxiety, liver transplant patients are particularly prone to organic brain syndrome post transplant (44). Although the rates of psychopathology in transplant patients appear higher than normal, these symptoms are often specific to time periods when the patient is particularly ill or undergoing graft rejection (21,36,60).

For children and adolescents receiving kidney transplants, there are mixed findings about long term psychiatric status. On the one hand, these children were found to score within the normal range on most subscales of the California Test of Personality one year following transplant, with somewhat more negative scores on scales of social adjustment, anxiety, and self esteem. Also, despite the apparent potential for family problems, family equilibrium appeared relatively normal for most in the absence of overwhelming medical problems (52,53,99). On the other hand, some children showed depression and problems dealing with parental overprotectiveness, donor-recipient conflicts, difficulties with non-affected siblings, unrealistic expectations of the transplant, and, especially in adolescents, acting out behaviors (12,81,99). One study estimated that perhaps 10% of children and adolescents manifest severe behavioral or emotional reactions (81).

Overall, most behavior disorders, noncompliance, diagnosable emotional maladjustment, trouble adjusting to peer relationships, and trouble coping with graft failure occurred in adolescents over 12 years of age while children under 12 years of age appeared to be free from behavior disorders (52,53,81,99). Most adverse psychological reactions among adolescents also appear to be associated with a medical crisis or complication (76,81).

One study of longer term adjustment in adolescent kidney transplant patients (2 to 10 years later) showed somewhat more negative results, with significant problems adjusting to school or job and in establishing heterosexual relationships (92). These authors also found that about half of these patients had made some kind of depressive statement and two of eighteen had made a suicide attempt. The majority of those old enough did not get a drivers license, reflecting their "blunted drive toward autonomy". In this longer term follow-up, extreme emotional dependence on the family was noted, especially within the symbiotic-like relationship between donor and recipient. This study showed that those adolescents who fared most poorly were those with poorer health, lower intelligence, and depressive symptoms interfering with adjustment.

Suicidal behavior occurs in about 0.5% of kidney transplant patients (21). Although higher than normal, suicidal behavior appears to be most prevalent in kidney transplant patients who have diabetes and therefore more physical problems than non-diabetics (21), and in patients who must return to renal dialysis following graft failure (98). It has also been noted that among kidney transplant patients, suicidal behavior is more prevalent in adolescents than either children or adults (21).

It should be noted that all psychiatric complications suffered during the post-discharge period are not necessarily caused by the transplant procedure itself. When symptoms experienced in reaction to medical complications are discounted, the percentage of psychiatric disorder in these patients may be no higher than that found in groups of other medical patients (87).

Finally, despite higher than average reported psychopathology in transplant patients, psychological testing showed that kidney and heart transplant patients improved in psychological health following transplant, with increased happiness and self esteem, and decreased anxiety and depression (21,50). However, even by one year post-transplant, MMPI profiles were not improved to the level of a control group (21).

Quality of Life. Moving beyond the specific category of psychiatric disorder leads to a consideration of the more general indicators of quality of life. These tend to fall into two categories: subjective quality of life including social and emotional well-being, and objective quality of life, most often reflected by physical status, vocational rehabilitation, and employment status (return to work). Quality of life in these two areas tend to be positively correlated, but the low correlations show that they tend to measure two separate aspects of the post transplant experience (100).

Subjective Quality of Life. Despite some early reports of poor subjective quality of life following kidney transplant (77,95), more recent reviews show that most transplant patients consider their post-transplant quality of life good (31,58,79,94). Approximately 82% to 91% of heart transplant patients reported a good quality of life an average of three and a half years post-transplant, and 95% of patients in one study answered that they would again have a heart transplant in similar circumstances (79). Heart transplant patients reported positive life changes in future outlook, feelings about self, social support, sense of achievement, decision making, sense of independence, and relationships with family, friends, and work associates (79). Negative life changes were reported by a minority (26%) in the areas of financial situation, physical appearance, and sexual functioning. Quality of life was poorer in patients who reported these negative life changes (79).

Kidney transplant patients have generally rated their physical, emotional, and social well-being, and life satisfaction and general affect significantly more favorably than their renal dialysis counterparts (21,100,101). Furthermore, they rate these as significantly improved over their own well-being when on renal dialysis (102,103). One study found that heart transplant patients had levels of subjective well being similar to that of kidney transplant patients and to a general population (104). Furthermore, kidney transplant patients had scores on subjective quality of life measures that were not significantly different from norms for the U.S. population from 1976 to 1978 (100). For these patients, subjective quality of life was not significantly affected by poor physical health (100).

Objective Quality of Life. Objective indicators of quality of life tend to focus on physical status, vocational rehabilitation, and return to work. All domains of self-perceived physical status, including restrictions caused by illness and physical mobility, appear to be improved by three months post-heart-transplant and this improvement is maintained at twelve months post-transplant (93,96,105). Furthermore, most of these physical ratings were equivalent to those of a normal population (93).

Rehabilitation success in transplant patients generally refers to employment, school, housework, or satisfaction with daily pursuits. A recent review showed that the occupational aspect of quality of life was generally improved following kidney transplant, and that up to 88% of non-diabetic patients were back to work or housework unless significant medical problems interfered (21,106). Furthermore, labor force participation rate for transplant patients was not far off national norms: 53.5%, compared to a 1981 statistic of 63.8% (100). whereas additional medical problems tended not to impact subjective quality of life, the presence of additional medical problems did have a significant impact on functional impairment and patients' ability to work.

Similar to the findings on kidney transplant patients, between 56% and 85% of heart transplant patients are able to resume normal life activities and return to work (4,13,94,96,105). For many, participation in fund-raising activities, hobbies, or sports was an acceptable alternative to paid employment. For some post-transplant patients, disability payments prevent return to full time employment (13).

In general, rehabilitation following transplant was found to be much better than that achieved with chronic hemodialysis. One study found that both heart and kidney transplant recipients had less functional impairment than hemodialysis patients and reported that they were more able to work, even with differing sociodemographic characteristics accounted for (104,107). Specifically, it appears that up to 74% to 83% of the transplant patients are working or in school compared to only 30% to 46% of dialysis patients (101). Kidney transplant recipients were somewhat more functional than heart transplant recipients in this study (104).

Children undergoing kidney transplantation appear to achieve good rehabilitation at one year post transplant, with at least average school participation and performance and a quite acceptable quality of life (52,53,81,99). However, long-term adjustment to school or work is more questionable (92). Exclusion from normal school and social activities for children appears to exacerbate any adjustment problems that children may be experiencing in this area (108).

Sexual Functioning. The level of sexual functioning can be an important indicator of medical adjustment as well as both subjective and objective quality of life. Sexual function is specifically emphasized in the kidney disease literature and deserves special attention here because it is so clearly related to both physical and psychological status. Sexual difficulties in kidney transplant patients are relatively prevalent in the post-transplant period, although not as severe as during hemodialysis (109). Frequency of intercourse, reduced potency, and reduced sexual interest during dialysis are improved following transplant, with younger patients and males having the better prognosis (109,110,111). For women, sexual problems are also prevalent during dialysis, but improvement following transplant is not as predictable. Some reports indicate that frequency of intercourse and sexual interest remain decreased following transplant for women (109,111), while one study specifically indicates that there is increased sexual satisfaction and frequency of intercourse following transplant for females, especially younger females (103).

Improvement in sexual functioning following kidney transplant is substantial, with 35% to 40% of male and female patients reporting increases in sexual activity. However, there still remains a significant level of impairment, with 20% to 22% of male and female patients reporting further decreases in sexual activity following transplant, and 43% to 52% of male patients considering themselves partially or totally impotent even after transplant (21,112). Sexual problems in these patients may be the result of physical problems such as physiological effects of uremia, hypertension medications, or hormonal imbalances. However, a number of psychological factors can also have a profound impact on sexual functioning. These include: demoralization, depression, and a reversal of family roles (109). We found no research to date on the effects of heart or liver transplant on sexual functioning.

Family Issues. Dynamic issues between patients and partners emerge during the post-transplant period, focusing on their sometimes conflicting goals. Patients may emphasize the present, wanting to withdraw from normal work activities and interrupt ongoing family processes to enjoy life's pleasures and spend their remaining time in close contact with their spouses. At the same time, spouses may need to focus on future security and survival, requiring movement toward independence and continuance of family processes (65).

INTERVENTION ISSUES IN THE POST DISCHARGE STAGE

Psychopathology. Treatment during this long term recovery period must deal with the manifestations of pre-existing psychopathology that occur following transplant. In particular, flareups in psychiatric conditions are expected around periods of stress that relate to exacerbations in medical complications, including biopsy, rejection, re-hospitalization, or severe effects of immunosuppression. Reactive anxiety may be treated behaviorally through relaxation techniques, cognitive behavioral techniques, or even biofeedback. Reactive depression may best be affected by cognitive behavioral techniques. Both types of symptoms may be affected by appropriate psychopharmacology. More severe psychopathology, including preexisting personality disorder, may need intervention primarily when it affects the management of the medical condition. In particular, psychopathology which affects the ability of the patient to comply with the medical regimen must be treated to ensure optimal medical outcome.

Compliance. Even where psychopathology is not a factor, it may be important for the psychosocial team to assist patients and their families in optimizing strategies for compliance with the relatively complicated medical regimen. The behavioral literature contains examples of strategies which have been successfully used to improve compliance in heart and surgical patients, as well as chronic illness patients.

Rehabilitation. When counseling for vocational rehabilitation, it should be kept in mind that for many transplant patients, active formal employment is not the goal. Sometimes disability payments preclude employment above a certain level under penalty of losing benefits. Sometimes, post-transplant patients reassess their priorities in light of shortened expected lifespan, with work taking a back seat to more interpersonal and family concerns. However, where active employment is the goal and issues such as dependency or "sick role" issues interfere, these may be dealt with in short-term counseling using relatively structured techniques, including behavioral and cognitive behavioral strategies.

Social rehabilitation focuses on relationships with others and may help the patient to give up the "transplant patient" status in order to enjoy more normalized relationships with others. This applies to a broad range of friends and acquaintances, but may be most important within the family. Within the family, the patient may need to be encouraged to resume former roles and give up sick role behaviors such as dependency, regressiveness, and "specialness". Sometimes, conjoint counseling may be an important adjunct to treatment and may be particularly important in helping patients and spouses negotiate their new roles vis-a-vis each other. Following discharge, one of our patients at first enjoyed the attention of friends and media, then temporarily became dysphoric. His greatly increased energy level and renewed interest in activities posed a problem for his wife, but this improved with individual and conjoint counseling. It took him and his wife about a year for the situation to normalize. He remains very involved in the transplant center as a volunteer peer counselor. Family counseling may be especially important with child or adolescent patients to facilitate family integration following discharge and to address parent-child relationship issues including overprotectiveness and donor-donee conflicts where applicable.

Sexual Dysfunction. Counseling with respect to sexual dysfunction in post-transplant patients should focus on encouraging patients to engage in sexual activity as soon as the surgical site is healed, as determined by the surgeon. Kidney transplant patients should be informed that it is probable that they will have improved sexual function compared with their time on dialysis. However, it should also be expected that some male transplant patients will continue to experience impotence, as well as continued diminished sexual interest. For female transplant patients, diminished interest in sexual activities or decreased sexual response may be more prevalent. Where there are sexual problems, consideration must be given to possible organic bases for these problems, including physical and pharmacological factors (112). Although little specific information is available concerning sexual functioning in heart transplant patients, it is suggested that individualized assessment of sexual problems will lead to similar proposed treatments for heart transplant patients with sexual problems, as follows.

In lieu of long-term psychotherapy aimed at discovering the origins of sexual difficulties, it is recommended that where sexual problems appear to be the result of depression or anxiety, treatment include appropriate medication or psychotherapy aimed at alleviating the depression or anxiety. Sometimes the long-term nature of the illness, the chronic run-down feelings, the loss of self-image (including masculinity or femininity), and shifts in the husband/wife roles that sometimes accompany the chronic illness may be at the root of sexual problems quite independently of depression. Where these factors appear important, general counseling with respect to quality of life issues may be conducted and may optimally include the spouse in the intervention. Where sexual problems have originated in one of these situations and continue to be maintained through such mechanisms as emotional distance between partners or performance anxiety, behavioral treatment of sexual dysfunction may be beneficial. (See Chapter 16)

CONCLUSIONS

Transplant patients go through a predictable pattern of psychological adjustment in response to transplant procedures. They go through a progression of stages which have unique, identifiable characteristics. A psychosocial team is required as a part of the larger transplant team in order to ensure a smooth medical and psychological course. During the transplant proposal stage, initial psychological reactions of the patient must be dealt with to ensure adequate decision-making and informed consent. Selection of appropriate transplant patients during the evaluation stage should consider the deleterious effects of severe psychiatric disorder, especially serious depression, psychosis, or personality disorder, significant family dysfunction or cognitive impairment, and potential for compliance problems. It should be further noted that personality disorder and chronic substance abuse appear to carry much stronger implications as obstacles to transplant than reactive symptoms of anxiety or depression (adjustment disorders).

The period of waiting for the donor organ appears to be a particularly stressful stage in the transplant protocol, requiring much support for the patient and family from the psychosocial team. A major issue during the perioperative period continues to be steroid-induced mental changes. Although there is some indication that these symptoms have decreased in recent years due to changes in the medication regimen, they still remain a problem requiring management, especially during more aggressive immunosuppressive treatment. During the recovery and post-discharge periods, psychological reactions to medical complications, biopsy procedures, and rejection episodes may need intervention. Patients may also need occasional assistance or intervention around compliance issues, as these often continue to be problematic due to the complexity of the medical regimen and th discomfort of the medication side effects. Following discharge, transplant patients can generally expect good long-term rehabilitation and quality of life in the absence of severe medical complications.

There are several issues that are common to the various stages of transplantation. Denial is a frequent and, to some extent, adaptive coping mechanism in transplant patients during all stages and should not be discouraged unless it interferes with decision-making or compliance. When rendering psychosocial services, it is important to consider the patient's pre-existing personality style and how it may exert itself at the various stages of the transplant protocol. When psychotherapeutic services are necessary, they may be most effectively and efficiently delivered through a brief psychotherapy model rather than a traditional psychotherapy model for most transplant patients. Finally, in addition to direct patient services, the psychosocial team should provide consultation to the larger transplant team to facilitate their understanding of these psychosocial issues.

REFERENCES

1. Merrill, J.P.; Murray, J.E.; Takacs, F.J.; et al. Successful transplantation of a human cadaver kidney. JAMA 185:347-353, 1963.

2. Starzl, T.E.; Groth, C.G., Brettschneider, L., et al. Orthotopic homotransplantation of the human liver. Ann Surg 168:392-415, 1968.

3. Barnard, C.N. Human heart transplantation. S Afr Med J 41:1271-1274, 1967.

4. Lesko, L.M.; Hawkins, D.R. Psychological aspects of transplantation medicine. New Psychiatric Syndromes - DSM-III and Beyond, Jason Aronson, Inc., New York, pp. 265-309, 1983.

5. Bentley, F.R.; Garrison, R.N. Organ donation in Kentucky. J Ky Med Assoc 86:243-245, 1988.

6. Solis, E.; Kaye, M.P. The Registry of the International Society for Heart Transplantation - Third official report - June 1986. J Heart Transplant 5:2-5, 1986.

7. Cascells, W. Heart transplantation - Recent policy developments. N Engl J Med 315:1365-1368, 1986.

8. Gil, G. Medicare to pay for heart transplants at Jewish - Hospital one of 18 on list, enhancing future of program. The Courier-Journal, Louisville, Kentucky, pp 1A, April 12, 1988.

9. Starzl, T.E.; Iwatsuki, S.; Shaw, B.W.; et al. Orthotopic liver transplantation in 1984. Transplant Proc, 17:250-258, 1985.

10. Boly, W. The chosen. Hippocrates 2:42-53, 1988.

11. Cramond, W.A.; Knight, P.R.; Lawrence, J.R. The psychiatric contribution to a renal unit undertaking chronic hemodialysis

and renal homotransplantation. Br J Psychiatry 113:1201-1212, 1967.

12. Kemph, J. Psychotherapy with donors and recipients of kidney transplants. Semin Psychiatry 3:145-158, 1971.

13. Christopherson, L.K.; Griepp, R.B.; Stinson, E.B. Rehabilitation after cardiac transplantation. JAMA 236:2082-2084, 1976.

14. Allender, J.; Shisslak, C.; Kaszniak, A.; et al. Stages of psychological adjustment associated with heart transplantation. J Heart Transplant 2:228-231, 1983.

15. Watts, D.; Freeman, A.M.; McGiffin, D.G.; et al. Psychiatric aspects of cardiac transplantation. J Heart Transplant 3:243-247, 1984.

16. McAleer, M.J.; Copeland, J.; Fuller, J.; et al. Psychological aspects of heart transplantation. J Heart Transplant 4:232-233, 1985.

17. O'Brien, V.C. Psychological and social aspects of heart transplantation. J Heart Transplant 4:229-231, 1985.

18. Kuhn, W.F.; Davis, M.H.; Lippmann, S.B. Emotional adjustment to cardiac transplantation. Gen Hosp Psychiatry 10:108-113, 1988.

19. Cummings, N.B.; Klahr, S. Chronic Renal Disease, Plenum Medical Book Co., New York, pp v-vii, 1985.

20. Busuttil, R.W. Liver transplantation today. Ann Intern Med, 104:377-389, 1986.

21. Simmons, R.G.; Klein, S.D.; Simmons, R.L. Rehabilitation and social-psychological adjustment of the post-transplant patient. Gift of Life - The Social and Psychological Impact of Organ Transplantation, John Wiley and Sons, New York, pp 45-88, 1977.

22. Gulledge, A.D.; Buszta, C.; Montague, D.K. Psychosocial aspects of renal transplantation. Urol Clin North Am 10:327-335, 1983.

23. Evans, R.W. The socioeconomics of organ transplantation. Transplant Proc 17:129-136, 1985.

24. Abram, H.S.; Wadlington, W. Selection of patients for artificial and transplanted organs. Ann Intern Med 69:615-620, 1968.

25. Kaye, M.P.; Elcombe, S.A.; O'Fallon, W.M. The International Heart Transplant Registry - The 1984 Report. J Heart Transplant 4:290-292, 1985.

26. MacDougall, B.R.; Williams, R. Indications and assessment for orthotopic liver transplantation. Liver Transplantation - The Cambridge-King's College Hospital Experience, Grune & Stratton, New York, pp 59-66, 1983.

27. Annas, G.J. The prostitute, the playboy, and the poet - Rationing schemes for organ transplantation. Am J Public Health 75:187-189, 1985.

28. Iglehart, J.K. Transplantation - The problem of limited resources. N Engl J Med 309:123-128, 1983.

29. Evans, R.W.; Manninen, D.L.; Garrison, L.P., et al. Donor availability as the primary determinant of the future of heart transplantation. JAMA 255:1892-1898, 1986.

30. Baumgartner, W.A.; Reitz, B.A.; Oyer, P.E.; et al. Cardiac homotransplantation. Curr Probl Surg 16(9):1-61, 1979.

31. Christopherson, L.K. Cardiac transplant - Preparation for dying or for living. Health and Social Work 1:58-72, 1976.

32. Lunde, D.T. Psychiatric complications of heart transplants. Am J Psychiatry 126:369-373, 1969.

33. Cooper, D.K.C.; Lanza, R.P.; Barnard, C.N. Noncompliance in heart transplant recipients - The Cape Twon Experience. J Heart Transplant 3:248-253, 1984.

34. Mai, F.M. Liaison psychiatry in the heart transplant unit. Psychosomatics 28:44-46, 1987.

35. Christopherson, L.K.; Lunde, D.T. Selection of cardiac transplant recipients and their subsequent psychosocial adjustment. Semin Psychiatry 3:36-45, 1971.

36. Penn, I.; Bunch, D.; Olenik, D.; et al. Psychiatric experience with patients receiving renal and hepatic transplants. Semin Psychiatry 3:133-144, 1971.

37. Freeman, A.M.; Watts, D.; Karp, R. Evaluation of cardiac transplant candidates: Preliminary observations. Psychosomatics 25:197-207, 1984.

38. Mai, F.M.; McKenzie, F.N.; Kostuk, W.J. Psychiatric aspects of heart transplantation - Preoperative evaluation and postoperative sequelae. Br Med J 292:311-313, 1986.

39. Kuhn, W.F.; Myers, B.; Brennan, A.F.; et al. Psychopathology in cardiac transplantation. J Heart Transplant 7:223-226, 1988.

40. House, R.; Dubovsky, S.L.; Penn, I. Psychiatric aspects of hepatic transplantation. Transplantation 36:146-150, 1983.

41. Kemph, J.P.; Bermann, E.A.; Coppolillo, H.P. Kidney transplant and shifts in family dynamics. Am J Psychiatry 125:1485-1490, 1969.

42. Kraft, I.A. Psychiatric complications of cardiac transplantation. Semin psychiatry 3:58-79, 1971.

43. Norvell, N.; Hecker, J.; Hills, H. Psychological and cognitive

assessment of candidates for heart transplantation. Presented
at the 94th annual meeting of the American Psychological
Association, Washington, D.C., 1986.

44. Surman, O.S.; Dienstag, J.L.; Cosimi, A.B.; et al. Liver
transplantation - Psychiatric considerations. Psychosomatics,
28:615-621, 1987.

45. Eisendrath, R.M. The role of grief and fear in the death of
kidney transplant patients. Am J Psychiatry 126:381-387, 1969.

46. Viederman, M. Psychogenic factors in kidney transplant rejection
Am J Psychiatry 132:957-959, 1975.

47. Ford, C.V.; Castelnuovo-Tedesco, P. Hemodialysis and renal
transplantation - Psychopathological reactions and their
management. Psychosomatic Medicine - Its Clinical Applications,
Harper & Row, Hagerstown, Md., pp 74-83, 1977.

48. Steinberg, J.; Levy, N.B.; Radvila, A. Psychological factors
affecting acceptance or rejection of kidney transplants.
Psychonephrology I - psychological Factors in Hemodialysis and
Transplantation, Plenum Medical Book Co., New York, pp 185-193,
1981.

49. Goldman, L.S.; Kimball, C.P. Psychiatric aspects of cardiac
surgery - A review. Cardiovascular Reviews and Reports, 6:1023-
1034, 1985.

50. Freeman, A.M.; Folks, D.G.; Sokol, R.S.; et al. Cardiac
transplantation - Clinical correlates of psychiatric outcome.
Psychosomatics, 29:47-54, 1988.

51. Yanagida, E.H.; Streltzer, J. Limitations of psychological
tests in a dialysis population. Psychosom Med, 41:557-567, 1979.

52. Fine, R.N.; Malekzadeh, M.H.; Pennisi, A.J.; et al. Long-term results of renal transplantation in children. Pediatrics, 61: 641-650, 1978.

53. Korsch, B.M.; Fine, F.N.; Negrete, V.F. Noncompliance in children with renal transplants. Pediatrics 61:872-876, 1978.

54. Frierson, R.L.; Lippmann, S.B. Heart transplant candidates rejected on psychiatric indications. Psychosomatics 28:347-355, 1987.

55. Kaplan de Nour, K.A.; Czaczkes, J.W. The influence of patient's personality on adjustment to chronic dialysis. J Nerv Ment Dis 162:323-333, 1976.

56. Lee, H.K. Psychiatric factors and non-compliant behavior in hemodialysis. Dial Transplant 6:1236-1241, 1978.

57. Yanagida, E.H.; Streltzer, J.; Siemsen, A. Denial in dialysis patients - Relationship to compliance and other variables. Psychosom Med 43:271-280, 1981.

58. Brennan, A.F.; Davis, M.H.; Buchholz, D.J.; et al. Predictors of quality of life following cardiac transplantation. Psychosomatics 28:566-571, 1987.

59. Ferris, G.N. Psychiatric considerations in patients receiving cadaveric renal transplants. South Med J 62:1482-1484, 1969.

60. Abram, H.S.; Buchanan, D.C. The gift of life - A review of the psychological aspects of kidney transplantation. Int J Psychiatry Med 7:153-164, 1976-77.

61. Simmons, R.G.; Klein, S.D.; Simmons, R.L. Gift of Life - The Social and Psychological Impact of Organ Transplantation, John Wiley and Sons, New York, 1977.

62. Levenson, J.L.; Olbrisch, M.E. Shortage of donor organs and long waits. Psychosomatics 28:399-402, 1987.

63. Mai, F.M. Graft and donor denial in heart transplant recipients. Am J Psychiatry 143:1159-1161, 1986.

64. Kraft, I.A.; Vick, J. the transplantation milieu, St. Luke's Episcopal Hospital, 1968-1969. Semin Psychiatry 3:17-23, 1971.

65. Mishel, M.H.; Murdaugh, C.L. Family adjustment to heart transplantation - Redesigning the dream. Nurs Res 36:332-338, 1987.

66. Greenberg, R.P.; Davis, G.; Massey, R. The psychological evaluation of patients for a kidney transplant and hemodialysis program. Am J Psychiatry 130:274-277, 1973.

67. Buchanan, D.C. Group therapy for kidney transplant patients. Int J psychiatry Med 6:523-531, 1975.

68. Jamieson, S.W.; Stinson, E.B; Shumway, N.E. Cardiac transplantation in 150 patients at Stanford University. Br Med J January:93-95, 1979.

69. Salvatierra, O.; Feduska, N.H.; Vincenti, F.; et al. Analysis of costs and outcomes of renal transplantation at one center. JAMA 241:1469-1473, 1979.

70. Tilney, N.L.; Strom, T.B.; Vineyard, G.C.; et al. Factors contributing to the declining mortality rate in renal transplantation. N Engl J Med 299:1321-1325, 1978.

71. Molisch, H.B.; Kraft, I.A.; Wiggins, P.Y. Psychodiagnostic evaluation of the heart transplant patient. Semin Psychiatry 3:46-57, 1971.

72. Castelnuovo-Tedesco, P. Transplantation - Psychological

implications of changes in body image. Psychonephrology I - Psychological Factors in Hemodialysis and Transplantation. Plenum Medical Book Co., New York, 1981.

73. Hotson, J.R.; Pedley, T.A. The neurological complications of cardiac transplantation. Brain 99:673-694, 1976.

74. MacDonald, D.J. Psychotic reactions during organ transplantation Can psychiatric Assoc J 17:SS15-SS17, 1972.

75. Wilson, W.P.; Stickel, D.L.; Hayes, C.P.; et al. Psychiatric considerations of renal transplantation. Arch Intern Med 122:502-506, 1968.

76. Bernstein, D.M. After transplantation - The child's emotional reactions. Am J Psychiatry 127:1189-1193, 1971.

77. Calland, C.H. Iatrogenic problems in end-stage renal failure. N Engl J Med August:334-336, 1972.

78. Muslin, H.L. On acquiring a kidney. Am J Psychiatry 127: 1185-1188, 1971.

79. Lough, M.E.; Lindsey, A.M.; Shinn, J.A.; et al. Life satisfaction following heart transplantation. J Heart Transplant 4:446-449, 1985.

80. Castelnuovo-Tedesco, P. Ego vicissitudes in response to replacement or loss of body parts - Certain analogies to events during psychoanalytic treatment. Psychoanal Q 47:381-397, 1978.

81. Bernstein, D.M. Psychiatric assessment of the adjustment of transplanted children. Gift of Life - The Social and Psychological Impact of Organ Transplantation, John Wiley and Sons, New York, pp 119-147, 1977.

82. Beck, A.L.; Nethercut, G.E.; Crittenden, M.R.; et al. Visibility of handicap, self-concept, and social maturity among young adult survivors of end-stage renal disease. J Dev Behav Pediatr 7:93-96, 1986.

83. Kay, J. Psychiatric qualifiers for heart transplant candidates. Psychosomatics 29:143-144, 1988.

84. Blazer, D.G.; Petrie, W.M.; Wilson, W.P. Affective psychoses following renal transplant. Dis Nerv Syst 37:663-667, 1976.

85. Buchanan, D.C. Psychotherapeutic intervention in the kidney transplant service. Psychonephrology I - Psychological Factors in hemodialysis and Transplantation, Plenum Medical Book Co., New York, 1981.

86. Freyberger, H. Consultation-liaison in a renal transplant unit. Psychonephrology I - Psychological Factors in Hemodialysis and Transplantation. Plenum Medical Book Co., New York, pp 255-263, 1981.

87. Fine, R.N.; Korsch, B.M. Renal transplantation in children. Hosp Pract 9:61-69, 1974.

88. Kemph, J.P. Psychotherapy with patients receiving kidney transplant. Am J Psychiatry 124:623-629, 1967.

89. Drotar, D. The treatment of a severe anxiety reaction in an adolescent boy following renal transplantation. J Am Acad Child Psychiatry 14:451-461, 1975.

90. Korsch, B.M.; Fine, R.N.; Grushkin, C.M.; et al. Experiences with children and their families during extended hemodialysis and kidney transplantation. Pediatr Clin North Am 18:625-637, 1971.

91. Eisendrath, R.M.; Topor, M.; Misfeldt, C.; et al. Service
     meetings in a renal transplant unit - An unused adjunct to total
     patient care. Int J Psychiatry Med 1:53-58, 1970.

92. Poznanski, E.O.; Miller, E.; Salguero, C.; et al. Quality of
     life for long-term survivors of end-stage renal disease. JAMA
     239:2343-2347, 1978.

93. Hunt, S.M. Quality of life considerations in cardiac
     transplantation. Quality of Life and Cardiovascular Care,
     September/October:308-312,316, 1985.

94. Pennock, J.L.; Oyer, P.E.; Reitz, B.A.; et al. Cardiac
     transplantation in perspective for the future. J Thorac
     Cardiovasc Surg 83:168-177, 1982.

95. Beard, B.H. The quality of life before and after renal
     transplantation. Dis Nerv Syst 32:24-31, 1971.

96. Wallwork, J.; Caine, N. A comparison of the quality of life of
     cardiac transplant patients and coronary artery bypass graft
     patients before and after surgery. Quality of Life and
     Cardiovascular Care, September/October:317-331, 1985.

97. Kalman, T.P.; Wilson, P.G.; Kalman, C.M. Psychiatric morbidity
     in long-term renal transplant recipients and patients undergoing
     hemodialysis - A comparative study. JAMA 250:55-58, 1983.

98. Stewart, R.S. Psychiatric issues in renal dialysis and
     transplantation. Hosp Community Psychiatry 34:623-628, 1983.

99. Lilly, J.R.; Giles, G.; Hurwitz, R.; et al. Renal
     homotransplantation in pediatric patients. Pediatrics 47:548-
     557, 1971.

100. Evans, R.W.; Manninen, D.L.; Garrison, L.P., et al. The quality of life of patients with end-stage renal disease. N Engl J Med February:553-559, 1985.

101. Simmons, R.G.; Anderson, C.R.; Kamstra, L.K.; et al. Quality of life and alternate end-stage renal disease therapies. Transplant Proc 17:1577-1578, 1985.

102. Sophie, L.R.; Powers, M.J. Life satisfaction and social function - Post-transplant self-evaluation. Dial Transplant 8:1198-1202, 1979.

103. Webb, S.M.; Powers, M.J. Evaluation of life satisfaction and sexual function in female patients post renal transplant. Dial Transplant 11:799-804, 1982.

104. Evans, R.W.; Manninen, D.L.; Maier, A.; et al. The quality of life of kidney and heart transplant recipients. Transplant Proc 17:1579-1582, 1985.

105. Baldwin, J.C.; Stinson, E.B. Quality of life after cardiac transplantation. Quality of Life and Cardiovascular Care September/October:332-335, 1985.

106. Taber, S.M.; Lee, H.A.; Slapak, M. A rehabilitation assessment of renal transplantees. Nephrology Nurse September/October:9-14, 1982.

107. Kaplan de Nour, A.; Shanan, J. Quality of life of dialysis and transplanted patients. Nephron 25:117-120, 1980.

108. Khan, A.U.; Herndon, C.H.; Ahmadian, S.Y. Social and emotional adaptations of children with transplanted kidneys and chronic hemodialysis. Am J Psychiatry 127:1194-1198, 1971.

109. Levy, N.B. What's new on cause and treatment of sexual

dysfunctions in end-stage renal disease. Psychonephrology I - Psychological Factors in Hemodialysis and Transplantation. Plenum Medical book Co., New York, pp 43-47, 1981.

110. Abram, H.S.; Hester, L.R.; Sheridan, W.F.; et al. Sexual functioning in patients with chronic renal failure. J Nerv Ment Dis 160:220-226, 1975.

111. Procci, W.R.; Hoffman, K.I.; Chatterjee, S.N. Sexual functioning of renal transplant recipients. J Nerv Ment Dis 166:402-407, 1978.

112. Levy, N.B. Sex and Intimacy for Dialysis and Transplant Patients, Virgil Smirnow Associates, Washington, D.C., 1973.

ORGANIC AND PSYCHIATRIC ASPECTS OF HEADACHE

BORIS KAIM, M.D.*

CONTENTS:

1) Clinical History of Headache

2) Differential Diagnosis of Headache

3) Classification of Headache

4) Treatment of Headache

5) Conclusion

6) Tables

7) References

*Neurologist and Psychiatrist
Associate Professor, Department of Psychiatry
Texas Tech School of Medicine, El Paso, TX

ORGANIC AND PSYCHOSOMATIC ASPECTS OF HEADACHE

Boris Kaim, M.D.*

The purpose in writing this chapter is 1) to call attention to the psychogenic origin of many cases of headache and 2) to stress organic causes of headaches and its differential diagnosis.

Here I give neurologic information with some detail for the benefit of psychiatrists. Headache is perhaps one of the most common causes of medical consultation. The causes of headache are multiple and they are related principally to neurological, medical and psychiatric problems (1).

The patient with headache must be studied not as having only one symptom but as an individual in which several factors (neurological, biochemical, medical, environmental and emotional) play a very important role. It is common to find patients with more than one type of headache. Headaches that previously were produced by certain factors or circumstances may reappear under other circumstances, probably through a conditioned reflex mechanism.

One of the most common causes of headaches is contraction headache that may be due to a direct or reflex muscle irritation or to psychogenic origin, which is related to frustration, depression and stress. Other types of headaches like migraine, at least in part, may be related to emotional tension.

Malingering is another cause of headache that has increased in the last years due to the present climate of litigation and easy compensation. In cases of hysteria or malingering a quick diagnosis must be made so that the situation is clarified and the individual returns as soon as possible to his or her usual occupation or activities. In headaches like in other disorders, the correct diagnosis of hysteria or malingering require a combination of neurologic and psychiatric skills, experience and resourcefulness. Stevens stated that the most conclusive proof of conversion hysteria is the successful removal of the symptom with sodium amytal hypnosis (2). For years I have used methohexital induced hypnosis in similar cases. However, at the same time I consider that it is necessary to do a good neurological evaluation including, according to the case, electroencephalograms, brainstem potentials, visual evoked responses, computerized cerebral map, radiological studies, to be sure that the patient's symptoms are not of organic origin and to help convince him of the nonorganic origin of his headache.

Many times the organic nature of the patient's symptoms is overlooked in part because they may have atypical or uncommon headaches: often those patients are labeled as "neurotic", "hysteric" or "hypochondriac". The other problem is that when patients with somatization disorders receive excessive medical attention, develop a "fixation" in their symptoms. Those patients may believe that because so many tests are done, they must have something wrong with them and it becomes very difficult to change their point of view afterwards. Many times during those extensive workups minor abnormalities are found and wrongly they may be blamed as the source of the patient's symptoms. In this way an iatrogenic disorder occurs.

Unwise commentaries contribute to the production of a psychosomatic pain disorder. As Platonov stated, "we must be very careful with the choice of our words to patients that are already in pain and under emotional stress because they may misinterpret the facts and with this misinterpretation, may magnify their symptoms" (3). During the physical examination, it is my custom to comment, for example, "the blood pressure is normal", "the examination of the eyes is totally normal", etc. and make suggestions in such a way that it helps to minimize the patient's concern about his symptoms. The words that are to be used in suggestion must be chosen very carefully and must be communicated in such a way as to avoid misinterpretation. The findings of the physical examination and laboratory tests must be clearly and thoroughly explained to the patient.

Patients with chronic pain may have distortions of their personality because the pain affects their life, work, emotions, social and sexual relationships. Head trauma, brain tumors and other medical disorders that act directly over the brain, principally when the lesions are on the left hemisphere, may produce depression, irritability and cognitive disorders. Lesions in the frontal and temporal lobes produce changes in the personality.

Some individuals are prone to complain of pain. Blumer and Hailbrunn studied 383 patients with "pain-prone disorder". The clinical features of this condition consists in continuous pain, desire for surgery or other procedures, denial of emotional and interpersonal difficulties. Those patients showed excessive passivity and depression (4).

It is very important for the clinician to know the different modalities of headaches before claiming that a given headache is of psychogenic origin. If the clinician rushes with a diagnosis of "psychogenic origin" many times he may be mistaken. Headaches that at times appear to be psychogenic may be due to organic factors.

Case #1

A 23 year old woman developed severe common migraine attacks at the time of her impending divorce. The neurological examination was normal. She had a dramatic improvement of her headaches with Limbitrol (chlordiazepoxide and amitriptyline). One month later, the headaches recurred and at that time a slight congestion of the optic discs was found at the funduscopic examination. A CT brain scan showed marked hydrocephalus due to stenosis of the aqueduct. After a ventricular shunt her headaches disappeared. This case illustrates that some headaches of organic origin may mimic a psychogenic headache and corroborates the need for neurologic follow up even in cases of disorders that appear "clearly" to be psychogenic.

Case #2

A 45 year old seamstress who 3 weeks prior to her consultation in my office, suffered from severe headaches. The examination done by her internist was reported as negative so he believed that her headaches were psychogenic and prescribed tranquilizers. Because the headache persisted a neurological consultation was requested. The neurological examination was normal except for a minimal sound of dragging the left foot while walking, although no actual defect in the gait was seen. The spinal tap disclosed subarachnoid bleeding and the radiological examination showed an intracerebral aneurysm. Due to incomplete neurologic examination a headache patient with a real organic lesion may be labeled as "nervous" or "hysteric".

Case #3

A 28 year old woman had a "terrible headache" for 3 weeks. She was studied in the hospital of a nearby city. The CT scan, EEG, spinal tap and neurological examination were normal. She was treated with numerous medications without any improvement at all. The neurological examination was normal. She had the "belle indifference". Persistently she denied any psychogenic problem that could be the cause of her headache. When asked if any relative or friend suffered from headaches she denied any knowledge of it. During the methohexital interview she said to be concerned about having a possible brain tumor. Her father had died of disseminated cancer with brain metastasis complaining of "terrible headache". After the methohexital hypnosis the situation was explained to the patient. She felt much relief and finally accepted the fact that she did not have any brain tumor. That same afternoon she requested to be discharged from the hospital.

This case illustrates the usefulness of methohexital hypnosis in the investigation of psychogenic headaches.

CLINICAL EXAMINATION

Like with any medical problem, a careful history must be obtained and it should include: (modified from Friedman (5) and Graham (6) 1. Type of headache (pressure, throbbing, burning, piercing, splitting). 2. Side of the headache (focal, generalized). 3. Precipitating factors. 4. Frequency and duration of the headache. 5. Time and mode of onset. 6. Aura and associated symptoms. 7. Conditions that make the headache worse. 8. Relieving factors and medications. 9. Age at onset of the headaches. 10. Family history of headache. 11. History of head trauma. 12. History of alcohol intake or use of drugs that may impair consciousness and facilitate, in any way, head trauma (the patient may be amnesic for the actual head trauma). 13. Does the patient know anybody who suffers from similar types of headaches? Some patients copy symptoms from relatives, friends, etc. 14. Is there any legal action or compensation involved? 15. Medical problems related to the headaches (arterial hypertension, renal disease, etc.) 16. Major stressful changes in life events such as going away from home, job, marriage, divorce, illness in the family, accidents, tragedies, death of a loved one, frustrations, menopause, depression, retirement, etc. 17. List of physicians and other therapists who have seen the patient.

DIFFERENTIAL DIAGNOSIS OF HEADACHES

A complete physical and neurological examination must be done. Special attention must be placed to the following conditions, that may indicate an organic origin of the headache and hint to the correct diagnosis.

1) Headache accompanied by photophobia. This may indicate migraine but also encephalitis or meningitis. In my experience, early cases of encephalitis always (except in two cases) were accompanied by photophobia and severe headache. Neck stiffness is not present in all the cases of early encephalitis and meningitis.

2) Headache associated with changes in the sensorium and agitation may indicate a meningeal syndrome (particularly acute meningitis, subarachnoid bleeding, subdural hematoma, brain tumor).

3) Nuchal pain and headache principally located in the occipital region, accompanied by stiff neck and incoordination: possible cerebrovascular accident or tumor in the posterior fossa, foramen magnum meningiomas, cervical pachymeningitis, herniated cervical discs, Arnold-Chiara malformation. Neuralgia of the major occipital nerve may produce severe pain in the nuchal area and posterior headache up to the vertex. The pain is worse while extending the neck.

4) Headache accompanied by unconsciousness. Very seldom common migraine or classical migraine are accompanied by unconsciousness, but it may occur. Basilar migraine, mostly in children, may be accompanied by unconsciousness although it does not happen frequently. The most common causes of unconsciousness and headache is cerebrovascular accident and seizure disorder.

5) Sudden severe headache: migraine, cluster headache, cerebrovascular accident, pheochromocytoma.

6) Headache in the presence of positive neurological deficit: tumors, CVA, complicated migraine (hemiplegic or opthalmoplegic migraine). A headache with hemiparesis may be due to a thromboembolic CVA, subdural hematoma, ruptured aneurysm or tumor. Hemiplegia and headache generally are due to a cerebrovascular accident. Opthalmoplegia is present in the Tolosa-Hunt syndrome.

7) Headache and fever: encephalitis, meningitis, brain abscess, subdural empyema, sinusitis.

8) Headache after the age of 50: CVA, arterial hypertension, cervical spondylosis, giant cell arteritis (temporal arteritis), brain tumor or metastasis. Depression could be another factor.

9) Headache that occurs with changes of position of the head: the most common cause if a sudden hydrocephalus produced by a colloidal cyst of the 3rd ventrical, or hydrocephalus due to aqueductal stenosis in which, in some cases, there is a valve mechanism due to glial or scar tissue.

10) Normal pressure hydrocephalus: headache, changes in the personality, dementia, spasticity in the lower extremities, lack of control of the micturition. Similar symptoms may be produced by transfalcial herniation of the cingulate gyrus due to a chronic subdural hematoma or tumor.

11) Headaches associated with mental changes and anosmia indicate a frontal tumor, like olfactory groove meningioma.

12) Headache associated with endocrine disorders: hypercalcemia, hypothyroidism, Cushing syndrome.

13) Headaches present after waking up: brain tumors, sleep apnea, cervical spondylosis, nocturnal bruxism.

14) Headaches related to the Valsalva maneuver (straining, bending, coughing, sneezing, lifting). Rule out increased intracranial pressure due to tumors, Arnold-Chiari malformation, subdural hematoma.

15) Headaches produced while bending the head, probably related to sinus disorders.

16) Headaches associated with nausea or vomiting: increased intracranial pressure, meningitis, migraine.

17) Headaches "in band" with a sensitive scalp: contraction headache. If the headache disappears after a local block with lidocaine this is the most possible diagnosis.

18) Throbbing headaches: Migraine, hypertension or febrile disorders; at times, encephalitis.

19) Headache and diplopia: multiple sclerosis, myasthenia gravis, intracerebral aneurysm; diabetes mellitus and other causes of neuropathy.

Most of the cases of monocular diplopia are hysterical but it may occur with eye diseases such as cataracts.

20) Headache related to neck movements probably are due to cervical spondylosis or muscle contraction headache. Headache related to reading, probably is due to eye strain.

21) Retrocular headaches, principally if associated to extraocular paresis may be related to intracerebral aneurysm.

22) Headache related to "belle indifferance": probably hysterical disorder.

23) Headache related to delusions ("pieces of the brain are coming out through a little hole in the back of my head") are due to a psychotic disorder, mostly schizophrenia.

24) Headaches related to chewing (chewing claudication): temporomandibular joint dysfunction, temporal arteritis.

25) Headaches related to pain in the face: cluster headaches, trigeminal neuralgia, pain of dental origin, neurosympathetic reflex dysfunction.

26) Headaches with pulsating proptosis: carotid artery-caverous sinus fistula.

27) Headache associated with intolerance to alcohol and certain foods: migraine, cluster headaches.

28) Headache during coitus: "benign" coital headache, headache secondary to arterial hypertension; ruptured intracerebral aneurysm.

TESTS TO BE DONE IN THE STUDY OF HEADACHE (Modified from 5, 6, 7)

Some of the following tests are to be done in cases of headache. They are not to be done on a routine basis but rather according to the circumstances, the clinical history, findings in the physical examination, mental status and social history.

1) Multimetabolic studies including thyroid function. Cortisol level.

2) Skull X-rays. Sinus series. X-rays of the cervical spine, radionuclide bone scan.

3) CBC, sedimentation rate, ANA and VDRL.

4) Noninvasive vascular studies.

5) Invasive vascular studies.

6) Electroencephalogram, computerized topographic cerebral map, visual evoked response, brainstem auditory evoked response, sleep apnea studies.

7) CT brain scan or MRI.

8) Spinal tap.

9) Block of a peripheral nerve (supraorbital nerve, occipital nerve, etc.); infiltration with local anesthetic of muscles or soft tissue: if the pain disappears it indicates that the origin of the pain is focal or superficial.

10) Interview with hypnosis or with methohexital or penthotal hypnosis: investigation of hysteria or malingering.

11) Psychological tests including MMPI, TAT, Luria-Nebraska, Bender-Gestalt.

MECHANISM OF HEADACHE

Ray and Wolff in 1940 demonstrated in neurosurgical patients that the pain sensitive structures of the head includes the skin, scalp, arteries, great venous sinuses and its tributories, the head and neck muscles, parts of the dura at the base of the brain, the dural arteries, the fifth and seventh cranial nerves and a minor component of the seventh cranial nerve and finally the cervical nerves. It is established that the parenchyma of the brain is not sensitive to pain (8, 9, 10, 11).

It is believed that the visual symptoms that occur during a migraine attack (aura) are secondary to ischemia of the occipital cortex (10, 11). During the intracerebral constriction there is inhibition of the cortical activity that spreads slowly (Leao inhibition). The extracerebral vasodilation is responsible for the pounding headache that occurs in migraine, fever and arterial hypertension.

CLASSIFICATION OF HEADACHES

(Modification of the Ad Hoc Committee on the classification of headache) (12)

A. Muscle Contraction Headache: 1. Cervical osteoarthritis, neck injuries. 2. Myositis. 3. Temporomandibular Joint Dysfunction. 4. Psychogenic muscular tension headache: a. Headache due to depression. b. Headache due to somatoform disorder. c. Headache due to anxiety and/or frustration.

B. Vascular headaches: 1. Classical migraine. 2. Common migraine. 3. Basilar migraine. 4. Opthalmoplegic migraine. 5. Hemiplegic migraine. 6. Hypertensive vascular headaches. 7. Toxic vascular headache. 8. Cluster headache. 9. Traction and inflammatory headaches (increased intracranial pressure, tumors, hematomas, intracerebral hemorrhage, edema, hydrocephalus, meningoencephalitis, meningitis, granulomatosis). 10. Arteritis. 11. Phlebitis. 12. Occlusive vascular disease.

C. Diseases of the eye, ear, nose, tongue, throat and teeth.

D. Retention of CO_2: sleep apnea, pulmonary diseases, brain tumor.

E. Neuralgias: 1. Trigeminal neuralgia. 2. Paratrigeminal neuralgia. 3. Glossopharyngeal neuralgia. 4. Supraorbital neuralgia. 5. Infraorbital neuralgia. 6. Sphenopalatine and vidian neuralgia. 7. Laryngeal neuralgia. 8. Herpes zoster neuralgia. 9. Sympathetic neurovascular reflex dysfunction (sympathetic dystrophy).

F. Atypical Facial Pain

G. Exertional headache.

H. Temperature and climate dependent headache: 1. Barometric headache. 2. "Ice cream headache"

I. Multiple sclerosis

J. Other types of headaches

HEAD TRAUMA AND HEADACHE

Head trauma is a very important cause of morbidity and mortality and one of the principal causes of headache. It is believed that there are more than ten million cases of head trauma in the United States every year. Forty five percent correspond to motor vehicle accidents; occupational causes account for 10%; recreational: 10%; falls: 30%; and assaults: 5% (13). It was estimated by different investigators that headaches may be present in 12-80% of the cases after mild head trauma. Post traumatic headache is not a single entity, it includes different types of headache, among them, vascular, muscle contraction headaches, supraorbital neuralgia, occipital neuralgia, temporomandibular joint dysfunction, post traumatic dysautonomic cephalalgia and finally, dysesthesias over scalp lacerations. Premorbid personality and other factors including compensation, disability, disruption of the social life, etc. play an important role. Because of the several types of post-traumatic headaches, different psychological, behavioral modification and drug treatment may be necessary.

MUSCLE CONTRACTION HEADACHE

Muscle contraction headache is the most common of the headaches. Most of the times the headache is perceived as a pressure, "like a band", principally in the frontal, temporal and occipital regions, and in the nuchal region. At times it may be present as a pounding sensation characteristic of vascular headaches. At other times it may be present as a combination of vascular and contraction headache ("mixed headaches").

Most of the authors have written that the muscle contraction headache is synonymous with "tension headache". My personal opinion is that the muscle contraction headache is the final pathway of different causes of headache. Among them: headaches secondary to lesions such as cervical osteoarthritis, neck injuries (including whiplash injuries) (14), myositis; referred headaches as in temporomandibular joint dysfunction. Stress is also a common cause of muscle tension and of muscle contraction headache.

Electromyographic studies of patients with muscle contraction headaches indicate that frequently there is a sustained muscular contraction that many times is focal. In cases of "psychogenic headache" the contraction of the muscles of the scalp and neck most of the times is generalized but also may be focal. Contrary to periodic headaches (migraine, cluster headache), the muscle contraction headaches don't have the same periodicity and may recur for days, weeks or months.

The criteria for the diagnosis of tension headache is imprecise and it has been used and abused as a "wastebasket entity" (15). The muscle contraction headache due to cervical lesions is aggravated by head movements and by pressure on the cervical paraspinalis muscles. This headache may improve with transcutaneous nerve stimulation, immobilization of the neck or physical therapy including local heat. Injections of local anesthesia may also block this type of pain.

Muscle contraction headaches frequently are due to spasm of the trapezius muscles and can be studied with surface electromyogram. With this test, in many instances the location of the offending muscle is determined and treatment with TENS unit or physical therapy are effective. In a few selected cases the patients can be treated with injections of local anesthesia (16). Bakal (17) described that some patients with migraine and patients with muscle contraction headache have higher amplitude in the EMG activity in the muscles of the neck than controlled subjects, which indicates that at least in some cases, contraction of the muscles of the neck may produce, or be related to, both migraine or muscle contraction headache ("mixed headaches"). Many reliable patients describe that their migraine headaches start by tension in the muscles of the neck and after that the visual symptoms develop followed by the typical pounding headache. Clifford et al (18) found, during the attack of migraine, that there is significant increased activity in the anterior temporal muscles which exceeds the patient's own baseline. Bakke, Tfelt-Hansen et al (19), in recording of the temporal, masseter, sternocleidomastoid and nuchal muscles, in four patients with attacks of common migraine described increased muscular activity. In two of their patients, the activity was sufficiently strong to account for a substantial part of their pain.

In many cases in which the patient complained of headache but was suspected of malingering, the EMGs were normal.

TREATMENT OF THE CONTRACTION HEADACHE

Muscle relaxants, physiotherapy, anti-inflammatory medications and amitriptyline are useful.

Muscle contraction headaches may be due to myofacial dysfunction secondary to local injury in the muscles. Local injections of lidocaine or procaine on the trigger points of the affected muscles may produce dramatic relief of the pain (20).

The post-traumatic headaches can be of several clinical types and are due to lesions on the cervical and head muscles, vertebrae, or ligaments (21). In those cases, generally the X-rays show a straightening of the cervical curvature. Post traumatic headaches may be accompanied by symptoms such as personality change, dizziness, vertigo, tinnitus, memory problems, mood alterations, reduced attention span, reduced motivation, asthenia, fatigue, and loss of libido.

In cases of head trauma the electroencephalogram may be slow but many times it is normal. The brainstem auditory evoked potentials may be abnormal, principally after the first week. The brainstem auditory evoked potential may demonstrate that a minor head or neck injury, with associated subjective symptomatology, has organic basis and is not psychogenic. (22) Added to the post traumatic headache itself, there is an emotional component. Many patients develop post traumatic phobic disorder. This condition responds relatively well to small doses of amitriptyline and/or alprazolam and behavior therapy.

PSYCHOGENIC HEADACHE

The term, "psychogenic headache" or "tension headache", implies that the headache is produced by emotional factors. They were made synonymous with "muscle-contraction headache". As previously described, muscle contraction headaches can be produced by numerous conditions that are related with muscle spasm of the cervical region, head or face secondary to focal pathology. I prefer to apply the term "muscle-contraction headache" in this context, and use the term "psychogenic headache" for those headaches that are primarily related to emotional problems. Many of the "tension headaches" or "psychogenic headaches" have, as a final pathway, a contraction of the muscles of the scalp, face or neck and are indistinguishable clinically and electromyographically of the "muscle-contraction headaches" due to organic causes.

There are many statistics that point that "tension headache" constitutes about 75% of the headaches in women (7). The clinical experience points that headaches of psychogenic origin are more common in women but they are also very common in men, and that muscle contraction headache of organic cause, including those secondary to head or neck trauma, are more common in men.

The psychogenic headache can be seen predominantly in hysterical, depressive, anxious, obsessive-compulsive individuals and finally in psychotic patients.

In the hysterical patient, the pain is a neurotic symptom and represents a symbolic attempt to resolve a mental conflict (5), or is due to neurotic identification with other people who suffer from headache. By definition, the hysterical headache is an unconscious disorder and it is not explained by any known physical or pathophysiologic mechanism. In this definition, the psychogenic pain is a conversion disorder (or hysterical disorder). Two mechanisms are suggested to explain the conversion symptoms (24). One is the "primary gain" by which the individual keeps an internal conflict or need out of his awareness. There is a temporal relationship between an environmental stimulus that is related to a psychological conflict or need and the initiation or exacerbation of the patient's symptom. The second mechanism is the "secondary gain". The symptom, no matter how disabling, is useful for the patient because he may get the support, attention, love and care from significant people and also have the opportunity to manipulate them.

In conversion (hysterical) disorders generally the symptoms, and in this particular case, the headache, appears suddenly during a period of psychological stress. "La belle indifference" is common: the patient shows lack of concern for his symptoms. Frequently, the patient complains of severe, disabling headache and at the same time smiles. Also, there is, many times, resistance to improve.

Some studies indicate that people with obsessive compulsive personality are prone to suffer from headaches (25) but other studies refute that observation. In hypochondriasis the patient has a fear of having a serious disease and in the case of the headache, principally of having a "brain tumor". In these cases, hypnosis or short acting barbiturate interview (26,27) are very useful to clarify the patient's problems and to make therapeutic suggestions. As Bleger described, the narcoanalysis ("penthotal interview") is useful in obtaining repressed information, establishing positive transference, interrupting as soon as possible the primary and secondary gain and treating the conversion symptoms; and releasing repressed hostility. Similar assertions were made by Stevens (2) and by many other authors.

Hypnosis is very effective in the removal of symptoms and treatment of patients with psychogenic pains and hysterical disorder (28, 29, 30, 31, 32, 33). The symptomatic hypnotic treatment is quite effective and very seldom, when used appropriately, has the drawbacks that the proponents of dynamic psychotherapy claim to have. The principal contraindication for hypnosis are: a. Paranoid patients; b. Individuals that are fearful of being hypnotized; c. Most psychotic, delusional individuals.

Hypnosis is practically free of complications except for a few dangerous induction techniques (34).

Hypnosis, or barbiturate induced hypnosis should be done early in the cases of conversion to relieve the symptoms, to avoid a fixation in the symptoms and any incapacity that may be produced by secondary changes (2).

VASCULAR HEADACHES

The most common of the vascular headaches are common migraine and classical migraine. Other vascular headaches are related to toxic states, febrile conditions, arterial hypertension, cerebrovascular accidents and vasculitis.

Generally there is a family history in migraine. In the common migraine the patient presents with a throbbing headache that could be unilateral or bilateral. As aura the patient may have some blurring of the vision, dizziness, nausea and changes in mood. Many patients are able to perceive a muscular contraction headache prior to the onset of the migraine, and this contraction headache generally is localized in the nuchal region. With the migraine there is increased urinary output (9), diarrhea, photophobia, sonophobia, pallor, and generalized weakness.

In the classical migraine, there is a period of aura characterized by visual phenomena such as positive or negative scotomas, scintillations and fortifications, many times of a hemianoptic nature. Typically, in migraine there is a gradual expansion of the scotomas. When the eyeball is displaced with the fingertip the visual abnormality will move with the eyeball if the origin of the visual abnormality is in the retina but not if it is in the calcarine cortex (35). The patient has a sensation of malaise and in about 15-45 minutes develops a severe pounding headache, generally unilateral (hemicranea); he prefers to rest in a dark room without any sensory stimulation. After sleeping for a few hours, generally, the headache goes away.

Migraine status is the condition in which a continuous migraine headache is present for over 24 hours. On occasions it may last for 3-4 days and even longer.

In migraine, olfactory aura may be present (36). In psychomotor seizures (partial complex seizures) and at times, in premenstrual tension disorder, olfactory hallucinations may also be present.

The visual symptoms that occur at the beginning of a migraine attack are due to ischemia of the occipital cortex and remain present even while the eyes are closed. In transient ischemic attacks affecting the circulation of the optic nerves, the visual symptoms disappear after closing the eyes (10).

In 1945, Leao and Morrison, indicated that the migraine aura is caused by spreading depression. In migraine, the scotoma begin near the macula and spread peripherally. The margin of the visual phenomena goes from the center to the periphery in about 25 minutes which covers a distance of 67 mm. in the visual cortex from the macular area to the periphery at the rate calculated in 3 mm./minute and corresponds to the Leao's spreading inhibition (37). Lauritzen et al (38) arrived to the same conclusion after studying 13 migraneurs with regional cerebral blood flow (rCBF) following intracarotid injection of xenon 131. A proof that the visual aura in migraine occurs in the occipital cortex and not in the retina was brought up by Peatfield and Rose (39) when they described a woman with eyes enucleated in childhood, presented with symptoms of classic migraine. The attacks included formed visual hallucinations in a hemianoptic field.

In transient ischemic attacks the amaurosis fugax lasts from a few seconds to 3-5 minutes, usually is monocular and seldom hemianoptic and it is not accompanied by hemianoptic fortifications (40).

The EEGs obtained during the visual aura and the actual migraine attack may show slowing over the involved occipital lobe (41).

In migraine, the vasospastic episode is followed by the throbbing headache which appears to be due to vasodilatation in the territory of branches of the external carotid artery. Graham thinks that the prodromal phase of the migraine is probably the basic phenomenon of this disorder and that the vasodilation, that produces the headache, probably represents an abnormal compensatory event (42). Some patients may develop brain infarctions secondary to migranous vasospasm (43).

Migraneur patients appear to have cycles of susceptibility during which they develop the migraine. During the susceptible phase, the migraine attack may be triggered by drinking alcohol, by eating certain foods or by stress (44).

Vasodilation is not the only mechanism of migraine. Many migraneurs may have vasodilation (as after a hot bath) without having headache. A migraine attack may be precipitated by hypoglycemia, stress, hormonal changes, smoking, exposition to bright lights or noises. Many types of food and beverages may produce migraine, among them the most common are cheese, beer, wine (principally red wine), cured meats (which contain nitrates), chocolate and monosodium glutamate. The same is true for reserpine and vasodilators like nitroglycerin and dipyridamole. There are several reports that tyramine which is present in beer, wine, pickles, etc. may produce migraine attacks (45). Ziegler and Stewart (46) studied 80 migraine patients and found that infusions of 200 mg. of tyramine precipitated migraine in 8 individuals. Retesting of 7 of these individuals did not reproduce the migraine. Placebo produced a severe headache as tyramine did. They concluded that tyramine alone is not a major cause of migraine attacks but perhaps tyramine, together with another factor, may precipitate the migraine episodes.

The most important theory about the pathogenesis of migraine is that it is due to a release of vasoactive substances from platelets and probably from other sources (11). Substances implied are serotonin, catecholamines, histamine, prostaglandines (47). During the migraine attack there is increased platelet hyperaggregability, release of serotonin from the platelets which causes release of histamine. Prostaglandin E1 produces vasodilation in the external carotid system and prostaglandin F2 induces vasoconstriction in the internal carotid system. Prostaglandin F2 also influences platelet hyperaggregability which perhaps is the first event in the genesis of migraine (48). At the onset of the prodrome phase of the migraine, there is increase in the plasma serotonin and in platelet aggregation. During the headache phase, there is decrease in plasma serotonin and in the platelet aggregation. Reserpine depletes the blood platelets of serotonin and in this way may induce the appearance of the migraine attack. Antihistaminics and antiserotonin compounds interfere with the action of vasoactive amines (11).

Arteriovenous malformations may be accompanied by migraine. In those cases, the migraine is always unilateral. Surgical removal of the arteriovenous malformation is followed by resolution of the patient's symptoms (49,50). Arteriograms done during a migraine episode showed vasospasm. It is known that patients with migraine may develop severe vasospasm and at times with tragic results. Lanzi described a correlation between mitral valve prolapse and migraine (51).

MIGRAINE EQUIVALENT

Several symptoms such as scotomas, scintillations, nausea, vomiting, abdominal pain may be due to a migraine syndrome but not always are accompanied by the headache itself, this situation is known as migraine equivalent. Prolonged migraine aura status was described (52).

PARAMENSTRUAL MIGRAINE

Paramenstrual migraine occurs principally during the premenstrual or menstrual period and perhaps is due to decreased estradiol levels. It is known that many women who suffer from migraine may be free of the migraine during pregnancy. Oral contraceptives may induce migraine in many women (53). On occasions the paramenstrual headache is not on endocrine basis but due entirely to emotional factors. I know of women who are so distressed of the menstrual flow that as soon as they see it they develop migraine.

CHRONIC PAROXYSMAL HEMICRANIA

Sjaastad and Dale described chronic paroxysmal hemicranea that consists in daily episodes of unilateral headaches accompanied by partial Horner's syndrome and rhinorrhea, that resembles cluster headache but occurs daily. This type of headache improves with indomethacin (54).

BASILAR MIGRAINE

In 1981 Bickerstaff described basilar artery migraine that consists in acute and transient visual loss, vertigo, ataxia, dysarthria, paresthesias, incoordination followed by severe headache and vomiting. Most of the patients have bilateral or homonimous hemianopsia (37).

Amit et al described global amnesia in a 9 year old girl who suffered from basilar migraine. It appears that the global amnesia may represent a variant of basilar migraine (55).

CYCLICAL MIGRAINE

Medina and Diamond described 27 migraneurs whose headaches occur in groups separated by headache free periods. In many patients the cycles were often accompanied by constant, low grade headache and depression. 22 patients were treated with lithium carbonate and of those 19 had a complete or partial control of the headache (56).

OPTHALMOPLEGIC MIGRAINE

Opthalmoplegic migraine generally occurs under 10 years of age and seldom after 20 years of age. The headache is unilateral and is followed by eyelid ptosis and paresis of the extraocular muscles with pupilary dilatation. Generally, there is a history of migraine (37). The differential diagnosis is with painful opthalmoplegia (Tolosa-Hunt syndrome). Prednisone (57) and flufenamic acid (48) are useful in the treatment of migraine opthalmoparesis.

HEMIPLEGIC MIGRAINE

Frequently many patients with migraine present numbness in the contralateral limbs to the headache. Some patients may have transient hemiparesis or hemiplegia but in some cases the hemiplegia is permanent. Zifkin et al (58) described an autosomal dominant syndrome of hemiplegic migraine, nystagmus and essential tremor in mother and son. Gastaut (59) stated that there are two forms of hemiplegic migraine: familial and sporadic.

TREATMENT OF MIGRAINE

The treatment of the migraine is prophylactic and symptomatic. Ergotamine is the medication of choice for the treatment of the attack. It is an alpha adrenergic blocking agent that produces direct stimulation on the smooth muscle of peripheral and cranial blood vessels (60).

Ergotamine is to be taken as soon as the patient presents the aura or in case of absence of aura, as soon as the headache begins. The dose for the sublingual preparation is 2 mg., to be given no more than 3 times a day or 6 times a week. It may be repeated in one hour if necessary. Ergotamine is available in combination with other medications, principally caffeine and barbiturates and also as spray. Ergotamine may induce nausea, vomiting, dizziness, drowsiness, and in some cases it will make the headaches worse and produce marked vasoconstriction. It may increase uterine contractions so abortions may occur. Gangrene of the tips of the fingers, the earlobes and arteritis and myocardial infarction may occur after the chronic use of ergotamine. Ergotamine is contraindicated in cases of cardiac disease, arterial hypertension, occlusive vascular disease, renal and hepatic diseases and pregnancy. Analgesics are to be used as soon as possible when the first symptoms of migraine appear. Aspirin, ibuprofen, acetaminophen, flufenamic acid (48) or propoxiphene are useful. In extreme cases, principally during migraine status, narcotics may help to control the headache but always there is a risk that patients with chronic pain, including migraine, may develop addiction to narcotics. In the rare occasions when narcotics are prescribed it should be under close supervision and for no more than 48 hours.

For the acute attack of migraine, oxygen 10 liters/minute, 100% concentration, administered for 15 minutes may abort many episodes of migraine (7, 60). Isoetheptene is a stimulant that is useful in some patients with migraine.

PROPHYLAXIS OF MIGRAINE

As prophylaxis for migraine I prescribe amitriptyline in small doses, generally 10-25 mg. one to two times a day. Seldom is it necessary to give higher doses. I keep the patients with this medication for 1-4 months depending on the severity of the migraine. Amitriptyline is to be taken again in case that there is a recurrence of the headaches. In anxious patients addition of a benzodiazepine is indicated.

Freidman and Mahloudji were the first to describe the use of amitriptyline as prophylactic agent in migraine in 1968. Couch and Hassanein (61) described in 1979 that nondepressed patients with severe migraine and depressed subjects with less severe migraine responded best to amitriptyline. It's action appears to be independent of the antidepressant activity. Methysergide is used for the prophylaxis of migraine but because of the risks of cardiopulmonary and retroperitoneal fibrosis I prefer not to prescribe it.

The beta blockers such as propranolol are very useful for the prophylaxis of migraine. Those are my second choice after amitriptyline. One of the drawbacks is the hypotension and bradycardia that the patient may develop.

Patti et al described that salmon calcitonin improved migraine in 30 patients. The dose was 100 units IM (62). Calcium channel blocking agents such as nifedipine, dilatiazem, verapamil produce dilatation of the arteries and are reported to be very useful for the treatment of migraine (63)and cluster headache (48).

Bonuso et al reported that sublingual flunarizine, a long acting calcium blocking agent, is very useful for the treatment and profilaxis of migraine attacks. This medication blocks the intracerebral vasoconstriction that probably is one of the first steps in the migraine attack (64).

A double blind study was done on the prophylaxis of migraine with flunarizine and pizotifen (an antiserotonin medication). Flunarizine was superior (65). Naproxen sodium is a prophylactic for migraine attacks probably because it is a potent inhibitor of prostaglandin biosynthesis and platelet aggregation (66).

Twenty six patients with migraine attacks were treated with flufenamic acid at a dose of 125 mg. 4-6 times per attack. The flufenamic acid is an inhibitor of prostaglandin synthesis. Of the 26 patients, 25 had symptomatic relief in 195 of 200 treated attacks (67).

Raskin (68) treated 55 migraine patients unresponsive to usual treatment with intravenous dehydroergotamine (DHE). Forty nine of the 55 patients became headache free within 48 hours and 39 of them had sustained benefits for up to 16 months.

HYPERTENSION AND HEADACHES

Hypertensive patients may suffer from headaches not only when the diastolic blood pressure is over 120 mm. (11,25) but also at lower ranges as it is observed over and over in clinical practice. The headache may be global or of the throbbing type. Headaches may be present during transient ischemic attacks.

Headaches are common during the end stage of renal disease. Those headaches are more apparent at the end of a dialysis session. Nephrectomy or a renal transplant many times abolishes those types of headaches (70).

PHEOCHROMOCYTOMA

Pheochromocytoma produce a release of catecholamines which induce paroxysms of arterial hypertension accompanied by throbbing headaches that last a few minutes, tachycardia, pallor and profuse sweating, perspiration, nausea, tremor and anxiety. The attacks may be induced during exercise (10,69).

CLUSTER HEADACHES

Cluster headaches are known by different names such as Sluder's syndrome, Bing's syndrome, vidian neuralgia, greater superficial nerve neuralgia, Horton's syndrome, etc. (70). Almost always the cluster headaches are episodic; may come suddenly and may last for days, weeks and at times months. Generally, the cluster headaches involve the periorbital region and the face.

The headaches may last from 15 minutes to 2 hours or more. Photophobia is unilateral and very severe. Injection of the conjunctiva and rhinorrhea also generally are unilateral. At times a partial Horner's syndrome may appear. It is typical for the patient with cluster headache to walk around holding his face, behavior which is different from the patient with migraine who prefers to lay down and avoids sensory stimulation. Attacks of cluster headaches may be precipitated by nitroglycerin, isosorbide dinitrate (71), histamine and alcohol and they are also worse during REM sleep (70, 72). Dalessio described an increase of serum histamine at the beginning of the cluster headache (11).

Facial thermography shows decreased temperature over the supraorbital areas in cases of cluster headache (72). For the acute attack of cluster headache the best treatment is 100% oxygen at 10 liters/minute for 15 minutes (73).

Kittrel administers local anesthesia for the treatment of cluster headache (74). He uses 4% lidocaine solution applied to the sphenopalatine fossa. The patient is placed in a supine position with the head extended backwards 45 degrees and rotated 30-40 degrees towards the side of the headache. One cc. of 4% lidocaine solution without epinephrine was slowly dropped into the ipsilateral nostril and the patient was kept in that position for several minutes.

The most common type of cluster headache is episodic and was described in 1947 by Ekbom. It responds well to lithium carbonate. The chronic paroxysmal hemicrania of Sjaastad responds well to indomethacin (75).

PROPHYLACTIC TREATMENT OF CLUSTER HEADACHES

Smoking and drinking may induce the headaches and should be avoided. Afternoon naps are not advised because the patient may have more tendency to have REM sleep early at night in which the cluster headaches are more common. Medications used in the treatment of cluster headache are lithium carbonate, ergotamine, corticosteroids, methysergide, indomethacin. Kudrow considers that prednisone prophylaxis is the treatment of choice in individuals under the age of 45 and lithium 300 mg. 3 times a day in patients over 45 (70).

Medina and Diamond describe a cluster headache variant in which there were atypical cluster headaches with multiple jabs and background vascular headaches. The headaches were localized and occurred several times daily, usually without any headache free periods. 83% of the patients responded to indomethacin. The 9 patients who did not respond to indomethacin were depressed and they responded well to tricyclic antidepressants (76).

Diamond treats patients with chronic cluster headaches who do not respond to the usual medications, with histamine desensitization (77). Bussone et al studied 16 patients who suffer from cluster headache. The brain auditory responses indicated prolongation of the I-V latencies ipsilaterally to the painful side. They suggested that perhaps there is a central pathogenesis of cluster headache (78). Boiardi et al (79) found that 20 individuals with cluster headaches had normal P100 latencies in the visual evoked response but the amplitudes were much lower than the controls. This finding also suggests that cluster headaches have a central origin.

The dexamethasone suppression test was normal in patients with cluster headaches which indicates that there is no hypothalamic-pituitary-adrenal dysfunction in those cases (80).

TEMPORAL ARTERITIS

Temporal arteritis or giant cell arteritis occurs generally after 65 years of age. Generally, the sedimentation rate is elevated. The headaches may be very severe principally in the temporal regions. It may be accompanied by chewing claudication and polymyalgia rheumatica and may be the cause of multiple cerebrovascular accidents. Temporal arteritis is one of the causes of multi-infarct dementia. It improves dramatically with corticosteroids (10,81).

NEURALGIAS AND OTHER ASSOCIATED PAIN DISORDERS

Cranial neuralgias such as trigeminal, paratrigeminal, glossopharyngeal, laryngeal, occipital and supraorbital neuralgias produce a severe, piercing and jabbing pain that generally lasts from a few seconds to minutes in the area of distribution of the affected nerve.

TRIGEMINAL NEURALGIA

The trigeminal neuralgia may be spontaneous or secondary to multiple sclerosis, brain tumors, epidermoid cysts and vascular anomalies (such as arterial loop and carotid aneurysm), pressure on the trigeminal nerve, secondary to fibrous bands across the petrous ridge, and chronic oral and dental disease (82). When the trigeminal neuralgia appears in a person under 50 years of age it is necessary to suspect multiple sclerosis. The brainstem evoked potentials and the trigeminal evoked potentials are useful (83,84).

Carbamazepine, phenytoin and baclofen are useful for the symptomatic control of trigeminal neuralgia (85,86). This condition can also be treated with radiofrequency rhizotomy (87), retrogasserian glycerol injection (88) and microvascular decompression (Janneta procedure (60).

PARATRIGEMINAL NEURALGIA (Raeder's neuralgia)

In the paratrigeminal neuralgia there is facial pain and oculosympathetic paresis (89). The pain of Raeder's paratrigeminal neuralgia is persistent and may last from weeks to months. Generally, the patient wakes up at night with severe unilateral supraorbital pain that can be throbbing or nonthrobbing. Photophobia is common and could be bilateral (60,90). At times the paratrigeminal neuralgia may be due to aneurysmal dilatation of the extracranial portion of the internal carotid artery and fibromuscular dysplasia, as described by Cohen (91).

GLOSSOPHARYNGEAL NEURALGIA

The symptoms of glossopharyngeal neuralgia are similar to the ones of the trigeminal neuralgia except that they are present in the tonsillar and pharyngeal area and in the ear but may radiate into the the vagal territory (92,93). They may be induced by swallowing, talking and yawning or by stimulation of the ear. I know of patients with glossopharyngeal neuralgia that were originally diagnosed as "hysterical".

SUPERIOR LARYNGEAL NEURALGIA

Superior laryngeal neuralgia occurs principally in middle aged men (94). The patient complains of severe paroxysms of pain in the lateral aspect of the neck and throat. The attacks are aggravated by swallowing, head turning and yawning. During the attacks there is an irresistible tendency to swallow that may temporarily alleviate the pain (95). Some patients are called "hysterical" because of this tendency to swallow.

GREATER OCCIPITAL NEURALGIA

This disorder is produced by inflammation or pressure of the greater occipital nerve which innervates the skin of the occipital region almost to the vertex and to the posterior border of the ear. The pain is severe and usually unilateral and is aggravated by touching the posterior area of the scalp, combing the hair, flexing or extending the head (95).

OCULAR ORIGIN OF HEADACHES

Frequent causes of headache are refractive errors, diplopia and disturbed accommodation (96). Other causes are uveitis (97) and glaucoma (98). Eyestrain may precipitate attacks of migraine (99) and muscle contraction headache (96).

In the painful opthalmoplegia (Tolosa-Hunt) syndrome the patient has severe facial pain, principally in the first division of the trigeminal nerve, in the periorbital and retroorbital regions and opthalmoplegia with dilatation of the pupil (100). The syndrome may be produced not only by granulomatouse tissue around the intracranial portion of the internal carotid artery but also by aneurysms (101), lupus erythematosus (102) and sellar erosion (103).

ENT CAUSES OF HEADACHE

In sinusitis the pain is unilateral and may be localized in the retroorbital, facial and seldom in the occipital regions. Lacrimation, rhinorrhea and photophobia may be present. Typically, the headache increases by changes in head position and may be worse by straining or by bending down (104).

The Ramsey-Hunt syndrome is due to unilateral lesion of the geniculate ganglion of the 7th cranial nerve produced by herpes zoster. The patient develops severe pain in the ear before the vesicles in the ear canal are apparent (95,104).

SPHENOPALATINE NEURALGIA (Sluder's Neuralgia)

In Sluder's neuralgia there is pain behind the eyes, upper jaw and may also involve the soft palate (95). Some authors believe that sphenopalatine neuralgia, vidian neuralgia and petrosal neuralgia are varities of cluster headache (105).

HEADACHE OR ORAL ORIGIN

Carious teeth, periodontitis and tooth abscess are well known causes of facial pain that at times may produce headache.

TEMPOROMANDIBULAR JOINT DYSFUNCTION

A not so rare cause of facial pain and headache is temporomandibular joint dysfunction. It becomes worse while chewing and eating. The patient may be aware of a clicking sound in the affected joint. At examination, it is common to find malocclusion in the teeth. The temporal, masseter and pterigoid muscles may be tender. Stethoscopic examination reveals a clicking and grinding sound on the affected joint. I know of several patients with temporomandibular joint dysfunction who originally were diagnosed as having psychogenic headache because the diagnosis of temporomandibular joint dysfunction was not considered.

Bell (106) classified the temporomandibular joint dysfunction as follows: 1) Masticatory muscle disorder; 2) Disc interference disorder; 3) Inflammatory disorders of the joint; 4) Chronic mandibular hypomobility; 5) Growth disorder of the joint.

BRAIN TUMORS AND HEADACHE

About 60% of patients with brain tumors may suffer from headaches and most of the times the headaches are localized in the same side as the tumor but this is not a constant finding. The headache may be due to displacement of the pain sensitive intracranial structures and also it may be due to increased intracranial pressure.

The headache produced by a brain tumor generally is constant but at times may be throbbing, and is worse while straining. It may occur during exertion, coughing, bowel movement or coitus. The headache of brain tumors is worse in the morning when the patient opens the eyes probably due to vasodilation secondary to an accumulation of CO_2.

PSEUDOTUMOR CEREBRI

In pseudotumor cerebri there is increased intracranial pressure Typically, headache and papilledema are present (107). The CT scan or MRI typically show small, narrow, slit-like ventricles. Pseudotumor cerebri may be produced by many causes, among them obesity, endocrine changes, intoxication with vitamin A, plumbism, ingestion of outdated tetracycline, lupus cerebritis, treatment with steroids, withdrawal of steroids, chronic respiratory insufficiency.

SLEEP APNEA HEADACHES

The most known symptoms of sleep apnea are loud snoring and diurnal hypersomnia. Other symptoms are decreased intellectual capacity, confusional states, personality change, intermittent nocturnal enuresis and headaches (108).

Sleep apnea is present in some cases of episodic cluster headache. It was found that most nocturnal attacks were preceded by oxygen desaturation and were REM related. A significant number of patients complain of severe nocturnal or early morning headaches (109).

ATYPICAL FACIAL PAIN AND HEADACHE

Some patients may have facial pain or headache that doesn't exactly fit one of the known patterns of headache. Some cases may be emotional in origin but in other cases the patient may suffer from conditions such as sympathetic neurovascular dysfunction, multiple sclerosis, temporomandibular joint dysfunction, etc. A rush judgment may label the patient as suffering from "emotional disorder".

Case #4

One of my patients with MRI proven multiple sclerosis developed episodes of facial pain that extended from the right to the left side of the forehead and from there obliquely through the left side of the face towards the right angle of the mandible to end in the left angle of the mandible. This is a "Z" pattern. Many times the pain is accompanied by ptosis of the superior left eyelid and rubral type of tremor in the right hand. The pain is lancinating and lasts for hours. She got relief with baclofen and carbamazepine. Initially, another neurologist thought that her pain was due to emotional reasons only.

HEADACHES AND CONVULSIVE DISORDER

Some patients with classical migraine, common migraine and basilar migraine may suffer from both convulsions and migraine attacks (110). It is difficult at times to differentiate between migraine and epilepsy based only on the EEG and clinical findings. Patients with migraine may present dizziness and loss of consciousness, and on the other hand, during the postictal state, epileptic patients develop a severe headache many times of a throbbing type (111). Many patients with headache may have EEGs with paroxysms of sharp waves and spikes. In these cases headaches are the only manifestation of a seizure disorder and constitute a "seizure equivalent"; generally this type of headaches are well controlled with antiepileptic medication.

Gastaut (112) described the benign epilepsy of childhood with occipital paroxysms (BEOP). This condition is characterized by:
1. Seizures with visual symptomatology frequently associated with other ictal phenomena and at times followed by postictal headache; 2. Interictal occipital rhythmic paroxysmal EEG appearing only after eye closure.

The sylvian spike epilepsy or benign Rolandic epilepsy is correlated with a high incidence of migraine in both the patients and his relatives (113). Confusional episodes are related at times with classical migraine and basilar migraine (114).

In "abdominal epilepsy" the patient who generally is a child presents with abdominal pain, many times of a colicky type, and with other symptoms such as dizziness, nausea and occasionally with headache. The EEG shows epileptogenic discharges.

EXERTIONAL AND COITAL CEPHALALGIA

Some individuals may develop headaches related to exercise. These patients must be investigated to rule out the possibility of increased intracranial pressure or vascular abnormalities. Indomethacin controls this type of headaches (115).

Vascular headaches may be associated not only with exercise but also with hypoglycemia, dehydration, increased environmental temperature and in some cases related to high altitude (69). Cerebral glucose hypometabolism (as measured by PET studies) was present in migraine headache induced by reserpine (116).

Coital headache is also called orgasmic headache and the first description was probably made by Hippocrates. The headache may be related to coitus and also to masturbation. Generally, these headaches are benign (117) and the headache in this condition (benign coital cephalalgia) may respond to propranolol (117,118) which probably indicates that this type of headache is a migraine variant.

SYMPATHETIC NEUROVASCULAR REFLEX DYSFUNCTION

Sympathetic neurovascular reflex dysfunction is synonymous with sympathetic dystrophy, reflex sympathetic dystrophy and with causalgia. Any injury may be associated with sympathetic neurovascular reflex dysfunction. Typically, the pain begins several days or weeks after injury and has a burning quality. The patient becomes very emotional and his complaints are disproportionate to the extent of the injury (119,120).

Jaeger et al (121) described two cases of reflex dystrophy of the face and made a review of the literature. They conclude that "there is a small but treatable group of patients with facial pain whose symptoms fall into the category of reflex sympathetic dystrophy". Blocks of the stellate ganglion can confirm the diagnosis and help to resolve the symptoms. A related type of headache is the post-traumatic dysautonomic cephalalgia in which vascular type of headaches are associated to autonomic dysfunction manifested initially by excessive sweating and pupillary dilatation (122).

Khurana and Nirankari described bilateral sympathetic dysfunction associated with traumatic headaches. After whiplash injury two patients developed generalized throbbing headaches, tenderness in the anterior neck and unilateral ptosis. There was supraorbital anhidrosis. The carotid artery studies were normal. The biochemical study of the pupils disclosed post ganglionic Horner's syndrome (123).

The sympathetic neurovascular reflex dysfunction improves with sympathetic blocks and in the case of the face, with blocks of the stellate ganglia. I had the opportunity to treat a few patients with sympathetic neurovascular reflex dysfunction affecting the face or the extremities, with oral papaverine and one with papaverine and TENS unit. This condition has also been treated with intravenous guanethidine and reserpine (119), antidepressants, anticonvulsants, calcium channel blocks, narcotics, physical therapy, blocks and surgery including neurolysis, neurectomy, rhizotomy and cordotomy. I want to call the attention that patients with sympathetic neurovascular reflex dysfunction develop marked alterations in their personality. Mimicking at times bipolar affective disorder.

MENINGEAL IRRITATION AND HEADACHES

Meningeal irritation may be produced by subarachnoid bleeding, meningitis, encephalitis, meningeal carcinomatosis and neurocisticercosis. It is accompanied by severe headaches.

MULTIPLE SCLEROSIS

Trigeminal neuralgia is the most common facial pain and headache related to multiple sclerosis, and it appears in people under 50 years of age. Other atypical headaches may appear in multiple sclerosis as previously described.

POST LUMBAR PUNCTURE HEADACHE

It is well known that many patients develop mild to severe headache after lumbar puncture, perhaps in 20 to 30% of the cases (124). The post spinal tap headache is believed to be related to seepage of spinal fluid through the hole in the dura made by the needle (hypoliquorrachia) and it is dependent on the spinal needle bore size (125).

UNCOMMON CAUSES OF HEADACHES

There are some unusual causes of headaches as: vasculitis (collagen diseases), hypersensitivity angitiitis (126), metabolic disorders (127).

THERMOGRAPHY AND HEADACHE

Kudrow (128) described an asymmetric, ipsilateral decreased in supraorbital temperature distribution in 67 to 75% of patients with cluster headaches, classical migraine, and hemiplegic migraine. This finding occurred with significantly less frequency in the common migraine group.

Twenty five percent of cluster headache patients and 14% of classical and hemiplegic migraine groups had a specific facial temperature pattern that was described as the "chai" sign named after the hebrew word for life. Kudrow's study showed that decreased temperature in the supraorbital region may significantly distinguish cluster, classical and hemiplegic migraine patients from patients with common migraine. Thermography is useful in the differentiating of some cases of organic and emotional headaches.

MEDICATION OVERUSE

Patients with chronic headache may easily become habituated to the use of tranquilizers and analgesics and narcotics, principally for those preparations with codeine and meperidine. It is important to try to avoid this situation by limiting the amount of medication and clearly establishing the correct diagnosis.

BIOFEEDBACK, TENS AND PHYSICAL THERAPY

Nonmedicamentose modalities for the treatment of chronic headache must be considered such as biofeedback and transcutaneous nerve stimulation. It is known that the application of EMG, biofeedback and relaxation techniques are useful for the control of pain (129). The techniques of Jacobson, Schultz and Wolpe are used to produce muscle relaxation (130,131,132) and are useful in the treatment of certain headaches. Deep muscle relaxation has autonomic effects that antagonize anxiety. Biofeedback is a special technique that trains the individual to control muscle tension, blood pressure, heart rate, brain wave activity and skin temperature and is based on operant conditioning (133).

The transcutaneous electrical stimulation is a well recognized treatment for the control of pain and headache and decreases the use and dose of medications (134,135). Not only contraction headaches, migraine, but trigeminal neuralgia and sympathetic reflex neurovascular dysfunction may be controlled with this type of treatment.

Oral splints are very helpful for the control of headache due to temporomandibular joint dysfunction and to chronic bruxism.

Physical therapy in the neck muscles may be helpful for some types of headaches, thus, decreasing the need for medication.

CONCLUSION:

For the successful treatment of headaches it is necessary to make a good neurological diagnosis, identify well the source of the pain and the modality of the headache disorder. Also, it is very important to assess the patient's emotional and environmental conditions and determine if the headache is of emotional origin, or at least if it is of mixed emotional and organic nature. An early treatment of the emotional factors is imperative in the therapy of headache. Almost all the patients with chronic and severe headache of organic nature develop emotional disorders that make the headache worse. Concurrent neurologic and psychiatric treatment is indicated in these cases.

Acknowledgments:

My thanks to Ruben Kaim for researching of the bibliography and to Elizabeth P. Figueroa, and Maria Eugenia Ramirez for typing of the manuscript.

TABLES

SUMMARY OF HEADACHE TREATMENT (note: not all the medications named in this list are available in the United States of America)

1. MIGRAINE

    A. Prophylactic   Treatment: Amitriptyline,   calcium   blocking channel agents; antiprostaglandins (naproxen, flufenamic acid)

    B. Acute Attack:

        1. Common   analgesics: acetaminophen,   ibuprofen,   propoxiphene, flufenamic acid, aspirin.

        2. Ergotamine, Dihydroergotamine subcutaneous or IV.

        3. Oxygen inhalation.

        4. Nonsteroid anti-inflammatory medications as flufenamic acid or indomethacin.

        5. Calcium channel blockers including flunarizine.

        6. Sedatives, hypnotics.

        7. Morphine or meperidine, IM, in few and selected instances for severe migraine status.

        8. Local anesthetic scalp blocks.

        9. Lithium carbonate: cyclical migraine.

        10. Salmon calcitonin

        11. Antiserotonin medications: methysergide, pizotifen.

2. CLUSTER HEADACHE

    A. Prophylactic medications: Prednisone, methysergide, ergotamine, lithium carbonate, calcium channel blockers; histamine desensitation.

    B. Acute attack:

        1. Oxygen therapy

        2. Lidocaine instillation in the sphenopalatine fossa: cocainization of the sphenopalatine ganglion. Indomethacin, tricyclic anti-depressants.

3. CHRONIC PAROXYSMAL HEMICRANEA: indomethacin

4. OPTHALMOPLEGIC MIGRAINE: prednisone, flufenamic acid, ergotamine

5. MUSCLE CONTRACTION HEADACHE: analgesics, muscle relaxants, amitriptyline, TENS unit, biofeedback. Blocking of specific nerves; intramuscular lidocaine block (myofascial pain syndrome) physiotherapy, biofeedback. As prophylactic: amitriptyline and small doses of benzodiazepime.

6. NEURALGIAS: TRIGEMINAL NEURALGIA, GLOSSOPHARYNGEAL NEURALGIA, carbamazepine, phenytoin, baclofen, surgery, blocks. Intranasal application of lidocaine or cocaine for glossopharyngeal neuralgia.

7. HERPES ZOSTER OPTHALMIC NEURALGIA: sympathetic block (stellate ganglion), prednisone, acyclovir, sympaticolytics.

8. COITAL HEADACHE: propranolol

9. EXERTIONAL HEADACHE: indomethacin

10. SYMPATHETIC NEUROVASCULAR DYSFUNCTION: sympaticolytics, sympathetic block, tricyclic antidepressants, anticonvulsants, TENS unit.

11. HEADACHE OF PSYCHIATRIC ORIGIN

    A. Psychotherapy, antidepressants, haloperidol, phenothiazines, benzodiazepines.

12. TEMPOROMANDIBULAR JOINT DYSFUNCTION: muscle relaxant, analgesics, bucal splint, possible surgery

13. TEMPORAL ARTERITIS: prednisone

BIBLIOGRAPHY

1. Packard, R.C.: Foreword, Symposium on Headache. Neurol Clin 1: 359-360, 1983.

2. Stevens, H.: Is it organic or is it functional, is it hysteria or malingering? The Psych Clin of N Am 9: 241-254, 1986.

3. Platonov, K.: La Palabra como Factor Fisiologico y Terapeutico. Ediciones en Lenguas Extranjeras. Moscow 1958.

4. Blumer, D., Heilbronn, M: The pain-prone disorder: A Clinical and Psychological Profile. Psychosomatics 22: 395-402, 1982.

5. Friedman, A.P.: Clinical Approach to the Patient with Headache. Neurol Clin 1: 361-368, 1983.

6. Graham, J.R.: Headache, in: Evaluation and treatment of chronic pain. G.M. Aronoff, Ed. pp 83-130. Urban and Schwarzenberg, Pub., 1985.

7. Lance, J.W., Anthony, M.: The cephalgias, with special reference to vascular and muscle-contraction headaches, in: Scientific Approaches to Clinical Neurology, pp 1959-1979. E.S. Goldenjohn, S.H., Appel, Eds. Leah-Febiger, 1977.

8. Dalessio, D.J.: Headache, in: Textbook of pain. P.D. Wall, R. Melzack, Ed. Churchill Livingstone, Pub. pp 277-292, 1984.

9. Graham, J.R.: Headache, in: Evaluation and Treatment of Chronic Pain. pp 83-130. G.M. Aronoff, Ed. Urban and Schwarzenberg, 1985.

10. Raskin, N.H.: Headache: The Symptom Disease. Sem in Neurol 2: 9-15, 1982.

11. Dalessio, D.J.: Classification and Mechanism of Migraine. Headache 19: 114-126, 1979.

12. Ad Hoc Committee on Classification of Headaches: Special report. JAMA: 717-178, 1982.

13. Evans, R.W.: Postconcussive Syndrome: An Overbiew. Texas Med 83: 49-53, 1987.

14. Ziegler, D.K.: Mechanism of pain in headache. Sem in Neurol 2: 52-58, 1982.

15. Saper, J.R.: Treatment of Chronic Daily Headache. American Academy of Neurology Annual Course #222, K.M. Foley, Director, April 5-1-1987.

16. Hay, K.M.: The treatment of pain trigger areas in migraine. J of the R C of Gen Pract 26: 372-376, 1976.

17. Bakal, D., Kaganov, J.: Muscle contraction and migraine headache: Psychologic and physiologic comparison. Headache 17: 208-214, 1977.

18. Clifford, T., Lauritzen, M., Bakke, M., et.al.: Electromyography of pericranial muscles during treatment of spontaneous common migraine attacks. Pain 14: 137-147, 1982.

19. Bakke, M., Tfelt-Hansen, P., Osesen, J., Moller, E.: Action of some pericranial muscles during provoked attacks of common migraine. Pain 14: 121-135, 1982.

20. Travell, J.G., Simmons, D.G.: Myofascial Pain and Dysfunction. The Trigger Point Manual. Williams and Wilkins, 1983.

21. Speed, W.G.: Post-traumatic headache, in: The practicing physician's approach to headache. Diamond, S., Dalessio, D., Eds. Williams and Wilkins, 1986.

22. Rowe, M.J., Carlson, C.: Brainstem Auditory Evoked Potentials in postconcussion dizziness. Arch of Neurol 37: 679-683, 1980.

23. Noseworthy, J.N., Miller, J., Murray, T.J., Regan, D.: Auditory Brainstem Responses in Postconcussion Syndrome. Arch of Neurol 38: 275-278, 1981.

24. American Psychiatric Association. Diagnostic and Statistical Manual of Mental Disorders (DSM-III-R), 1987.

25. Friedman, A.E.: Symposium on Headache and Related Pain Syndrome. Med Clin of N Am 62: 443-450, 1978.

26. Bleger, J.: Teoria y Practica del Narcoanalisis. El Ateneo, 1952.

27. Torres, J.: Terapeutica por el sueno prolongado. Crespillo, 1959.

28. Rosen, H.: Hypnotherapy in Clinical Psychiatry. Julian Press, 1960.

29. Teitelbaum, H.: Hypnosis. Induction Technics. Ch.C.Thomas, 1980.

30. Campos, M.H.: Hipnosis moderna. Vasquez, 1960.

31. Haley, J.: Advanced Techniques of Hypnosis and Therapy. Selected papers of Milton H. Erickson, M.D. Grune Straton, 1967.

32. Scheneck, J.M.: El Hipnotismo en Medicina Moderna. Diana, 1962.

33. Gindes, B.C.: New Concepts of Hypnosis as an Adjunctant to Psychotherapy and Medicine. George Allen and Unwin, Publishers, 1953.

34. Kaim, B.: Some Dangerous Techniques of Hypnotic Induction. Am J of Clin Hypn 5: 171-176, 1963.

35. Atkinson, R., Appenzeller, O.: Classical, Complicated and Common Migraine: Clinical Features. Sem in Neurol 2: 16-29, 1982.

36. Diamond, S.: Letters to the Editor. Olfactory Aura in Migraine. New Eng J of Med 312: 1390-1391, 1985.

37. Hedges, T.R.: An Opthalmologists View of Headaches. Headache 19: 151-155, 1979.

38. Lauritzen, M., et.al.: Ann of Neurol 13: 633-641, 1983.

39. Peatfield, R.C., Rose, F.C.: Migranous Visual Symptoms in a Woman Without Eyes. Arch of Neurol 38: 466,1981.

40. Friedman, A.P.: Migraine, in: Pathogenesis and treatment of headache. O. Appenzeller, Ed. pp 69-79. Spectrum Publication, 1976.

41. Westmoreland, B.V.: EEG in the evaluation of headaches, in: Current practice of clinical electroencephalography. D.W. Klass, D.D. Daly, Publishers, pp 381-394. Raven Press, 1979.

42. Graham, J.R.: Migraine Headaches: Diagnosis and Management. Headache 19: 133-141, 1979.

43. Dorfman, L.J.: Cerebral Infarction and Migraine, Clinical and Rasiological Correlation. Neurol 29: 317-322, 1979.

44. Lance, J.W., Curran D.A., Anthony M.: Investigations into the mechanism and treatment of chronic headaches. The Med J of Aust 2: 909-914, 1965.

45. Diamond, S., Dalessio, D.J.: The Practicing Physician's Approach to Headache. S. Diamond, D.J. Dalessio. Williams and Wilkins, 1986.

46. Ziegler, D.K., Stuart, R.: Failure of Tyramine to Induce Migraine. Neurol 26: 725-726, 1977.

47. Meyer, J.S., Hardenberg, J.: Clinical effectiveness of calcium entry blockers in prophylactic treatment of migraine and cluster headaches. Headache 23: 266-277, 1983.

48. Rabey, J.M., Vardi, Y., Van Dyck, D., Streifler, M.: Opthalmoplegic Migraine: Amelioration by Flufenamic acid. A Prostaglandin inhibitor. Opthalmologica 175: 148-152, 1977.

49. Troost, B.T., Mark, L.E., Maroon, J.C.: Resolution of Classical Migraine after Removal of an Occipital Lobe AVM. Ann of Neurol 5: 199-201, 1979.

50. Kattah, J.C., Luessenhop, A.J.: Resolution of Classical Migraine After Removal of an Occipital Lobe AVM. Ann of Neurol 7: 93, 1980.

51. Lanzi, G., Grandi, A.M., Gamba, G., et al: Migraine, Mitral Valve Prolapse and Platelet Function in the Pediatric Age Group. Headache 26: 142-148, 1986.

52. Haas, T.C.: Prolonged Migraine Aura Status. Ann of Neurol 11: 197-199, 1982.

53. Kudrow, L.:   Hormones, Pregnancy and Migraine, in: Pathogenesis and Treatment of Headache.   pp 31-41.   O. Appenzeller, Ed.   Spectrum Publications, 1976.

54. Price, R.W., Posner, J.B.:   Chronic Paroxysmal Hemicrania: A Disabiling Headache Syndrome Responding to Indomethacin.   Ann of Neurol 3:   183-184, 1978.

55. Amit, R., Shapiro, Y., Flusser, H., Aker, M.:   Basilar Migraine Manifested as Transient Global Amnesia in a 9 year old child.   Headache 26:   17-18, 1986.

56. Medina, J.A., Diamond, S.:   Cyclical Migraine.   Arch of Neurol 38:   343-344, 1981.

57. Smith, C.D., Reeves, A.G.:   Amelioration of Opthalmologic Migraine by Prednisone: A Case Report.   Headache 26:   93-94, 1986.

58. Zifkin, B., Andermann, E., Andermann, F., Kirkhamt: An Autosomal Dominant Syndrome of Hemiplegic Migraine, Nystagmus and Tremor.   Ann of Neurol 8:   329-332, 1980.

59. Gastaut, J.L., Yermenoi, E., Bonnefoy, M., Cros, D.:   Familial Hemiplegic Migraine: EEG and CT Scan Studies of 2 Cases.   Ann of Neurol 10:   392-395, 1981.

60. Dalessio, D.J.:   Headache and Face Pain.   American Academy of Neurology: Annual Course #222, Pain and Headache.   K.J. Foley, Director.   April 1987.

61. Couch, J.R., Hassanein, R.S.: Amitriptyline in Migraine Prophylaxis. Arch of Neurol 36:   695-699, 1979.

62. Patti, F., Scapagnini, U., Nicoletti, F., et.al.:   Calcitonine and Migraine.   Headache 26:   172-174, 1986.

63. Gelmers, H.J.:   Nimodipine, a New Calcium Antagonist, in the Prophylactic Treatment of Migraine.   Headache 23:   106-109, 1983.

64. Bonuso, S., DiStasio, E., Marano, E., et.al.: Sublingual Flurarizines: A New Effective Management of the Migraine Attack, Comparison Versus Ergotamine. Headaches 26: 227-230, 1986.

65. Rascol, A., Montastruc, J.L., Rascol, O.: Flunarizine vs. Pizotifen: A Double Blind Study in the Prophylaxis of Migraine. Headache 26: 227-230, 1986.

66. Welch, K.M.A., Ellis, D.J., Keenan, P.A.: Successful migraine prophylaxis with Naproxen Sodium. Neurol 35: 1304-1310, 1985.

67. Vardi, Y., Rabey, I.M., Streifler, M.: Migraine Attacks: Alleviation by an Inhibitor of Prostaglandin Synthesis and Action. Neurol 26: 447-450, 1976.

68. Raskin, N.H.: Repetitive Intravenous KiHydroergotamine as Therapy for Intractible Migraine. Neurol 36: 995-997, 1986.

69. Appenzeller, O.: Cerebrovascular aspects of headache. Med Clin of N Am 62: 467-480, 1978.

70. Kudrow, L.: Cluster Headaches: A New Concept. Neurol Clin 1: 360-384, 1983.

71. Bernat, J.L.: Cluster Headaches from Isosorbide Dimitride. Ann of Neurol 6: 554-555, 1979.

72. Couch, Jr., J.R.: Cluster Headache: Characteristics and Treatment. Sem in Neurol 2: 32-40, 1982.

73. Fogan, L.: Treatment of Cluster Headaches. Arch of Neurol 42: 362-363, 1985.

74. Kittrell, A.P., et.al.: Cluster Headache. Local Anesthetic Abortive Agents. Arch of Neurol 42: 496-498, 1985.

75. Medina, J.L., Fareed, J., Diamond, S.: Lithium Carbonate Therapy for Cluster Headache: Changes in Number of Platelets and Serotonine and Histamine Levels. Arch of Neurol 37: 559-563, 1980.

76. Medina, J.L., Diamond, S.: Cluster Headache Variant Expectant of a New Headache Syndrome. Arch of Neurol 38: 705-709, 1981.

77. Diamond, S., Freitag, F.G., Prager, J., Gandhi, S.: Treatment of Intractable Cluster. Headache 26: 42-46, 1986.

78. Bussone, J., Sinatra, M.G., Boiardi, A., et.al.: Brainstem Auditory Evoked Potentials (BAERPs) in Cluster Headache (CH). New Aspects for a Central Theory. Headache 26: 67-69, 1986.

79. Boiardi, A., Carenini, L., Frediani, F., et.al.: Visual Evoked Potentials in Cluster Headaches: Central Structures Involvement. Headache 26: 70-73, 1986.

80. Devoize, J.L., Rigal, F., Eschalier, A., Tournilhac, M.: Dexamethasone Suppression Test in Cluster Headaches. Headache 26: 126-127, 1986.

81. J.R. Saper, Ed.: Temporal Arteritis: The atypical may be the normal. Topics in Pain Management 1: 18-19, 1985.

82. Fromm, J.H., Terrence, C.F., Maroon, J.C.: Trigeminal Neuralgia: Current Concepts Regarding Etiology and Pathogenesis. Arch of Neurol 41: 1204-1209, 1984.

83. Iraguii, V.J., Wiederholt, W.C., Romine, J.S.: Evoked Potentials in Trigeminal Neurolgia Associated with Multiple Sclerosis. Arch of Neurol 43: 444-446, 1986.

84. Stohr, M.D., Petruch, F., Scheglemann, K.: Somatosensory Evoked Potential Following Trigeminal Nerve Stimulation in Trigeminal Neuralgia. Ann of Neurol 9: 63-66, 1981.

85. Tomson, T., Tybring, G., Bertilsson, L., et.al.: Carbamazepine Therapy in Trigeminal Neuralgia. Arch of Neurol 37: 699-703, 1980.

86. Fromm, G.H., Terrence, C.F., Chattaha, A.S., Glass, J.D.: Baclofen in Trigeminal Neuralgia, Its Effects on the Spinal Trigeminal Nucleus: A Pilot Study. Arch of Neurol 37: 768-771, 1980.

87. Tew, J., Keller, J.:   Percutaneous Rhizotomy in the treatment of intractable facial pian, in: Pain Management.   Synmposium on the Neurosurgical Treatment of Pain.   pp 145-165.   Lee, J.F., Ed.   The Williams and Wilkins Co., 1977.

88. Landsford, L.D., Bennet, M.H., Martinez, J.:   Experimental Trigeminal Glycerol Injection: Electrophysiologic and morphologic effects. Arch of Neurol 42: 146-149, 1986.

89. Mokri, B.: Raeder's Paratrigeminal Syndrome. Arch of Neurol 39: 295-299, 1982.

90. Atkinson, R., Appenzeller, O.: Classical, complicated and common migraine: Clinical Features. Sem in Neurol 2: 16-29, 1982.

91. Cohen, D.N., Zakove, Z.N., Salanga, V.D., Dohn, D.:   Raeder's Paratrigeminal Syndrome. Am J of Opth 79: 1044-1049, 1975.

92. Davis, J.N., Thomas, P.K., Spalding, J.M.K., Harrison, M.S.:   "Diseases of the ninth, tenth, eleventh and twelfth cranial nerves", in: Peripheral Neurology (chapter 29).   P.J. Dyck, P.K. Thomas, E.H. Lambert, Eds.   W.B. Saunders Co., 1975.

93. Adams, R.D., Victor M.:   Headache and other craniofacial pains. Principles of Neurology, McGraw Hill, 95-111, 1977.

94. Bruyn, G.W.: Superior Laryngeal Neuralgia.   Cephalalgia 3:   235-240, 1983.

95. Frank, R.A.: Cranial Neuralgias, in: Neurologic Clinics, W.B. Saunders Co., Publishers, 1: 501-509, 1983.

96. Carter, J.E.: Opthalmic and neuro-opthalmic aspects of headache and neck pain. Neurol Clin 1: 415-443, 1983.

97. Behrens, M.M.: Headaches Associated with Disorders of the Eyes. Med Clin of N Am, 507-521, 1978.

98. Vaughan, D., Sahbury, T.:   General opthalmology.   Lange Medical

Publications, 1974.

99. Smith, J.L.: Migraine, in: Neuro-opthalmology update. J.L. Smith, Ed. Masson Publishing Co., 1977.

100. Walsh, F.B., Hoyt, W.B.: Clinical Neuro-opthalmology. The Williams and Wilkins Co., 1969.

101. Coppeto, J.R., Hoffman, H.: Tolosa-Hunt Syndrome with Proptosis Mimicked by Giant Aneurysm of Posterior Cerebral Artery. Arch of Neurol 38: 5455, 1981.

102. Evans, O.B., Lexow, S.S.: Painful opthalmoplegia in systemic lupus erythematosus. Ann of Neurol 4: 584-585, 1978.

103. Polsky, M., Janicki, P.C., Gunderson, C.H.: Tolosa-Hunt Syndrome with Sellar Erosion. Ann of Neurol 6: 129-131, 1979.

104. Joseph, D.J., Renner, G.: Head pain from diseases of the ear, nose and throat. Neurol Clin 1: 399-414, 1983.

105. Ross, G.S., Wolf, J.K., Chipman, M.: The Neuralgias, in: Clinical Neurology, Chapter 52. A.B. Baker, R.J. Joynt, Eds. Harper and Row, Publishers, 1985.

106. Bell, W.T.: Temporomandibular Disorders. Yearbook Medical Publishers, 1986.

107. Hart, R.G., Carter, J.E.: Pseudotumor cerebri and facial pain. Arch of Neurol 39: 440-442, 1982.

108. Martin, R.J., Block, A.J., Cohn, M.A., et.al.: Indications and standard for cardiopulmonary sleep studies. Sleep 8: 371-379, 1985.

109. Mathew, N.T., Glaze, D., Frost, J.: Sleep apnea and other sleep abnormalities in primary headache, in: Migraine, clinical and research advances. F.C. Rose, Ed. pp 40-49, Karger, 1985.

110. Andermann, F., Lugaresi, E.:   Clinical Features of Migraine-Epilepsy Syndrome, in: Migraine and Epilepsy. pp3-30. Butterworth Publishers, 1987.

111. Panayiotopoulos, C.P.: Difficulties in Differentiating Migraines and Epilepsy Based on Clinical and EEG Findings. pp 31-46 in: Migraine and Epilepsy. Andermann and Lugaresi. Butter worth Publishers, 1987.

112. Gastaut, H., Zifkin, B.G.: Benign Epilepsy of childhood with occipital spike and wave complexes.   pp 47-81 in: Migraine and Epilepsy. Andermann and Lugaresi, Eds. Butterworth Publishers, 1987.

113. Bladin, P.F.: The association of benign Rolandic epilepsy with migraine, in: Migraine and Epilepsy. pp 145-152. Andermann and Lugaresi, Eds. Butterworth Publishers, 1987.

114. Sacquegua,   T.,   Cortelli,   P.,   Valdrati,   A.,   et.al.: Electroencephalographic observations on migraine and transient global amnesia, confusional migraine, and migraine and epilepsy, in: Migraine and Epilepsy: 153-161.   Andermann and Lugaresi, Eds.   Butterworth Publishers, 1987.

115. Diamond, S.: Recurrent Exertional Headache. JAMA 237:   580, 1977.

116. Sacks, H., Wolf, A., Jerome, A.G., et.al.:   Effect of Reserpine on regional cerebral glucose metabolism in control and migraine subjects. Arch of Neurol 43:   1117-1123, 1986.

117. Porter, M., Jankovic, J.:   Benign Coital Cephalgia.   Differential Diagnosis and Treatment. Arch of Neurol 38:   710-712, 1981.

118. Johns, D.: Benign Sexual Headache within a Family. Arch of Neurol 43: 1158-1160, 1986.

119. Payne, E.R.:   Reflex Sympathetic Dystrophy Pain.   American Academy of Neurology Annual Course #222. Pain and Headache, K.M. Foley, Director. April, 1987.

120. Tabira, T., Shibasaki, H., Kuroiwa, Y.: Reflex Sympathetic Dystrophy, (Causalgia): Treatment with Guanethidine. Arch of Neurol 40: 430-432, 1983.

121. Jaeger, B., Singer, E., Kroening R.: Reflex Sympathetic Dystrophy of the Face. Arch of Neurol 43: 693-695, 1986.

122. Vijayan, N., Dreyfus, P.M.: Post-traumatic Dysautonomic Cephalgia. Clinical Observations on Treatment. Arch of Neurol 32: 649-652, 1975.

123. Khurana, R.K., Nirankari, U.S.: Bilateral Sympathetic Dysfunction in Post-Traumatic Headaches. Headaches 26: 183-188, 1986.

124. Cole, M.: Examination of the cerebrospinal fluid, pp 30-47, in: Special Techniques for Neurologic Diagnosis. J.F. Toole, Ed. Contemporary Neurology Series. David, 1969.

125. Kovanen, J., Sulkava, R.: Duration of postural headache after lumbar puncture: Effect of needle size. Headache 26: 224-226, 1986.

126. Henry, G.G., Little, N.L.: Headache, (chapter 7), in: Neurologic Emergencies, McGraw-Hill Book Co., 1985.

127. Hatfield, W.B.: Headache associated with metabolic and systemic disorders. Med Clin of N Am 63: 451-458, 1978.

128. Kudrow, L.: A distinctive facial thermographic pattern in cluster headache. The "chai" pattern sign, in: Medical Thermology, pp 50-55. M. Abernathy, S. Vematsu, Eds. American Academy of Thermology, 1986.

129. Basmajian, J.V.: Anatomical and Physiological basis for Biofeedback of Autonomic Regulation Biofeedback, in: Principles and Practice for Clinitians. Williams and Wilkins, 1983.

130. Brenneke, H.F.: Autogenic training in: Handbook of innovative psychotherapies, (chapter 5). R. Corsini, Ed. Wiley-Interscience Publication, 1981.

131. Wolpe, J., Salter, A., Reyna, L.J.: The conditioning therapies. Holt, Reinhart and Winston, Eds., 1964.

132. Wolpe, J.: Psychotherapy by reciprocal inhibition. Stanford University Press, 1958.

133. Diamond, S.: Biofeedback and Headache. Neurol Clin 1: 479-488, 1983.

134. Long, D.M.: Transcutaneous Electrical Stimulation in the treatment of chronic and acute pain, pp 54-64, in: Pain Management. J.F. Lee, Ed. Williams and Wilkins, 1977.

135. Mannheimer, J.S., Lampe, G.N.: Clinical Transcutaneous Electrical Nerve Stimulation. F.A. Davis Company, 1984.

PSYCHOSOMATIC ILLNESS AND THE GERIATRIC PATIENT

Jary Lesser, M.D.

Assistant Professor of Psychiatry

University of Texas

Health Science Center At
Houston

PSYCHOSOMATIC ILLNESS AND THE GERIATRIC PATIENT

Part I

    A.   Factors influencing symptom presentation

        1.   Sociocultural

        2.   Psychodynamic

        3.   Cognitive Status

        4.   Perceptual and Propioceptive

        5.   Normal Physiology

    B.   Ambiguous presentations of psychiatric disorder

        1.   Dementia, pseudodementia, and pseudo-depression

        2.   Other atypical depressions

Part II

Psychosomatic and somatopsychic

    A.   Chronic pain

    B.   Hypochondriasis

    C.   Psychosomatic disorders per se

Conclusion

PSYCHOSOMATIC ILLNESS AND THE GERIATRIC PATIENT

Jary Lesser, M.D.

INTRODUCTION

Elderly patients are frequently puzzling and frustrating to clinicians. The older person may present with a variety of physical and emotional symptoms which seem to multiply and become less well defined as the examination proceeds. In this connection, it is important to recognize that many elderly persons conceptualize and communicate differently than do their younger counterparts. Words such as "fever," "numbness," "depression," and "nerves" may have a variety of meanings, and the clinician may be easily misled. Cognitive impairment, may further impair communication and increase ambiguity. When one adds to this multiple illnesses and medications, the diagnostic problems may be formidable.

In this chapter, I would like to cover two broad areas: First, the general problem of the intermingling of psychic and physical symptomatology in the elderly, and, second, psychosomatic illness per se as it presents in old age.

FACTORS INFLUENCING SYMPTOM PRESENTATION

Sociocultural Factors

It is well known that the elderly are the most heterogeneous of human groups, yet certain generalizations are possible. The existing cohort of persons aged 65 to 75 in the U.S. have 7.5 years of education as opposed to 11.3 years for those 55 to 65 (1). There are qualitative as well as quantitative differences, as education has changed radically, and this is even more dramatic for persons over 75 years of age. The effect of this educational gap is reflected in vocabulary, general knowledge, and conceptions of mental and physical health. Limited education seems to be associated with a greater tendency to attribute symptoms to physical illness and to code psychic distress as somatic complaint although the matter is far from clear (2). Elderly persons have, in many cases, also grown up in settings where emotional problems and expression of feelings are stigmatized. In some cases the older person has only the vague conceptualization of emotions such as sadness, fear and anger. Consequently it is common for both the clinician and the patient to be confused about the nature of symptoms.

Psychodynamic Factors

It has been suggested that the senium may be associated with limited regression and strengthening of narcissistic tendencies (3). Regression may take the form of recathexis of oral and anal needs and preoccupation with digestion and elimination (4), as well as a general withdrawal of investment from the external world with concomitant egocentricity. The result of this is a tendency to express all distress as somatic complaint and to invest the clinician with magical powers, expecting him to make a diagnosis with minimal data.

Cognitive Status

A substantial fraction of elderly people have some degree of cognitive impairment, this being especially common in the physically ill and in the group over 75 (5). This cognitive loss may be subtle, and may be clinically discernible only as deficit in judgment and in abstracting ability and as circumstantiality. Cognitive impairment is often associated with personality change, and the use of more primitive defense mechanism. Defenses often seen in cognitively impaired elderly include projection, denial, and somatization (6). This last becomes particularly obvious and transparent in patients with manifest dementia (case vignette).

CASE VIGNETTE

Mrs. L was a 73 year old polish born woman with a fifth grade education, brought to outpatient clinic by her sister. The patient's chief complaint was "my head, my stomach, and my vagina. They hurt." The patient had been having fluctuating memory problems for about two years coupled with intermittent somatic complaints for the same period. The patient had been evaluated at a medical clinic within the last month and no physical basis for her somatic complaints could be found. However, a dementia workup was done and a tentative diagnosis of primary degenerative dementia was made. Significantly, she was not described as particular scored 8 of 10 correct on the pfeiffer scale. Digit span was 5 forward and 2 reverse. She remembered two of three objects at 5 minutes. Subtraction of serial these was done with two errors but she could not perform serial sevens. She was concrete both in discussing the details of the last two years. She frequently could not remember significant events and became confused in the order of occurrence of events. She was not overtly psychotic. She stoutly maintained that her memory was perfect and insisted that there was nothing wrong with her mind. The problem being her head, stomach and vagina.

It was noted that the patient was taking at least seven different medications unpredictably and irregularly and because of this polypharmacy as well as for further evaluation, she was hospitalized.

In the hospital a full scale dementia work-up was done including C.T. scan, EEG, blood chemistries, thyroid function, B 12 and folate screen, serology, chest X-ray and EKG. All of this was noncontributory with CT. Findings of mild atrophy and EEG findings of generalized slowing.

An OB-Gyn consultation was requested for evaluation of vaginal and abdominal pain. The consultant's opinion was chronic pain secondary to pelvic adhesions and atrophic vaginitis, and Premarin cream per applicator was prescribed. Biofeedback treatment was instituted for the chronic pain and the patient was begun on low-dose doxepin and haloperidol. On this program, her somatic complaints receded but again peaked as discharge approached. At follow-up she was less hostile but still multiply somatic. Although complaining less. Final impression was of probable primary degenerative dementia with exaggerated response to chronic pain.

Subsequent follow-up of this patient over an 18 month period has demonstrated progressively more obvious cognitive impairment with frank disorientation and perseveration.

Physical Illness

Clearly, the elderly are at greater risk for chronic disease and are attuned to respiratory, cardiac, arthritic and gastrointestinal symptoms. Preoccupation with such symptoms and need for reassurance may result in the older person's communication being largely restricted to physical complaints, so that these contaminate even unrelated issues.

Physical Signs and Symptoms of Disease

The localization and specificity of pain may become impaired in the elderly. For example, documented myocardial infarction was found to be associated with chest pain in only 19% of cases of elderly persons. (7). The acute abdomen is also often pain free in the elderly (8).

Other signs and symptoms of disease may become muted or aberrant in old age. The aging body is less capable of mustering a febrile response to infection so that pneumonia, pyelonephritis and even subacute bacterial endocarditis can be afebrile (8).

On the other hand, there are certain general responses to dysfunction that serve as a subtle, if nonspecific message that all is not well. Mental confusion may be literally the only symptom of disturbances as various as sepsis, coronary occlusion, malignancy, and simple dehydration (8). It is as though the aged brain is the most sensitive indicator of changes in the internal milieu.

SLEEP

In the elderly, complaints of frequent awakening, and of general sleep disturbance tend to increase, as does use of sedative hypnotic agents (9). These complaints are more common in women, in the physically ill, and in persons with manifest psychopathology (9). In their 1980 review Miles and Dement point out that polysomnographic studies of the elderly consistently reveal specific patterns. Total time in bed is both subjectively and objectively increased whereas total sleep time tends to be reduced. Further, there is both an absolute and relative reduction in time spent in stage IV sleep. Rapid eye movement (REM) sleep, on the other hand, tends to be fragmented in the elderly with characteristic awakenings roughly every 90 minutes.

All of these changes while variable, are considered to be normal for the senium. However, the patterns described are greatly exaggerated in demented persons with marked decrements in stage 4, REM and REM density (9, 10, 11). Also, while elderly persons may complain of insomnia through ignorance of normal age changes in sleep, it is noteworthy that documented sleep apnea and/or nocturnal myoclonus exist in many subjects in a sample of healthy, asymptomatic elderly (9). Clearly disturbed sleep may be an important symptom of an underlying psychiatric or medical problem.

Specific psychiatric conditions associated with sleep disturbance include dementia, anxiety disorders, and depression. In dementia, regardless of cause, there is an exaggeration of normal age changes in sleep architecture with commonly associated nocturnal confusion and agitation. In severe dementia, the sleep wake cycle is virtually reversed with excessive daytime napping and minimal nocturnal sleep (9). Major depression is classically associated with initial, middle, and terminal insomnia (12).

Sleep studies reveal shortened REM latency in major depressives, and attempts are being made to use this as a biological marker for endogenous depression (13). Anxiety disorders, on the other hand, have much more variable sleep symptomatology probably reflecting their heterogeneity (14).

While it is beyond the scope of this chapter to consider the organic and medical causes of disturbed sleep, some of the more important entities should be discussed. Physical illnesses contributing to sleep disturbance include arthritis, congestive heart failure with paroxysmal nocturnal dyspnea, nocturnal angina, hypothyroidism and chronic obstructive pulmonary disease (13, 16). Clearly, the major management of this kind of sleep difficulty is treatment of the underlying disorder. The specific sleep pathology I would like to consider in greater detail is sleep apnea.

The sleep apnea syndrome consists of three subtypes; upper airway obstructive, central, and mixed (16). The upper airway variety is due to any lesion or process which compromises the patency of the upper airway. Such conditions include obesity with pickwickian syndrome, acromegaly, amyloydosis, poliomyelitis and the Shy-Drager syndrome (16). The etiology of central sleep apnea is uncertain.

Symptoms include loud snoring, restlessness during sleep, and morning headaches (16). Clearly the diagnosis is tricky and can only be made definitively in a sleep laboratory. The need for proper diagnosis is underscored by evidence linking sleep apnea with sudden death, cardiac decompensation, and cognitive impairment (16). Treatment must be individualized and since the majority of sleep apneas are obstructive, treatment of the underlying condition may ameliorate the problem. Tracheostomy is always an alternative to be considered (17) [Table I]. There is evidence that sedative hypnotic agents may increase the number of apneic episodes and for this reason are contraindicated. Again, it should be stressed that occult sleep apnea can be found to exist in 40% of asymptomatic elderly, so that routine use of sedative hypnotics in this population is a questionable practice.

Nocturnal myoclonus is a disorder often found in East-European and Mediterranean Jews, consisting of repetitive myoclonic movements of the lower extremities, often associated with disturbed sleep. The incidence that tricyclic antidepressants can worsen such movements and clearly are contraindicated in this condition (18).

In terms of management of geriatric insomnias, it is important to rule out conditions such as depression, dementia, and undiagnosed medical problems. In dementia, for example, use of a sedative-hypnotic is likely to cause increased confusion and agitation whereas low dose antipsychotic medication is the treatment of choice.

If one must use a sedative-hypnotic agent in the elderly lower dose and shorter acting non-barbiturate agents are recommended (19).

SEXUALITY

Much remains to be learned about sexual function in the healthy older adult. There is a general consensus that sexual interest and activity continue throughout the lifespan, that slowed sexual activity is to be expected with advancing age and that there is tremendous inter-individual variability (1,20). The older male requires a greater (minutes rather than seconds), time to achieve erection, and time to ejaculation (plateau phase) is also increased.

The refractory period (length of time required to restore ability to achieve a subsequent erection) also increases significantly (20). Finally, the erection in old age is less full and it is not uncommon for the erect penis to point down rather than up.

Less is known about consistent changes in sexual function in the healthy older woman. The two most important factors leading to reduced sexual interest and behavior seem to be absence of an available partner and dyspareunia secondary to atrophic vaginitis (20). Needless to say, this second problem is remediable.

Impotence is a not infrequent complaint in elderly males and should never be dismissed as trivial. Though some of such cases are psychogenic, the clinician should not overlook organic causes such as diabetes mellitus, cord lesions, alcoholism, post-prostatectomy and, iatrogenic impotence. (guanethidine, reserpine, thioridazine). Post myocardial infarct and post-cerebrovascular accident status, often make the affected male functionally impotent via his fear of precipitating another vascular accident. In this case, appropriate information and counselling may help the problem. Nonorganic cause of impotence run the gamut from cultural attitudes and misinformation to major psychiatric illness.

As an example of the former many elderly people have been indoctrinated with the idea that with age people become asexual and that sexual activity in the senium is indecent, unnatural and shameful. Society and adult children tend to reinforce these ideas with stereotypes of the "dirty old man" and the like. Considerable time and effort may be required to modify these attitudes. Added to these problems are concerns with appearance and changes in body image, again largely generated by societal propaganda.

The most significant major psychiatric illness associated with impotence is depression. As described in a later section, depression in the elderly may not present with classic symptoms and may go undiagnosed. Major depression is certainly one of the treatable causes of impotence.

GASTROINTESTINAL COMPLAINTS

Constipation is a nearly ubiquitous complaint of the elderly but it can be both a genuine problem and symptom of disease, but other possibilities must be considered first.

First, there is definitely some decline in bowel motility with age (20). In addition to this, however, many elderly people have grown up with the belief that one must evacuate one's bowels every day and that failure to do so will lead to absorption of "poisons." This leads many older people to abuse laxatives and enemas to the point of actually reducing bowel motility. A third element is exercise. With age, many persons become sedentary and this may be accentuated by arthritis, claudication or other impairment.

Diet also contributes with insufficient fiber. Finally, the effect of medication must not be minimized; many preparations have considerable anticholinergic effect and can worsen constipation. Tricyclic antidepressants, lower potency phenothiazines and antiparkinson drugs are special offenders.

Another element contribution to the ubiquity of complaints of constipation is the psychology of the aging process. For many (though certainly not all) people, the senium is a period of regression. This regression probably exists in part, as a response to the stresses and losses of aging; decreased physical well-being, decreased or slowed ability to process information, feelings of being out of touch with society, and losses of friends and relatives. Regression is a retreat to earlier, or more primitive psychological modes of coping. A preoccupation with the gastrointestinal tract can be one expression of this regression and elimination has symbolic connections with issues of control and of mastery. Thus the older person who feels powerless, frustrated and defeated may focus on constipation and other bowel complaints, becoming almost obsessively preoccupied with them.

AMBIGUOUS PRESENTATIONS OF PSYCHIATRIC ILLNESS

Dementia, pseudodementia and pseudodepression. While it is clear that major depression may coexist with dementia (21, 22) there is still much confusion about the relationship of these two syndromes. Problems arise because the two entities may mimic each other, because of the difficulty of eliciting subjective mood descriptions from demented patients, and because of the clinician's tendency to view one illness as "primary."

In line with the bias towards making a single primary diagnosis, very little has been written about incidence and frequency of these coexisting disorders. Riefler, et al, (23), in a study of geriatric out patients with cognitive deficits found coexisting depression in 30%, with a tendency for depression to develop early in the course of the dementia. Ron and co-workers (24) in a sample of 33 patients, found significant depression in 30%. Unfortunately, in both studies, it is impossible to know how many of these patients had presumptive dementia of Alzheimer's type (DAT).

It is accepted lore that cognitive impairment reduces one's ability to recognize and report subjective mood. Very little systematic work has been done examining symptoms of depression accompanied by dementia, and confirmation of a true depressive state may depend upon a successful therapeutic trial.

In general, depression is more commonly atypical in the elderly. Atypical presentations may take the form of hypochondriasis, pseudoconfusion, and failure to thrive without subjective sadness. It is logical that a coexisting dementia would increase the probability of such an atypical picture. To our knowledge, however, this question has been addressed only in anecdotal reports. This is not to say that depression is invariably difficult to recognize:

Mrs. W., and 89 year old woman residing in a nursing home, had been followed for one year in an outpatient geriatric psychiatry clinic. She had a 5-6 year history of progressive dementia and was disoriented to time, and demonstrated impaired recent memory, and judgment. She had multiple somatic complaints that tended to increase as her memory was tested. There was no insight into her memory was defect. Her mood was cheerful and sleep and appetite good. Very little past history could be obtained but there was a vague suggestion of previous episodes of depression.

Shortly after she entered the clinic, it was noted that she had been receiving thioridazine 25 mg q a.m. and amitriptyline 25 mg at H.S. Concerned about the anticholinergic effect with already compromised cognition, the treating psychiatrist discontinued both psychotropic agents. At the patient's next clinic visit, one month later, she was noted to be tearful, withdrawn and irritable, sleep and appetite were both impaired. She had also developed a mood-congruent delusion that she had become blind. In addition, there was a clear diurnal variation. Cognitive functioning on mental status was no different than on her previous visit. Both the thioridazine and amitriptyline were restarted and two weeks later, the tearfulness and withdrawal had largely disappeared, and the delusional thinking was much attenuated. While she was slightly less preoccupied, her cognition remained essentially the same. The case vignette illustrates the differentiability of depressive and dementia symptoms, and the existence of classic symptoms of melancholia in an at least moderately demented patients. The case also raises another important point: that of the value of reliable past psychiatric history. If documentation could have been obtained, it might have been established that this patient had been subject to recurrent episodes of depression and needed her maintenance medications.

Pseudodementia is a syndrome that describes symptoms of organic brain syndrome which are in fact due to a functional illness, usually depression. Pseudodementia may also be found in brief reactive psychoses, hysterical conversion and dissociative reactions. Intrinsic to the concept is the idea that the functional illness is primary and the cognitive symptoms completely reversible with its resolution. In various series, 18-57% of patients initially labeled demented have been found to be misdiagnosed and, in fact, have pseudodementia (25). Wells (26) lists important clinical features relatively specific to pseudodementia as vigorous complaint of poor memory, clear detailed responses to open-ended questions coupled with "I don't know" responses to directive questions, prominence of depressive or anxious as opposed to shallow affect, absence of nocturnal worsening, and inconsistencies of performance. Wells also notes in his sample a great component of dependency in premorbid functioning.

McAllister (21) stresses that the syndrome is not homogenous with depressive pseudodementia closely resembling a diffuse OBS and hysterical syndromes producing a more dramatic "caricature." He also makes the point that coexisting previous organic brain syndrome seems to predispose to development of pseudodementia. Several authors have concluded that the concept is not helpful in that clinicians are encouraged to dichotomously regard patients as either "demented" or "pseudodemented" with no shades of gray. Folstein et al. (27), argue that a trial of antidepressant medication in an elderly patient may improve some cognitive functioning, but that some residual impairment may remain.

Depressive pseudodmentia as well as depression coexisting with DAT are responsive to all of the currently available pharmacologic modalities. Clearly, an important factor in choice of tricyclic, with such a patient, is anticholinergic effect. In this regard, the secondary amines, desipramine and nortriptyline, are preferred to tertiary amines, such as amitriptyline and imipramine. The usual cautions observed in geriatric patients, cardiac conduction defects, orthostatic hypotension, and urinary retention, of course, also apply. [Table II]

OTHER ATYPICAL DEPRESSIONS

The current criteria on mood disorders of the diagnostic and statistical manual of the American Psychiatric Association (DSM-III-R) is discussed elsewhere in this book.

Not surprisingly, in the elderly, depression is rarely this clear cut. In addition to pseudodementia, several other atypical presentations are found. Essentially, these consist of 1.) masked depression 2.) hypochondriasis and 3.) paranoid or psychotic depression. Masked depression and hypochondriasis are each treated elsewhere in this chapter. Psychotic and paranoid depressions merit some discussion.

Elderly persons are at great risk for the development of persecutory ideas. These can be found in association with dementia, hearing impairment, and isolation (29). The very real vulnerability and dependency of many elder also lends it self to a paranoid stance. Finally the social stigmatization of western societies can contribute to feelings of worthlessness with corresponding desperate (if primitive) efforts to preserve self esteem via use of projection (30, 31). With all these factors, it is fairly easy for paranoid delusions to contaminate geriatric depression. Sometimes this contamination is so extreme that is is unclear whether one is dealing with an affective disorder or a paranoid disorder.

Of course, when psychotic manifestations accompany depression, whether mood congruent or incongruent, consideration should be given to use of a neuroleptic with the antidepressant, or to electro-convulsive therapy.

Finally, occasionally it is difficult to distinguish depression from an anxiety disorder in the elderly. Once again, the major problems seem to be poor verbal skills and/or psychological-mindedness, and the vagueness of symptoms and signs that comes with age. Words used to describe the feeling state are "worried," "nervous," or "afraid." There is often a component of anxiety in geriatric depression, but usually the mood is clearly one of sadness. Occasionally where the mood state is bland, one may need to pay more attention to neurovegetative signs to make the correct diagnosis.

HYPOCHONDRIASIS

The third edition of the diagnostic and statistical manual of mental disorders (DSM III-R) defines hypochondriasis as preoccupation with the fear or belief of having a serious disease based on an unrealistic interpretation of physical signs or sensations as abnormal. This unrealistic fear or belief persists despite medical reassurance, and causes impairment in social or occupational functioning. The disorder must not be due to any other mental disorder (schizophrenia, affective disorder, somatization disorder). Additionally, of course physical disorders must be ruled out as causing the patient's symptoms. While controversy continues regarding the validity of the specific diagnostic entity, it has been found useful to divide hypochondriasis into primary and secondary categories (32). Primary hypochondriasis would represent the DSM III criteria as described above whereas secondary hypochondriasis is the syndrome as either a manifestation of another of another psychiatric illness or as a transient situational adjustment reaction.

The primary hypochondriac typically has a history extending back over many years and is more likely to come from a lower socioeconomic background. Complaints often involve the musculoskeletal, gastrointestinal, or central nervous systems. These patients tend to present certain personality features such as obsessionality, anxiety proneness and dependency (32). Indeed, it has been suggested that the hypochondriacal complaints offer the patient an unconscious solution to dependency/autonomy conflicts by providing an acceptable avenue for dependent status (32).

Secondary hypochondriacal symptoms may be associated with depression, organic brain syndromes with or without coexisting psychosis, and with the functional psychoses, particularly schizophrenia.

In the elderly, hypochondriacal complaints are, of course, quite common. In the evaluation of the elderly hypochondriacal patient, it is crucial to make this distinction between primary and secondary syndromes, as management will be quite different. The most important bit of information in doing this is the past psychiatric history. Primary hypochondriacs have a long history of multiple somatic complaints, multiple physician contacts disability and, often, dependent behavior. Secondary hypochondriacs give a history of somatic complaints either beginning with the present illness or as an intensification of previous patterns. Secondary hypochondriasis in the elderly can be broken down into the following categories: 1). masked or atypical depression, 2). manifestation of dementia 3). symptom of schizophrenic or schizophreniform psychosis 4). transient adjustment reaction. These categories are, of course, not mutually exclusive. Each of them will be discussed briefly below.

Masked Depression represents depressive illness with little or no subjective or objective mood disorder (33).
In these cases, patients manifest their depression through somatization. Emotional symptoms are either denied or presented vaguely with words such as "worry" and "nervousness," but with little ability to describe what these words mean. Neurovegetative signs of depression, however, are usually prominent and patients frequently report middle and terminal insomnia, decreased energy and interest, poor appetite and weight loss. There may even be crying spells which the patient is at a loss to explain.

It is felt that a major factor in this clinical picture is sociocultural and childhood learning (33). Many of these patients seem to have grown up in settings where emotional expression is devalued or where perception of physical and mental phenomena are poorly differentiated. Since many elderly people of the current cohort have come form this sort of situation, it is not surprising that masked depression is quite common in geriatrics.

The treatment of masked depression does not differ from that of the classic variety except that compliance may be a problem. While some patients are receptive to education, others may strenuously resist any suggestion that theirs is an emotional problem. General speaking, it is more productive to focus on the neurovegetative signs and general sense of well-being. These patients, of course, should be treated by a psychiatrist.

Hypochondriasis as a symptom of dementia has been addressed earlier. The only thing that should be added is that somatic complaints are occasionally the early symptoms of a developing dementia. Later, of course, cognitive impairment is clearer.

As a symptom of schizophrenia. A percentage of schizophrenic patients may have hypochondriacal complaints sometimes to the point of bizarre somatic delusions. These features reflect the primitive defenses and archaic thought processes in schizophrenia. Diagnosis is usually simple and the clinician will find prominent delusions, hallucinations, and fragmented thinking, as well as a long history of mental illness. An unusual syndrome is the entity of paraphrenia. This is a late appearing psychosis clinically resembling paranoid schizophrenia and often associated with hearing loss (34). Paraphrenia is much more common in women, generally appears in the late fifties to seventies and shows a moderate response to neuroleptic. As with schizophrenia, hypochondriacal complaints can be found but are clearly part of the psychosis (35).

Adjustment Reactions

In the elderly adjustment reactions often take the form of increased bodily concern. There may or may not be a previous pattern of hypochondriasis but the complaints are found to have worsened and exploration will usually uncover significant life stresses. Simple ventilation coupled perhaps with short term antidepressant medication may be sufficient. continued focussing on, and medical evaluation of somatic complaints can be counter productive as a pattern is set and ventilation of feelings discouraged (36).

It must be remembered that the aging organism has reduced functional reserve capacity (37). In addition, the quality of stress is different in old age, the major stressors being illness, loss, and financial difficulty (38, 39). Thus, the older person is both constitutionally and situationally less able to mount an active, effective response to stress.

Chronic Pain

Chronic pain as a presenting problem seems to be less common in the elderly than in those aged 40-60. This is odd in a group so attuned to physical complaint but may be partly attributable to altered pain perception in the senium. There is also very little literature addressing this problem in the elderly.

One of the problems for the clinician in dealing with the chronic pain patient is the question of whether the pain is organic ("real") or functional ("imaginary"). In truth this this is a nonquestion. The diagnosis of causes of obscure pain is not easy, communication skills of patients vary greatly, and many personality styles (dependent, histrionic, obsessional) lend themselves to negative stereotyping. It is very easy for the frustrated clinician to label a difficult patient's pain supratentorial and to treat the problem inappropriately; probably with the exception of malingering; all pain is "real" in the sense that there is subjective discomfort.

Hendler (40) subdivides chronic pain syndromes into four groups; objective pain, undetermined pain, exaggerated pain, and associative pain. Objective pain patients have good premorbid adjustment and organically demonstrable lesions. Undetermined pain patients, show good premorbid social and psychological adjustment post onset life difficulties in proportion to the reported pain, but an obscure etiology for their pain. Exaggerated pain patients have a prior history of emotional problems along with an objective organic etiology of the pain and a seemingly exaggerated affective response and disability. Finally, associative pain patients have a past psychiatric history, often severe, and no definable organic cause of pain. This last group tends to attribute all their problem to the pain. Hendler recognizes that these groups are diagnostically impure but suggests that they may share common pain etiologies, dynamics and clinical course. The author feels that this conceptualization may be useful in considering geriatric chronic pain where cause is even more ambiguous.

Chronic pain syndromes are often associated in the elderly, with intellectual impairment and/or depression. The presence of cognitive impairment is frequently associated with an exaggerated pain syndrome (40) indeed, the patient's use of the pain to attract attention or avoid responsibility may be transparently obvious to the examiner as well as the family. That it is not so obvious to the patient this is something that must be repeatedly borne in mind and carefully explained to relatives and caregivers. The use of the pain in such a primitive fashion, and the lack of insight are reflections of the general coarsening of personality in dementia.

Depression is uncommonly expressed as chronic pain; the so-called depressive equivalent, common sites are the head, musculoskeletal system and abdomen. Since malignancy may cause both pain and depression, a label of depressive equivalent must be applied cautiously.

It is never easy to know how far to push diagnostic procedures, nor where to draw the line in physical treatments. The best guides to these questions are 1.) premorbid adjustment and 2.) the quality of the patient's reaction to the pain. Relevant features of premorbid adjustment include nature of personality style, interpersonal and occupational problems, history of specific psychiatric diagnoses, marital and sexual adjustment and previous response to illness. Significant elements to be assessed in the patients's reaction to the pain include convergence between subjective and objective distress, convergence between disability and actual organic impairment, willingness to verbalize anxiety or depression, and presence of secondary pain. In essence, the poorer the premorbid adjustment and the greater the disparity between disability and demonstrable pathology, the greater should be caution in using aggressive or invasive techniques such as nerve blocks and facet denervations (40, 41). Where there is evidence for a strong psychiatric component, referral to a pain clinic is indicated. This is generally better received by the patient than

specific psychiatric referral as he feels that the existence of his pain is
validated (40, 41, 42).

Psychosomatic Disorders

Psychosomatic illnesses are physical ailments with demonstrable
physiologic or tissue pathology whose cause is wholly or partly psychic. The
concept has always been a troublesome one and has undergone much revision. In
the 1920's and 30's when psychoanalytic theory was influential, the concept of
specificity was widely held the idea that a specific intrapsychic conflict was
responsible for a specific illness (43). This is no longer seriously
entertained. The field of psychosomatics is handicapped by the methodological
variables, and well controlled studies are few. This problem is, of course,
more difficult in the elderly.

Six illnesses had classically been labelled psychosomatic; hypertension,
asthma, rheumatoid arthritis, Graves' disease, peptic ulcer, and ulcerative
colitis (44).

Hypertension is the most common of these six in the senium.
Psychoanalytic theory postulates hostile – dependent characteristics in
hypertensives with many prohibitions against direct expression of anger and
this inhibited and or being channelled into autonomic mechanisms resulting in
elevated blood pressure (45), it has been argued that industrialized societies,
particularly in the west, place the older person in such a hostile-dependent
position (46). Certainly, in our society, the elderly are in danger of falling
progressively more out of step. At the same time their dependent status may
discourage open expression of resentment. In support of these ideas are the
findings of Cruz-Coke (47) wherein low blood pressures are found in elderly
living in societies which venerate wisdom and tradition and accord them a
higher status. Of course, other factors underlie hypertension, but one is left

with the question of just how "physiologic" is the age-related rise in blood pressure.

The situation is much more clouded for the other diseases listed and while one suspects a role for emotional factors particularly in asthma and peptic ulcer disease, these have not been conclusively demonstrated (48, 49, 50). The whole field of stress related illness is still in it's infancy and much remains to be learned of the relationship of psychic factors and the immune system, the cardiovascular system and the gastrointestinal tract.

Conclusion

It is clear that the geriatric patient presents unique challenges to the busy clinician. It has been suggested that the greatest barrier to satisfactory management of the elderly psychosomatic patient is the clinicians preconceptions. It is all too easy to dismiss such patients as "crocks" or as persons suffering the irreversible inroads of the aging process. It is hoped that this chapter has demonstrated that many psychosomatic and somatopsychic syndromes of the elderly are treatable, and that, sometimes, minor interventions can produce major improvement.

TABLE 1

Suggested guidelines for evaluating and treating
Patients with possible obstructive sleep apnea (OSA)

Clinical Situation	Sleep Laboratory Evaluation	Treatment
Obese, normotensive, asymptomatic except for snoring. Hypoxemia abscent, or minimal.	Not indicated initially	Weight loss*, counseling (includes explana- of risks of obesity, possible consequences of sleep apnea, avoid- ance of alcohol and other CNS depressants at bedtime, avoidance of supine position, etc).
Normotensive. Bed partner gives a his- tory compatible with OSA, degree of daytime impairment due to somnolence difficult to quantitate clini- cally.	PSG+ if the patient is hypoxemic on room air in the awake state. MSLT+ is a consideration in some patients to assess the severity of sleep- ness. PSG	Weight loss if obese. Counseling May require nasal CPAP+, UPPP+, or protriptyline.
Moderate to serve impairmentdue to the effects of suspected OSA.	Nasal CPAP trial on same or subsequent night.	Weight loss if obese. Nasal CPAP until desired weight is achieved, clinical and laboratory revaluation then. UPPP is a con- sideration.
Obesity hypoventilation syndrome.	PSG Nasal CPA trial	Weight loss. Nasal CPAP. Tracheostomy in life- threatening disease, if intolerant of nasal CPAP or unreliable. Medroxpyrogesterone acetate may be useful.

*While most patients with OSA, the disease can occur in thin patients as
well.
 PSG, nocturnal polysomnography; MSLT, multiple sleep latency test
(objective measurement of exccessive somnolence); nasal CPAP, nasal
continuous positive airway pressure; UPPP uvulopalatopharyngoplasty.
 A gastric reduc tion operation should be considered in patients with
severe OSA and OHS that have failed serious efforts to lose weight.

TABLE II

Important Side-Effects of Tricyclic Antidepressants

Source: Geriatric Psychopharmacology by Jenike

	Clinical Signs	Causative Factors	Prevention and Treatment
Behavioral	excitement; "manic shift"	stimulating effect	lower dose or change drug
	exacerbation of psychotic symptoms	underlying paranoid or schizophrenic disorder	use antipsychotics in combination or alone
Central Nervous System	EEG changes	large doses, parenteral admin.	lower dose, avoid parenteral admin.
		family history of epilepsy	do not combine with MAOI
	seizures	history of CNS injury, combination with MAOI or phenothiazines.	wait 1-2 weeks after one drug before starting another.
	Parkinosonism; tremors	unclear; rare	lower dose or change drug; don't use antiparkinson drugs
	Central anticholinergic syndrome: acute confusion, hallucinations, agitation, short term memory loss	anticholinergic effects, combination with antipsychotics or antiparkinson drugs	differential diagnosis: Karsakov, transient ischemic attacks, etc.
			check peripheral anticholinergic signs treatment: physostigmine.
Neurological	hypertonus hyper-reflexia ataxia neuropathies tremors, fasciculations	anticholinergic or adrenergic effects, combination with MAOI; old age; vitamin deficiency	lower dose or stop drug avoid polypharmacy give vitamins
Cardiovascular	EKG changes; hypotension	pre-existing CVD	do pretreatment EKG
	myocardial infarcts (- CVA)	adrenergic & anticholinergic effects	monitor cardiovascular indices
	increased blood pressure in hypertensive patients	blocking of guanethedine	stop drug or use other antihypertensive, e.g., hydralazine
Ocular	glaucoma, blurred vision, accomodation paralysis	anticholinergic effects	lower dose or stop drug
Genitourinary	urinary retention; delayed ejaculation	prostate hypertrophy	lower dose or stop drug
Gastrointestinal	dry mouth, constipation fecal impaction		lower dose or stop drug; stop drug

REFERENCES

1. Busse, E.W., and Blazer, D., Disorders related to biological functioning in Hand Book of Geriatric Psychiatry, E.W. Busse and D. Blazer (Eds.) Van Hostrand-Reinhold, 390-414, 1980.

2. Wolff, E.B. and Langley, S. Cultural factors and the response to pain: A review. American Anthropologist, 70:494-501, 1968.

3. Verwoerdt, A. Clinical Geriopsychiatry, E. Williams and Wilkins (Eds.) Baltimore, 11-21, 1976.

4. Zinberg, N.E., and Koffman, I. Cultural and personality factors associated with aging: An introduction in Normal Psychology of the Aging Process, N.E. Zinberg and I. Kaufman (Eds.), International Universities Press, N.Y., 7-56, 1978.

5. Katzman, R. and Terry, R. Normal aging of the nervous system in The Neurology of Aging, R. Katzman and R. Terry (Eds.), F.A. Davis CO., Philadelphia, 15-50, 1983.

6. Reisberg, B. Brain Failure, Macmillan Publishing Co., New York, London, 8199, 1981.

7. Pathy, M.S. Clinical presentation of myocardial infarction in the elderly. Brit. Heart J., 29:190, 1967.

8. Agate, J. The natural history of disease in later life. In Clinical Geriatrics, I. Rossman (Ed.), J.B. Lippincott Co., Philadelphia, 115-120, 1971.

9. Miles, L.E. and Dement W.C. Sleep and aging. Sleep, Vol. 2, No. 38, 1980.

10. Prinz, P. and Raskind, M. Aging and sleep disorders. In Sleep Disorders, Diagnosis and Treatment, R. Williams and I. Karakan (Eds.), John Wiley and sons, New York, 303-321, 1978.

11. Feinberg, I., Koresko, R. and Shaffner, I. Sleep electroencephalographic
     and eye movement patterns in patients with chronic brain syndrome. J.
     Psychiat. Res., 3:11-26, 1965.

12. Freedman, D.X. Introduction, In Depression Biology, Psychodynamics and
     Treatment. Plenum Press, 1-12, 1976.

13. Nowlin, J.B. et. al. The associations of nocturnal angina pectoris with
     dreaming. Annals of Internal Medicine, 63:140, 1965.

14. Lehmann, H.E. Affective disorders, clinical features. In Comprehensive
     Textbook of Psychiatry, H.I. Kaplan and B.J. Sadock (Eds.), Williams &
     Wilkins, 786-811, 1985.

15. Nemiah, J.C. Anxiety states. In Comprehensive Textbook of Psychiatry,
     H.I. Kaplan and B.J. Sadock (Eds.), Williams and Wilkins, 883-894, 1985.

16. Guilleminault, C. and Dement, W.C. Sleep apnea syndromes and related
     sleep disorders. In Sleep Disorders, R.L. Williams, I. Karakan and
     C.A. Moore (Eds.), John Wiley & Sons, 47-71, 1988.

17. Perez-Guerra, F. The treatment of obstructive sleep apnea, Texas
     Medicine, 83:30-33, 1987.

18. Moore, C.A. and Gurakar, A. Nocturnal myoclonus and restless legs
     syndrome. In Sleep Disorders, Diagnosis and Treatment, R.L. Williams, I.
     Karacan, and C.A. Moore (Eds.), John Wiley & Sons, 73-88, 1988.

19. Vitello, M.V. and Prinz, P.N. Aging and sleep disorders. In
     Sleep Disorders, Diagnosis and Treatment, R.L. Williams, I. Karacan, and
     C.A. Moore, (Eds.), John Wiley & sons, 293-312, 1988.

20. Goldman, R. Decline in organ function with aging. In
     Clinical Geriatrics, I. Rossman (Ed.), J.B. Lipincott Co., 19-48, 1971.

21. McAllister, T.W. and Price, T.R.P. Severe depressive pseudodementia with
     and without dementia. Am. J. Psychiatry, 139:626-629, 1982.

22. Morstyn, R., et.al. Depression vs. pseudodepression in dementia. J. Clin. Psychiatry 43:197-199, 1982.

23. Reifler, B., Larson, E., and Hanley, R. Coexistence of cognitive impairment and depression in geriatric outpatients. Am. J. Psychiatry 139:623-626, 1982.

24. Ron, M.A., Toone, B.K., Garrazda, M.E. et al. Diagnostic accuracy in presenting dementia. Br. J. Psychiatry, 134:161-168, 1979.

25. Blazer, D.G. Depression in late life. C.V. Mosby Co., 136-148, 1982.

26. Wells, C.E. Pseudodementia, Am. J. Psychiatry, 136:896, 1979.

27. Folstein, M.F., Folstein, S.E. and McHugh, P.R. "Mini mental state" A practical method for grading the cognitive state of patients for the clinician. J. Psychiat. Res. 12:189, 1975.

28. Spitzer, R.L. and Williams, J.B.W. Diagnostic and Statistical Manual of Mental Disorders, Third Edition, Revised. American Psychiatric Association, Washington, 1987.

29. Roth, M. The natural history of mental disorder in old age. J. Ment. Sci. 101:281-301, 1955.

30. Kay, D.W.K. and Roth, M. Environmental and hereditary factors in the schizophrenias of old age (Late Paraphrenia) and their bearing on the general problem of causation in schizophrenia. J. Ment. Sci., 107:649-686, 1961.

31. Raskin, A. Signs and symptoms of psychopathology in the elderly. In Psychiatric Symptoms and Cognitive Loss in the Elderly, A. Raskin and L.F. Jarvik (Eds.), Hemisphere Publishing Co., 3-18, 1979.

32. Nemiah, J.C. Somatoform disorders. In Comprehensive Textbook of Psychiatry, IV, H.I. Kaplan and B.J. Sadock, (Eds.), Williams and Wilkins, 924-942, 1985.

33. Hamilton, M. Symptoms and assessment of depression. In Handbook of Affective Disorders, E.S. Paykel, (Ed.), Guilford Press, N.Y., 3-11, 1982.

34. Post, F. Persistent Persecutory States of the Elderly. Pergamon Press, Oxford, 1966.

35. Turk, D.C., and Holzman, A.D. Chronic pain: Interfaces among physical, psychological and social parameters. In Pain Management a Handbook of Psychological Treatment Approaches, A.D. Holzman and D.C. Turk (Eds.), Pergamon Press, 1-9, 1986.

36. Fish, F. Senile Schizophrenia, J. Ment. Sci., 106:938-948, 1960.

37. Gaitz, C.M. and Varner, R.V. Adjustment disorders of late life: Stress disorders. In Handbook of Geriatric Psychiatry, E.W. Busse and D. Blazer (Eds.), Van Nostrand Reinhold, 381-389, 1980.

38. Comfort, A. The Biology of Senescence. New York, Holt Rinehart & Winston, 1956.

39. Dohrenwend, B.P. and Dohrenwend, B.S. The conceptualization and measurement of stressful life event: An overview of the issues. In Origins and Course of Psychopathology, J.S. Strauss, H.M. Babigan, and M. Roff (Eds.), New York, Plenum, 93-115, 1977.

40. Zetzel, E.R. Metapsychology of aging. In Geriatric Psychiatry, M.A. Berezin and S.H. Caths (Eds.), International Universitities Press, N.Y. 21-72, 1965.

41. Hendler, N. Diagnosis and Nonsurgical Management of Chronic Pain, Raven Press, 1981.

42. Gentry, W.D. and Owens, D. Pain groups. In Pain Management, a Handbook of Psychological Treatment Approaches, A.D. Holzman and D.C. Turk (Eds.), Pergamon Press, 100-112, 1988.

43. Mersky, H. Psychiatry and Pain. In The Psychology of Pain, R.A. Sternbach, (Ed.), Raven Press, 97-120, 1985.

44. Alexander, F. Psychosomatic Medicine, New York, Norton, 1950.

45. Kaplan, H.I. History of psychosomatic medicine. In Comprehensive Textbook of Psychiatry, 4th Edition, H.I. Kaplan and B.J. Sadock (Eds.), Williams & Wilkins, 1106-1112, 1985.

46. Palmore, E. The social factors in aging. In Handbook of Geriatric Psychiatry, E.W. Busse and D.G. Blazer (Eds.), Van Hostrand Reinhold, 222-248, 1980.

47. Cruz-Coke, R. Environmental influences and arterial blood pressure. Lancet, 2:885, 1960.

48. Weiner, H. Psychobiology and Human Disease. New York, Elsevier, 1977.

49. Sklar, M. Functional bowel distress and constipation in the aged. Geriatrics, 27:79, 1972.

50. Gebves, K. and Bossaert, H. Gastrointestinal disorders in old age. Aging, 6:197, 1977.

DISORDERS OF SPHINCTER CONTROL IN CHILDREN

ENCOPRESIS

Roy Julian, Ph.D.
Assistant Clinical Professor, Psychiatry
Texas Tech University
El Paso, Texas

CONTENTS:

ENURESIS

Gwendolyn Lee-Dukes, M.D.
Assistant Professor, Psychiatry
University of Texas Medical Branch
Department of Psychiatry and Behavioral Sciences
Galveston, Texas

CONTENTS:

ENCOPRESIS

Roy Julian, Ph.D.

DEFINITION

Encopresis can be broadly defined as the voluntary or involuntary passage of feces that results in the soiling of clothing in individuals whose chronological age exceeds the age at which bowel control is normally attained. There is a considerable degree of variance among definitions; however, as can be seen by a review of 110 articles done by Fitts and Mann (1) which reported no firm consensual agreement among them on definition. Most clinicians would agree; however, that encopresis is truly a psychosomatic disorder in which both psychosocial and physiological elements interact in the development and maintenance of this problem.

Historically, fecal soiling was first dealt with as a specific disorder by George Fowler (2) in 1882. He was able to successfully treat two cases of encopresis using a combination of psychological and physical treatment.

The term "encopresis" was first coined by Potosky (3) and later used in 1926 by Weissenberg (4) to parallel the term enuresis which was seen as a disorder with similar etiological factors at that time. From a more modern perspective, the DSM III defines encopresis as "repeated voluntary or involuntary passage of feces of normal or near normal consistency into places not appropriate for that purpose in the individual's own sociocultural setting" (5).

There are a variety of synonyms which have been used in place of the term encopresis such as psychogenic megacolon, colonic inertia, incontinentia alvi, functional fecal incontinence, or idiopathic incontinence. As can be seen, the terms voluntary and/or involuntary have been used to define encopresis in a variety of literature sources, (6,7) and refer to whether the soiling is done consciously or is a result of the involuntarily passage of fecal material around an impacted stool. The term fecal incontinence is now used primarily for soiling caused by organic lesions or abnormalities of the rectum, sphincter, or other spinal or cerebral diseases. This issue will be further discussed in the section on etiology.

Any definition of encopresis should incorporate the three following general definitional categories according to Groves (8), age, defecation patterns and etiology.

Age criterion for diagnosis of this disorder have varied anywhere from three years (9) to four years of age (10). Other authors have used more generalized age-related criterion which refer to elimination beyond the acceptable age for acquisition of bowel control (11). It is important to note that this age varies across cultures from about two years in America and British cultures (7) to three years in French and Scandinavian countries to as much as six years in some primitive cultures (12). Due to peer pressure and increased knowledge, most children will cure themselves by age 14 to 16 (13).

Defecation patterns (8) as a definitional criterion refer to the various forms and consisting of which the stool may take. Some authors insist that the fecal matter must be of normal consistency to be considered encopresis (14) (DSM III, 1980), (14) while others (10) have a broader definition of consistency which includes "formed, semi-formed or liquid stools"., (p 412). This issue is important in that it relates directly to the underlying cause of the soiling, whether from voluntary passage of feces with normal stool (15), or the passage of thin, ribbon-like or liquid stool in the case of children with constipation and impaction.

The final definitional category, etiology, (8) ties in well with the above concepts in that encopresis is no longer seen as a strictly organic vs psychogenic phenomenon (1). Rather, it is recognized today that nearly all forms of encopresis, with the exception of certain organic cases such as Hirschsprung's Disease, represent an interwoven combination of physical, physiological, psychological, and social-familial causes (13,16,17). A multicausal view of encopresis has been accepted by many clinicians who have researched the problem (18) and an eclectic approach to treatment utilizing knowledge from the various disciplines of pediatrics, (6), child psychiatry (16) and psychology (19,20) is advocated by this paper.

A final aspect of the definition process is to clarify

the distinction between primary and secondary encopresis. Primary encopresis refers to continuous, soiling from birth due to failure of ever achieving bowel control (21). Secondary encopresis, of course, describes children who have managed bowel control for some distinct period of time and then have reverted to incontinence at a later date (10).

EPIDEMIOLOGY incidence of encopresis in the general pediatric population ranges from 1.5% (22, 18) to 3% (10,16). As with many childhood developmental problems, encopresis is much more prevalent in males than females, with ratios ranging anywhere from 3.5:1, male to female, in Bellman's (1966) (22) study to as high as 6:1 in Levine's (1975) (10).

It is quite important to realize that the frequency of psychogenic encopresis is as much as twenty times as great as that of strictly organic cases, (23), making the purely organic forms a relatively rare occurrence. Bellman (22) and Walters (24) indicate that 50% to 60% of encopretic children suffer from the secondary forms of encopresis which is usually psychogenic in nature. It can be seen that of the remaining 40% who never achieve full bowel control, a significant proportion are also psychogenic in nature although it is with this group that most organic cases are found.

The disorder appears to cross most socioeconomic and cultural boundaries (12), with no significant differences found among various racial groups in the literature surveyed.

ETIOLOGY: ORGANIC

A wide variety of organic or physiological disorders can cause or contribute to the development of encopresis. Of these organic causes, perhaps the most frequently cited and most feared in terms of missed diagnosis by pediatricians is Hirschsprung's Disease, (13) or aganglionic colon. This disorder results from the congenital absence of ganglionic cells in the wall of the rectum or colon. The bowel is then unable to respond to the pressure exerted by normal amounts of fecal material and initiate a defecation reflex. Chronic constipation and/or diarrhea results and the fecal soiling pattern begins.

Cavanaugh (6) suggests that encopresis is usually secondary to constipation which in turn can be caused by a host of organic related conditions. These conditions may relate to neurologic, endocrinologic, metabolic, or anatomic sources.

Groves (8) gives an extensive list of more specific potential organic causes of constipation and hence encopresis. These conditions include "dehydration, diabetes insipidus, idiopathic hypercalcinemia, redundant rectosigmoid colon, and infantile renal acidosis" (p. 283) further possible causes of constipation have been outlined by Fitzgerald (1975)

(25) to include cerebral palsy, hypothyroidism, infections, polyneuritis, congenital absence of abdominal wall muscles, and amytomia congenita. Dietary factors, such as soft, low leakage food, have also been implicated by a number of researchers (11), as well as allergic reactions (1975) (26) and even some types of intestinal tract infections. Finally, it is well known that certain medications have a constipating propensity such as imipramine, ritalin, anticholinergics, and certain antihistamines and narcotics such as codeine.

The basic pathophysiology for all of these syndromes with regard to encopresis is the same. The organic condition produces constipation due to its particular effects and the constipation in turn leads to fecal impaction and eventual soiling or leakage. The impacted fecal mass may produce overflow diarrhea which oozes around the impaction, or small stool of loose consistency may break off from the mass and produce soiling. It is clear that the fecal soiling represents a symptom of the underlying disorder, rather than the disorder itself in these organic cases.

As the colo-rectal impaction continues, the child may suffer from abdominal distention and wall to wall stool reaching as much as 6 to 10 cm across (13). The chronic distention of the rectosigmoid colon leads to a numbing of the rectal distention triggers, necessary for normal defecation. As a result, the child soon loses the normal urge to defecate and may become detached from the whole process. At this point, the disorder can become chronic and even life-threatening if appropriate measures are not taken.

ETIOLOGY-PSYCHOGENIC

One of the important aspects of assessing etiology from a psychogenic standpoint is that constipation and impaction can also come to play an important role in the maintenance of this disorder. What changes is the cause of the development of the impaction in the first place? These psychogenic or functional causes will be examined from psychoanalytic and behavioral viewpoints.

PSYCHOANALYTIC

Classical analytic theory views encopresis as a symptom of some deeper unconscious conflict, perhaps originating during anal phase of sexual development (27), although this approach is received as largely nonproductive by modern clinicians (9). Freud (28) suggested that anal fixation and conflicted toilet training experiences were positive contributors. It seems that either coercive and early training, or neglectful and late training may equally lead to its development. Fenichel (32) further postulated that excessive gratification, frustration, or an alteration of these as related to toilet training can lead to anal fixation and hence encopresis. The unconscious mind of the child may equate feces with gift, infant, or penis (28), and use them in working out various unconscious conflicts with parents or with their own impulses.

For example, if the child subconsciously regards his

feces as a valuable possession, he may wish to retain them, particularly if the child has animosity towards his mother and does not wish to please her by depositing the gift in the toilet (7).

Excessive parent-child power struggles over toilet training, use of coercive toilet training methods, or excessive demands for perfection have also been implicated in psychoanalytic causation (29). In this case, the encopretic symptoms may represent anger or rebellion toward parents, and over reaction by parents demonstrates to the child the effectiveness of this weapon.

Sexual gratification has also been suggested as a causative factors in encopretics (28). Some children may equate their stool to sexual pleasure - Freud mentions children who retain their excreta until they can derive voluptuous sensations from their evacuation.

From a less exotic standpoint, psychoanalyst also feel that negative family relationship can contribute to encopresis. Bemporad (1971) (31) and Hoag et al (1971) (30) have implicated a rigid, controlling, unempathic mother and a passive, unavailable or absent father in the genesis of this disorder. Obviously, those types of family dynamic could significantly contribute to conscious or unconscious feelings of anger, rage, abandonment, or rebellion and lead to encopresis as one symptom, not to mention a host of other symptoms.

ETIOLOGY: BEHAVIORAL

A behavioral approach to the etiology of this disorder would parallel the learning theory description of how most behavior is acquired. Both normal and abnormal behavior is acquired through the conditioning received in life by means of reinforcement and punishment.

More specifically, behaviorally oriented practitioners would point to such learned behavior as pot phobia, fears of using school bathrooms, (22) improper parental toilet training techniques, or desire to regain parental attention after the birth of a sibling. Children who have been accustomed to defecating each day in the privacy and comfort of their own home may receive a rude shock upon finding that most school toilets are neither private nor comfortable. Many times there is no door in front of the stall and as Levine (1982) (10) points out, "the school lavatory is the theater for a varied program of humiliating scenarios. (p. 320)."

From the standpoint of parent-child interactions, the child may be reinforced for his encopretic behavior in a great variety of ways. Gaining parental attention and love seems to be an almost universal, powerful reinforcer in cases of functional encopresis. If a child feels unloved or neglected, he may go to great lengths to regain parental attention, including soiling his pants. Even punishment or strict discipline may have a paradoxically reinforcing effect on encopretic behavior if it gains parental attention.

This type of problem can easily be exacerbated by the birth of a younger sibling (22), thereby causing the older sibling to feel loss of parental attention. Encopresis develops from a vicarious learning viewpoint (33), when the older child sees all the attention and affection which is showered upon the infant when it messes its pants.

Encopresis can be a very powerful source of negative reinforcement or punishment in its own right, and learning theorists have observed that once this association develops it gives the child a powerful, although abnormal, tool in dealing with and controlling parents. The initial soiling "behavior" may have been a true accident. But once the child learns of the parents (over) reaction, it may become further reinforced and maintained by the inadvertent reinforcement given by the parents.

It is important to remember that even from a behavioral standpoint, the inappropriate soiling itself may be caused by either the retention of stool (and the vicious cycle of constipation and impaction that implies) or by the deliberate expulsion of them. Retention of stool is the most common direct cause (13). As the impaction is formed, the colon, rectum, and finally anus become dilated and fecal material seeps out.

Behaviorally, the retentive (involuntary) type is more likely associated with phobias, self-consciousness at school, pain in defecation (creating a conditioned reflex against defecating), or poor toilet training techniques. The deliberate type of soiling is in an entirely different class and suggests quite different contingencies in its acquisition and maintenance. The latter type is more likely to be associated with direct operant conditioning of increased parental attention, desire to control or manipulate parents, punishment, or vicarious learning from a sibling.

From a behavioral view, the important point is that regardless of the actual physical mechanism involved it is the covert and overt reinforcement the child receives which initiates and maintains the encopretic behavior.

This brings out a final interesting contribution from the learning viewpoint. Encopresis is of the type of disorder which can be initially acquired by reinforcement, punishment, etc., but which can be perpetuated by megacolon long after the psychogenic problems have been ameliorated. This is important to know in terms of the type and extensiveness of treatment used. If the behavioral contingencies which caused its acquisition in the first place are no longer in existence, then simple retraining and colon decompression may be all that is necessary. If, however, the original contingencies still exist, then more extensive behavioral work is indicated.

TREATMENT

ORGANIC

It is beyond the scope of this paper to deal with all physiological treatments in detail and the interested student is referred to the excellent pediatric literature dealing more with this area (13,7,8).

In specific cases of anatomical abnormalities such as in true Hirschsprung's Diesease, imperforate anus, or bowel obstruction, surgery may be required to delete the aganglionic portion of the bowel or repair the affected area. As these conditions represent less than 5% of encopretic children (23), we will focus the remainder of this section on the treatment of functional encopresis.

PEDIATRIC

Pediatric approach to the treatment of functional encopresis has generally focused on bowel evacuation for any impaction and the subsequent establishment of regular defecation patterns (6,17).

A complete physical examination is essential (6) to rule out organic etiology, including a rectal examination. Some physicians recommend hospitalization (16), with complete blood work and radiologic investigation (34) while others feel that such extensive examinations are unnecessary (35). A simple abdominal radiograph to rule out significant colonic impaction seems to be acceptable (36).

Levine and Bakow (37) have proposed the following type of pediatric approach which is representative; (1) orientation counseling; (2) vigorous bowel catharsis with enemas and laxatives; and (3) a maintenance phase using daily mineral oil and regular counseling. These methods were said to achieve, at one year follow-up, results of complete remission in 50% with marked improvement in 27%.

Another non-hospital pediatric approach as advocated by Schmitt (13) feels that no routine laboratory studies barium enemas, or rectosigmoid manometric studies are generally indicated unless Hirschsprung's disease is strongly suspected. Schmitt (13) advocates that retentive and nonretentive encopresis should be separated because treatment of the two types is quite different. Retentive or encopresis associated with chronic constipation and impaction, is treated with enemas to remove the impaction (Fleets hyperphosphate usually one ounce for every 20 pounds, with a second enema given one hour after the first) mineral oil to keep bowel movements soft (for as long as three months or more if necessary), a nonconstipating diet (raw fruits and vegetables), regular sitting on toilet for ten minutes three times a day, and positive reinforcement for staying clean. Schmitt further suggests a gentle response to accidents, avoidance of punishment, and seeking cooperation from the child's school, which are all excellent.

For non-retentive encopresis (non-impacted) Schmitt indicates initial exclusion of organic causes, although makes the point that these represent less than one percent of cases. Following this, he suggests use of (1) ventilation about the crisis; (2) restoring the child's confidence before retraining; and (3) retraining mainly through use of positive social reinforcement. Also recommended is discontinuance of any harsh child-rearing practices and an increase in positive time spent with the child's parents.

Using these approaches, Schmitt (13) indicates excellent results with an 80-90% cure rate.

Hospital approaches to the treatment of this disorder (38,16) have indicated the benefits of having a variety of treatment modalities available including individual and group therapy, occupational therapy, family therapy and behavior modification techniques, in addition to traditional medical modalities. There is more complete control over the child's environment and a temporary removal of the child from any pathological family relationship.

These are certainly desirable features of a treatment program and may by needed in certain selected cases of severe, intransient encopresis. However, with DRG's[*] a reality the necessity of keeping the child in the hospital for 15 to 52 days (16) or as long as three months (38) must be highly selective at best! Most clinicians would agree that hospitalization is not necessary for the vast majority of functional cases and simply not economically feasible for many families.

A fairly recent addition to the medical treatment of encopresis has been with the use of pharmacological agents, particularly antidepressants such as Imipramine. Geormaneanu and Voiculescu (39) claim that little benefit has accrued from therapeutic management of encopresis (a charge many clinicians would vigorously oppose), but that small doses of imipramine and diazepam brought about rapid cures in the two cases they report on. These authors describe the therapeutic effect of imipramine as increasing the amount of noradrenaline in the synaptic cleft by blocking catecholamine reuptake. No follow-up on these two cases was reported.

Schmitt (13), on the other hand, urges caution in the use of drugs to treat encopresis. He notes that many psychotropics have side effects which can accentuate constipation and hence impaction, leading to an exacerbation of the problem in cases of retentive encopresis. It may be that imipramine has its uses in cases of non-retentive encopresis where stool is normal, but it is clear that careful diagnosis is needed before using it to avoid the above complications. In addition, more long-term follow-up studies are needed with this drug to assess its lasting effects.

PSYCHOANALYTIC

Psychoanalytic approaches to treatment of encopresis center on the uncovering of unconscious conflicts or impulses, relief from castration, anxiety (40), and amelioration of disturbed family dynamics (30). Many analysts (14) consider the discontinuous type of encopresis to be a sign of deep disturbance requiring lengthy psychotherapy coupled with protection from the mother. Some clinicans (32) have used this hypothesis to advocate actual physical separation of the child from the mother through the use of hospitalization. As they put it: "The hospitalization was Toby's first separation from his mother and allowed him also to separate from his stool" (p. 269). It is instructive to note that in this case study it took the child two months to accomplish his first bowel movement in the toilet.

Classical psychoanalytic theorists would suggest that the pediatric approach to treatment of functional encopresis with the use of drugs, enemas, laxatives, suppositories, etc. are simplistic and avoid the real root of the problem, which is some unconscious psychic disturbance. Furthermore, the use of enemas, digital excavations and suppositories may actually be detrimental by causing the child to become further fixated on the anal region of the body and thereby interfere even more with normal psychosexual development. If these means work at all, according to the analyst, it is by suggestion, coercion, or fears of further punishment while the basic problem has not been dealt with at all.

To avoid these exacerbations of the problem, Anthony (14) recommends the use of analytic play therapy free association, and uncovering of unconscious attitudes towards feces and defecation through the use of pictures drawn by the child. He describes one case where the child was beset by unconscious anger and hostility toward the mother. The child perceived his feces as collecting in his body and becoming as "hard as cannon balls." "One day" he remarked cheerfully, "it will come out with such a pop that it will knock mummy right over and kill her." As Anthony (14) remarks: "The battle of the bowel is not waged without ammunition on the child's side." (p. 162).

As can be seen, family dynamics of the encopretic child are frequently interpreted as having a rigid, covertly hostile, controlling mother coupled with a passive, unavailable or absent father (31). The family pathology may be pervasive, with conflicted toilet training techniques merely being one aspect of the disturbance. Once a sadomasochistic relationship between mother and child has been fully established, the encopretic symptom may become quite intractable to treatment (14).

The level of parental disgust is critical, according to the analyst, and disappearance of this exaggerated reaction during therapy is the first healthy sign. With the "discontinuous" type of encopresis, a negative fixation presents a very difficult treatment prospect with prognosis being rather poor for this type case.

On the other hand, Whiting and Child (12) believe that the "continuous" type with a positive fixation may not need lengthy therapy at all and may respond to simple unlearning of bad habits and reinforcing of good ones. Prognosis is much better in this type of case than with the discontinuous type, and severe family pathology is usually not encountered.

BEHAVIORAL

Behavioral approaches to the treatment of encopresis follow basic learning theory (33) guidelines. These would include such learning theory principles as positive and negative reinforcement, punishment, contingency management, use of token economies, vicarious learning, and self-charting (41,42). Others (43), report success by means of extinction procedure alone.

Behavioral treatment methods are at times unconcerned with organic factors and may use learning techniques without resorting to enemas, laxatives, mineral oil, etc. in the treatment regimen with good success reported (44). The reason for this success rate without paying particular attention to factors involving constipation or impaction is that most of the above behavioral studies have dealt with cases of nonretentive or voluntary encopresis where there is no impaction, as the child defecates regularly into his clothes (45).

On the other hand, some clinicians (46) report successfully treating a case of encopresis due to Hirschsprung's Disease solely through behavioral treatment methods in toilet training.

However, most practitioners using behavioral methods, whether psychologists or physicians, have employed them with case of both retentive and nonretentive encopresis (19), using cathartics where appropriate.

Waksman (19) used a combination of positive reinforcement, such as extra time spent with parents, glycerin suppositories to elicit proper defecating behavior, record keeping, diet changes and mineral oil. Self charting by the child was also utilized as recommended by Plachetta (47). It was noted that no punishment or token economy devices were used in this particular case study because the child was well motivated. The entire treatment procedure consisted of three office calls and a couple of telephone follow-ups. Thirty weeks and 22 months follow-up revealed no remission of constipation or soiling behavior. Waksman felt that psychologist-pediatrician cooperation was an important contribution to the success of this case and advocates this approach.

There is equivocation on whether use of punishment or aversive techniques is indicated. Some researchers feel that positive reinforcement is the most effective approach and that the negative side effects of punishment limit their usefulness. Particularly of concern is the possibility of engendering further hostility or power struggles between parent and child.

On the other hand, some clinicians (48) have quite successfully employed punishment procedures such as having the child clean up his own mess and be sent to a time-out room after soiling incident, with good results.

DISCUSSION

It is apparent that the different theoretical and philosophical schools of thought approach the etiology and treatment of encopresis from very different standpoints.

The pediatric view tends to focus on concrete physical and medical factors with some allowance for psychological and familial influences by the more eclectic minded physicians. Outcomes from this approach have been fairly good, ranging in the 60-80% level, although much of the research design is somewhat unsophisticated and at times lacking in adequate follow-up. A two to three year follow-up would be desirable with this type of disorder.

Another potential problem with the medical-pediatric approach is that it can rapidly become too time consuming and expensive, particularly if hospitalization is advocated. Except for those few true organic cases or cases of severe impaction, encopresis would appear to be a disorder best handled on an outpatient basis. The need for a two or three month hospital stay in today's world of $150 plus hospital rooms appears hard to justify, except perhaps for the most intractable of cases.

From a positive standpoint, the contributions of pediatrics to a thorough physical examination and diagnostic work-up appear imperative. Even though true organic causes of encopresis may be rare, the necessity of discovering whether an impaction exists or whether there are other physical concomitants is a medical necessity and should be done by the physician. Medical expertise in dietary factor, cathartics where needed, and the use of enemas, are also very important contributions to the successful treatment of this disorder.

Psychoanalytic theory tends to rely heavily on unconscious factors in the etiology and maintenance of encopresis. Dynamic treatment focuses on these factors with the hypothesis that the lifting of repression or bringing material to consciousness will be curative. The dynamic view of the pediatric or behavioral approach is that these methods only deal with surface symptomatology, rather than with the true underlying "conflict." Furthermore, the analytic approach asserts that unless these "deeper" issues are addressed and resolved the patient will suffer from symptom substitutions. If this happens, the encopretic symptom will merely manifest itself in some other form. Recent research into this possibility (50) does not support this contention, rather the opposite would appear to be the case. Once the embarrassing and demeaning aspects of soiling behavior are eliminated the child appears to gain self-confidence and experience a reduction of anxiety and depression.

Analytic contributions and better understanding family dynamics can be useful in some cases, particularly where parental pathology is clearly implicated in the soiling process. One must be careful with generalizations, however, as many encopretic children clearly do not have the stereotypic "detached, hostile, unempathic" mother or the "aloof, distant" father.

Psychoanalytic theory tends to do what research is done on the basis of a simple case studies rather than with groups of individuals and statistical data. This has both positive and negative aspects. From a positive perspective case studies certainly allow a much more involved, in depth understanding of the particular individual and problem. On the other hand, results obtained from one encopretic child may have poor generalization to other cases. Outcomes studies from a psychoanalytic perspective usually indicate a 50-60% success rate with poor follow-up reporting.

Behavioral approaches to this disorder lean heavily on

learing theory to support their contention that encopresis is merely a learned behavior, like any other behavior, and that its treatment should focus on "unlearning" the behavior. Behaviorists feel there is no need to rely on unconscious conflicts, repressed impulses, or castration anxiety to explain the genesis of this disorder. Nor does treatment need to be a lengthy, expensive affair to achieve significant results.

Instead, behavioral practitioners prefer to focus on the target behavior, encopresis, and identify powerful reinforcers which will be contingent on the child staying clean. Contingency management is frequently, however, just a subtle way of altering the parent's attitudes and behavior toward the child. This is something which "born-again" behaviorist would not particularly want to consider.

The behavioral approach does make significant contributions to the treatment of this problem in helping to specify behaviors, contingencies, and reinforcers which can help shape more appropriate behavior. Emphasis of self-charting and self-reinforcement can also increase the child's feelings of mastery of the problem and enhance self-esteem as well. On the negative side, some behaviorists become excessively caught up with minute behavioral acts to the exclusions of everything else such as physiology, emotions, and cognitive processing. The behavioral practitioner ignore organic concomitants to encopresis at their own risk.

CONCLUSIONS

This paper is strongly supportive of an eclective, integrated, multimodel approach to the treatment of encopresis (42). Close cooperation between pediatrics, psychiatry, and psychology leads to the most effective and successful outcomes as advocated by Waksman (19), and Stabler (20).

Multimodel treatment is normally accomplished on an outpatient basis in a matter of weeks. Hospitalization is rarely necessary. Organic concomitants are recognized and attended to by the pediatrician. Behavioral contingencies, family interaction patterns, self-monitoring schedules, and supportive therapy is provided by psychology. Psychiatry provides an important consultative function regarding medications, dynamics, and where more severe underlying childhood disturbances such as psychosis, may be present.

Outcome studies for this eclectic type of approach have been quite favorable (42); in the 85-90% range with 6 months to 2 year follow-ups. When appropriately treated, with cooperation and consultation among professionals rather than interdisciplinary pettiness, encopresis is an eminently treatable disorder with good prognosis.

* Diagnostic Related Groups

ENURESIS
Gwendolyn Lee-Dukes, M.D.

Enuresis is documented as a source of concern to parents and healers as far back as 1550 B.C. In a historical-cultural review, Glicklich reports that treatments were designed to fit the cultural beliefs about the etiology of enuresis. A common belief was that there was a defect in the bladder innervation or musculature. Burning the sacral area was thought to increase the efficiency of the sacral nerves. The bladder neck muscle was thought to be strengthened by having the child ingest pulverized animal organs, or by applying them directly to the child's body. To prevent "leaking" of urine into bedding or clothing; penile yokes were applied to boys, and vaginal bags to girls. Elevating the bed, and tilting the pelvis were also used in an effort to prevent the gravitational loss of urine. (51)

Other commonly held theories were that children slept too deeply, and could not wake up to void, or that they drank fluids beyond the capacity of their bladders. These theories are still held to some degree today, and the same treatments that were used then are used now. Often, prior to seeking professional intervention, parents have tried restricting a child's fluid intake before bed, or have insisted on their going to the bathroom before going to bed. Sometimes they will have made a schedule to awaken the child at midnight to go to the bathroom.

Although day and/or night time wetting can occur at any age, the highest incidence of this disorder is found in the pediatric population. This is because functional enuresis often spontaneously remits, with most children achieving dryness by the adolescent years. Also, adult-onset enuresis is usually associated with organic illnesses, such as diabetes mellitus, diabetes insipidus, seizure disorder, severe obstructive sleep apnea, severe mental retardation, sickle cell anemia and renal tubular disease. (52,53)

DEFINITION

Enuresis is defined as "repeated involuntary or intentional voiding of urine during the day or at night into bed or clothes, after an age at which continence is expected". Expectations for achievement of day and night bladder control vary according to cultural norms. The DSM-III-R, and most investigators have found that age to be about five years old in American children. (54,55)

Primary and secondary enuresis are classified according to whether the child had ever achieved dryness, or whether there had been at least one year of continence prior to the occurrence of inappropriate day and/or night wetting. (Table 1)

In nocturnal enuresis, wetting usually occurs more than one time during the night. Although some earlier investigations had associated enuresis with REM sleep, later sleep laboratory studies have shown that wetting is more related to the time of night than stage of sleep. Most incidents occur in the early part of the night, between midnight and 3:00 a.m., during non-REM sleep. Few children actually awaken during the episode, but may incorporate the wetness into a dream during the next REM period (53,55). When primary nocturnal enuresis persists into adolescence and adulthood, the enuretic episode shifts to a later part of the night. (56)

The onset of secondary enuresis is usually between the ages of five and eight years. (54,55) Stressful events, such as the birth of a sibling, a move to a new home, death of a parent, physical abuse, or even starting school, have been implicated as precipitants of relapse of wetting after a period of being dry. In spite of this association, there is not a higher rate of psychiatric disturbance among secondary enuretics than among those children with primary enuresis. (53,55,52,57)

EPIDEMIOLOGY

Most children with enuresis have never been dry and fall into the category of primary enuretics. It is estimated that approximately 25% of three year olds wet their beds at least once a week. Of this group, 80% will remain enuretic by their fourth birthday. Another 94% of these will still not have achieved dryness by their fifth birthday. (55)

Girls generally achieve continence at an earlier age than boys do. Among five year olds, the prevalence rate for primary enuresis is approximately 7% in males and 3% in females. By the age of ten years, it has dropped to 3% in males and 2% in females. And by the age of 18, the prevalence is almost zero in females and only 1% in males. (54)

Secondary enuresis is not often seen before the age of five years. Again, this is more often seen im males.

In contrast to nocturnal enuresis, daytime wetting is more common in girls than in boys. (58) It is estimated that 2% of five year olds are wet during the day once per week. As many as 8% are wet at least monthly. Daytime wetting can occur in toddlers when they are too busy playing to stop and go to the bathroom appropriately, or during naps. Children with urinary tract infections who wet the bed are also more likely to wet their clothes during the day. (59) As many as 60 - 80% of children who wet during the day also wet their beds at night, (52,60) while only 8% of bedwetters have incontinence in the daytime as well. (61) As children grow older, the condition becomes less common, with only 1% of twelve year olds reporting daytime wetting once or more per month.

In the National Health Examination Survey of 1967, enuresis was found more frequently in families from the lower socioeconomic classes. A higher prevalence was also found in children with two or more siblings. "Only" children had a much lower prevalence of enuresis. The class difference was postulated to have been the effect of less effective toilet training, or of low birth weight and concomitant developmental delays.

In comparing prevalence rates among western countries, it was found that the United States has a higher rate than that found in Great Britain or the Scandinavian countries. (62) Differences in toilet training, and expectations for dryness were said to account for the rate differences.

ETIOLOGY

In infancy, the urinary bladder is completely under reflex motor control. The detrusor muscle of the bladder, and the internal sphincter are composed of smooth muscle, innervated by the parasympathetic nerves from the sacrospinal cord. The external sphincter, composed of voluntary muscle, is innervated by the pudendal nerve. As the bladder fills, the walls stretch until there is enough tension to elicit the "micturition reflex", an automatic spinal cord response. The desire to urinate is felt, but can be inhibited by centers in the brain. Usually the brain maintains constant tonic contraction of the external sphincter, while keeping the micturition reflex partially inhibited. In enuresis, there is a failure to maintain the inhibition of the reflex, but rarely is spinal cord injury or a higher brain center deficit found. (52) Bladder control is developed in stages, beginning with the child being aware of the sensations that signal bladder fullness. This is physiologically possible between the ages of 12-24 months. At 36 months, the child can retain urine by voluntary control of her muscles. At age four, she can voluntarily initiate voiding, and by age 6 years, voiding is under voluntary control.

Learning theorists and psychoanalysts have focused on toilet training, either too early and too strict, or too late and not strict enough, as the underlying cause of enuresis. Learning theorists point to inconsistent reinforcement or too little reinforcement during toilet training as leading to habit patterns that are inconsistent or ineffective. Psychoanalysts have characterized toilet training as a battleground between parents and child for authority and dominance over the child's body. When the child achieves mastery over elimination, this is a symbolic representation of achieving autonomy. Conflicts and anxieties regarding sexual identity have also been identified as causative factors in enuresis. While the exact relationship between the timing and method of toilet training, and success in preventing enuresis is not clear, (62) there are basic guidelines agreed upon by most developmental specialists. A child is ready for toilet training when she can: (1) recognize when her bladder is full, (2) control her sphincter muscles, (3) pay attention to, and follow instructions, and (4) When she shows some interest in toileting activities. For many children, this occurs between the ages of 18 - 24 months. Initiating training prior to this time can be difficult at best, and totally ineffective at worst. (63) Parents and caretakers are urged not to punish children for failures, but to reward them with praise and small treats when they succeed. Pediatricians and psychiatrists can be helpful to parents in explaining these guidelines. Often the issue of toilet training raises parental anxiety, and reassurance is needed.

Constipation has been associated with enuresis. Some investigators have noted that wetting stops after a child receives treatment for, and relief from, the constipation. The causal relationship is hypothesized to be compression of the bladder wall by an overly full rectum. (64)

The psychoanalytic literature has additionally viewed enuresis as a disorder of impulse, or a symbolic representation of wishes. The bedwetting episode was assumed to occur during dreaming. The dream's manifest or latent content was said to portray the child's unconscious conflict. Children have been described as using wetting in passive-aggressive, or directly aggressive ways. Fantasies of genital damage, distortions of body image, and sexual identity conflicts have all been noted in the analyses of patients with enuresis. (65,66,67)

There is a familial pattern of incidence of nocturnal enuresis. Almost 75% of enuretic children have first degree biologic relatives who have, or have had, the disorder. (68) Monozygotic twins were found to be concordant for enuresis twice as often as dizygotic twins. The evidence for a familial pattern is not as strong when analyzing the data from studies of children with only diurnal enuresis.

Historically, and currently, it has been assumed that one of the causes of nocturnal enuresis was difficulty with sleep arousal. (69,51,62) Actual comparison of sleep arousal times in enuretics with matched controls has failed to show any significant differences (70). Sleep EEG studies have shown enuresis to occur randomly through the night, with no particular association to any stage of sleep. (62)

Maturational delay has been proposed as the biological factor underlying enuresis. Evidence for this in studies from England is the finding of concomitant delays in enuretics, such as late onset of walking and talking, and slower growth in height and physical sexual development. While these findings have not been confirmed in all studies, they would help to explain finding an increased prevalence of enuresis among males, since they are slower in their rate of physical development throughout childhood and adolescence. (62)

Bladder size and function are considered by most investigators to be important etiologies in some enuretic children. Functional bladder capacity, which is a measure of the largest amount of urine the child can tolerate retaining before voiding, is said to be limited or diminished. On the average, enuretics are found to have a smaller functional capacity than non-enuretics. There is some overlap however, between enuretics and non-enuretics of the same age. (62,69,71) In one study, comparing the true bladder capacity of continent vs. enuretic children, there was no significant difference found. (72) So while some enuretic children void with only small amounts of urine, the exact biological/physiological mechanism is unknown. Urine retention training has been practiced with some success in eliminating daytime wetting but authors are not in agreement as to whether this actually results in an increased bladder capacity. (55,60,62,71)

Other non-organic, or functional causes of daytime wetting may be secondary to a chronic or persistent stress, such as parental fighting, going to a new school, or the birth of a new sibling. Incontinence may occur at school if a child is too shy or frightened to request bathroom privileges or to use the public restroom when others are present. A child with a small bladder capacity may not, because of strict rules, gain permission to use the bathroom as many times as he needs to, and so have "accidents".

Organic etiological factors are not common in enuresis. When they are present, they are usually associated with diurnal and/or secondary enuresis rather than the nocturnal or primary type.

Urinary tract infection is up to five times more prevalent in enuretic girls than in a control population. And, enuresis is more often associated with urinary tract infections. It is not clear, however, whether the presence of infection causes enuresis, or the other way around. Sometimes enuresis stops when the infection is treated but this is not always the case. (62,52,73)

Obstructive lesions in the bladder neck and urethra can lead to symptoms of dribbling, or a small urinary stream. An ectopic ureter can cause a child to be continually wet. This is associated with diurnal enuresis. (61)

Lumbosacral disorders can affect bladder innervation, causing so-called "neurogenic bladder". Spina Bifida and myelomeningocele may have associated a gait disturbance and inadequate bowel control.

Urethrovaginal reflex of urine may occur after normal voiding. The child stands up, and urine continues to seep out for up to 20 minutes. Risk factors in females are obesity and anterior displacement of the posterior labial frenulum. Instability of the detrusor muscle of the bladder is the most common cause of incontinence in adolescents and adults. The majority of these patients are also female, and they suffer from nocturnal enuresis as well. (61)

TREATMENT

As stated before, there have been multiple treatment approaches to the child with enuresis, often tailored to a specific belief about etiology. Popular and long standing treatments have been limiting fluid intake prior to bedtime, or waking the child during the night to get up and go to the bathroom. When the cause is suspected to be a problem of lack of arousal from sleep, "light" sleep has been encouraged by administering cold sitz baths, or conversely, warm baths, at bedtime. Special diets have been advocated, with the restriction of tea, coffee, alcohol, and salt. Historically, even nitrate of potash has been given to children to increase the irritating quality of the urine, and thereby lead to more frequent voiding. (51) The extreme measures used are an indication of how frustrating enuresis can be for children and their caretakers.

Fluid restriction continues to enjoy popularity among parents as a method of controlling wetting. It may be tried prior to seeking the physician's help, and, if successful, that child may not be seen in treatment. There has been one controlled study, with a group of psychiatric inpatients, that showed an initial decrease in the frequency of night time wetting, but a return to baseline frequency after three months. (74).

In spite of the finding that enuresis often spontaneously remits, most physicians agree that treatment is in the child's best interest. It is generally believed that even enuretic children without other psychiatric problems experience an increase in social confidence and independent behavior after treatment. Only one study, by Wagner & Johnson, found no significant differences in improvement of psychological functioning after treatment, or being left on a waiting list. Other studies have re-affirmed a possible increase in children's self-esteem, and a decrease in family tension when treatment succeeds. (75,76,77,78,79)

According to Shaffer, approximately 10% of enuretics will show a decrease in bedwetting episodes after one physician visit. In this study, parents and children were asked to begin systematic recording of wet nights, (55) and given some reassurance that they could be helped with their problem. Other studies have confirmed this finding, with some proportion of "cures" among children on a waiting list for treatment.

Psychotherapy is generally not the sole modality of a treatment plan. It is helpful for addressing the child's self-esteem and guilt issues, and the parental issues of anger and frustration. In general, psychotherapy will be used in conjunction with a behavioral modality.

Hypnosis, has been studied by two investigators. For children who were able to achieve a hypnotic trance, a high degree of success was attained. These have not been replicated, and the relapse rate was unclear. (55,62,80)

Current practitioners have several treatment modalities from which to choose for those enuretics who are brought to clinic. Schmitt has compared their effectiveness, and concludes, as do most authors, that enuresis alarms lead to the highest success rate. (81,79,55,60) Of special note is that approximately 15% of enuretics show spontaneous remission.

In "motivational counseling," the physician talks with the child and parents, and suggests that the child's problem is due to a small bladder, or some other physiologic problem. The purpose is to minimize shame and guilt feelings. The parents and child are given a behavioral contract to follow: dry nights are rewarded with praise, or some tangible reward that is agreed on ahead of time. The child must restrict fluids for 3 hours prior to her/his scheduled bedtime, and empty the bladder just before going to bed. The physician provides frequent follow-up appointments, encouraging both the child and the parents to maintain the contract. This type of treatment may be referred to as supportive therapy and behavioral contracting. This is associated with a 25% success rate.

Treatment to increase functional bladder capacity, sometimes called urine retention training or bladder exercise, is another form of behavior therapy. The child is asked to drink increasing amounts of fluid, and to delay urination for increasing amounts of time daily. The child is reinforced with praise or other rewards for delaying urination, and should learn to tolerate an increased bladder fullness. This learning is said to carry over into the night time, so that bladder fullness can be tolerated without voiding.

Schmitt's review shows an overall success rate of 35% (Table 2) In comparison to the enuresis alarm, this method is not as effective. Also when functional bladder capacity has been measured before and after treatment, there has been no significant increase following treatment. This intervention does have the advantage of not involving any equipment or disruption of sleep for the family. It does require strict compliance from the parent and child, and has a high possibility of relapse.

Dry bed training, a relatively new treatment procedure, relies on intensive behavioral training in a highly motivated family. Azrin and Fox have incorporated elements of positive practice, positive reinforcement, retention control training, night time awakening, negative reinforcement, and full cleanliness training. (63,82) Treatment begins with explaining the full program to the child and parents. On the first night, the child must start with 20 positive practice trials. Each trial consists of lying in the bed for a brief period of time, rising, going to the bathroom, displaying the appropriate toileting behavior, then returning to bed. After this practice, the child is to drink his favorite liquid, verbally repeat the training instructions, and go to bed. The parents must then awaken the child every hour. Each time, the child must walk to the bathroom, where he is encouraged to void or inhibit urination depending on his age. If the bed is dry, parents are to praise the child and give him a small amount of liquid to drink. If the bed is wet, the child is directed to change his night clothes and the bed, wash himself, (full cleanliness training) and perform several positive practice trials.

Following the initial night of intensive training, children are awakened and taken to the bathroom once during the late or mid evening. This is gradually done less and less as progress is made. Dry nights are reinforced with verbal praise, and encouraging the child to share his success with other relatives and friends. When wetting occurs, the child must again change his night clothes and bed, and wash himself. The next night, he must repeat the positive practice trials at bedtime. This phase is called "posttraining supervision".

The "normal routine" phase of training begins after a child has been dry for seven consecutive nights. Full cleanliness training is conducted only in the mornings following a wet night. Positive practice trials are performed in the evening following a wet night. If two or more wet nights occur within any seven consecutive days, the post training supervision phase is re-introduced. (82,83,84)

This method was reported to be effective in over 85 percent of cases with retarded children. Later, in a matched control series comparing efficacy with an enuresis alarm, remission rates were higher and occurred more rapidly than when the alarm was used alone. (82,83,63,62) This method requires a great deal more parent commitment and parent-child interaction than others. It can be effective if the family is able to learn and follow through with the procedures.

Medications have been used to treat enuresis with varying results. Desmopressin has been used as it is effective, rapid acting, and has few side effects. In a double-blind, cross-over study, it was found to be more effective in children aged 9 years or older, who were inconsistent night time enuretics (that is, children who were not wet every night). Relapse was significant, with less than half of the children remaining dry after the medication was stopped. (85)

In comparing desmopressin to the conditioning alarm system, both were effective, but the relapse rate after discontinuation of the medicine was significantly higher. Desmopressin is postulated to work through its antidiuretic action of increasing the reabsorption of water in the renal collecting duct. (86)

Oxybutynin is an antispasmodic agent that works by reducing detrusor muscle contractions. Some child and adult enuretics have achieved good results with this.

Tricyclic antidepressants, most notably imipramine, have been established in clinical trials as effective in treating enuresis. It is usually effective within one week, at doses lower than those used for the treatment of depression. Rapaport et al., found that there is no cumulative effect on wetting if the dose of imipramine remains constant. Those children for whom it was effective showed immediate improvements, with none of them having a delayed response. (87,88) In a more recent study, Fournier found that there was not one specific dose of medication or serum level associated with improvement. (79) Relapse rates after discontinuation of the medication is high. The presence of wetting and its frequency both relapse. And neither abrupt nor slow cessation of medication alters the outcome. (89)

In studies that compare Imipramine with the conditioning alarm treatment, the bell and pad is always found to be significantly more effective, with a much lower relapse rate. Because of the relapse rate, and the danger of possible overdosing, Imipramine is not considered to be the first treatment of choice. It may be considered in those instances in which a family cannot tolerate the long time, and sustained effort to achieve results with the conditioning alarm device.

Mowrer and Mowrer, in 1938, described a device to alert children and parents when wetting occurred during sleep. (90) Known variously as a conditioning alarm, enuresis alarm, or bell and pad system, it continues to use the same basic design with a few technical refinements. The apparatus usually has perforated metal or foil sheets separated by a cloth sheet. When urine comes into contact with the two sheets, a buzzer or bell is activated, and the child is to awaken and go to the bathroom. It has a high success rate, and when utilized correctly, a low relapse rate.

A number of theories have been proposed to explain the effectiveness of the alarm system. It has been suggested that the alarm sound is aversive, and the child learns to avoid this by delaying urination. (91) Turner pointed out that using the alarm system focuses parental attention on the child's wetting, and may lead to an increased likelihood of their rewarding dry nights. (92) Macaulay et al. suggest that sleeping on the wire mesh of the apparatus causes the child to move around more during the night. Further, they theorize that this increased motility is associated with the cessation of wetting. (93)

Success rates, as stated before, are high. Difficulties encountered have been faulty devices, false alarms, and occasionally, erythema with ulcerations of the skin and perineum. (52,60) Treatment dropout is another problem. When families discontinue treatment before the child is dry, it is often due to frustration with the length of time required for initial success. The bell & pad aparatus should be used until the child has achieved dryness for 21 consecutive nights. This may require use for 6-12 weeks. If relapse occurs, defined as a wet bed more than once in 7 nights, re-training with the bell and pad should occur.   (81,69,75,94)

Daytime enuresis can also be treated with alarms and/or medication. When the etiology is not organic, this is easier to treat than night-time wetting. Various studies have compared treatment modalities. One such study, by Meadow & Berg found no significant difference between Imipramine and placebo for daytime wetting. Random alarm devices, that is, those that rang or buzzed at intervals during the day were found to be equally as effective as those that sounded off when the child was wet. (58) In a study by Holliday and Meadow, more than half of the children achieved daytime dryness by the twelfth week of treatment using either method. There was no significant connection between achieving daytime dryness and improvement in bedwetting. (95)

SUMMARY

Enuresis is a fairly common problem in the pediatric population, and may present to the pediatrician or psychiatrist. Left untreated, there is a remission rate of 10 to 20 per cent of cases per year. Since most children will have neither an organic nor psychiatric illness, overinvestigation and overtreatment should be avoided.

The first step is to gather a complete developmental history, including medical conditions and a description of wetting history. The latter should include details of onset, whether the child had ever achieved dryness, the severity and frequency of wetting, and a toilet-training history. Birth weight and developmental milestones should be documented. Parents should be asked if there is a family history of enuresis, diabetes, allergies, sickle cell trait or disease, or convulsive disorders. Examination of a first morning voided specimen of urine by the laboratory can help to rule in or out the conditions frequently confused with enuresis. Contrast studies, and/or further consultations with a urologist are not necessary unless there is evidence of pathology found during the history and complete physical examination.

Treatment of functional enuresis begins with reassurance of the parents and child. The next step then depends on the family's ability to learn and follow through with various modalities, as well as their proven efficacies. The conditioning alarm will be appropriate for a majority of children. Medications may be appropriate when it is important to obtain an immediate short-term effect, or the bell and pad method is unacceptable to, or unusable by, the family. They are also useful in families in which the symptom is the focus of intense hostile conflict between child and parents, preventing their ability to use the conditioning device.

Practitioners and patients can feel assured that treatment is usually successful, that the cessation of symptoms will benefit the child socially and emotionally.

TABLE 1

DIAGNOSTIC CRITERIA FOR 307.60 FUNCTIONAL ENURESIS

A. Repeated voiding of urine during the day or night into bed or clothes, whether involuntary or intentional.

B. At least two such events per month for children between the ages of five and six, and at least one event per month for older children.

C. Chronologic age at least five, and mental age at least four.

D. Not due to a physical disorder, such as diabetes, urinary tract infection, or a seizure disorder.

SPECIFY PRIMARY OR SECONDARY TYPE.

PRIMARY TYPE: the disturbance was not preceded by a period of urinary continence lasting at least one year.

SECONDARY TYPE: the disturbance was preceded by a period of urinary continence lasting at least one year.

SPECIFY NOCTURNAL ONLY, DIURNAL ONLY, OR NOCTURNAL AND DIURNAL.

- from DSM-III-R, American Psychiatric Association, 1987, p. 85

COMPARISON OF TREATMENTS FOR ENURESIS

TABLE II (from Schmitt, 1982 B)

Spontaneous Cure Rate	15%
Motivational Counseling	25%
Bladder Exercises	35%
Enuresis Alarms	70%
Medication (Imipramine)	25%

(Schmitt, 1982 b, p. 22)

REFERENCES

1. Fitts M.A., Mann R.A. Encopresis: An historical and behavioral perspective of definition. Pediatric Psychology, 4 (1), 31-33, 1976.

2. Fowler G.B. Incontinences of feces in children. Amer J Abstet, 15:984-988, 1882.

3. Potosky C. Dic Encopresis, Psychogenase and Psychotherapic Korperlicher Symptome. Schwarz O. Ed., Springer, Berlin, 1925.

4. Weissenbey S. Uber Encopresis. Z Kinderh., 40:674-677, 1926.

5. DSM III: American Psychiatric Association, 49, 1980.

6. Cavanaugh R.M., Jr. Encopresis in children and adolescents. Am Fam Physician, 27 (5): 107-9, May, 1983.

7. Fritz G.K., Armbrust J. Enuresis and Encopresis. Psychiatric Clin North Am, 5 (2):283-96, Aug, 1982.

8. Groves J.A. Interdisciplinary treatment of encopresis in individuals with developmental disorders: need and efficacy. Monog Am Assoc Ment Defic, (5):279-327, 1982.

9. Doelys D.M., Schwarty M.S., Cisninero A.R. Elimination problems: Enuresis and encopresis. In EJ Marsh and LG Terdal (Eds.), Behavioral assessment of childhood disorders NY: The Guilford Press, 1981.

10. Levine M.D. Children with encopresis: A descriptive analysis. Pediatrics, 56 (3):412-416, 1975.

11. Walker C.E. Toilet training, enuresis and encopresis. In

PR Magrab (Ed.), Psychological management of pediatric
problems. Vol I. Early life conditions and chronic
diseases. Baltimore: University Park Press, 1978.

12. Whiting J., Child I.L. Child Training and Personality.
New Haven, Yale University Press, 1953.

13. Schmitt B.D. Encopresis. Primary Care. 11 (3):497-511,
Sep, 1984.

14. Anthony E.J. An experimental approach to the psychopathology of childhood encopresis. Brit I Med. Psych.
30:146-175, 1957.

15. Werry J.S. Psychosomatic disorders, psychogenic symptoms
and hospitalization. In HC Quay and JS Werry (Eds.),
Psychological Disorders of Childhood (2nd ed) NY: Wiley
and Sons, 1979.

16. Ringdahl I.C. Hospital treatment of the encopresis
child. Psychosomatics 21 (1):65, 69-71, Jan, 1980.

17. Crowley A.A. A comprehensions strategy for managing
encopresis. MCN, 9 (6):395-400, Nov-Dec, 1984.

18. Halpern W.I. The treatment of encopretic children. J Am
Acad Ch. Psychiatry, 12 (4):641-659, 1973.

19. Waksman S.A. A multimodal treatment for secondary
psychogenic encopresis: a case study. Psychol Rep.
53 (1):271-3, Aug, 1983.

20. Stabler B. Emerging models of psychologist-pediatrician
liaison. J Ped Psychol, 4:307-313, 1979.

21. Easson W.M. Encopresis. Can. Med. J., 82:624-628, 1960.

22. Bellman M. Studies on encopresis. Acta Pediatrician

Scandinaria (supplement #70), 1-137, 1966.

23. Wright L. Handling the encopretic child. Professional Psychol, 4:137-144, 1973.

24. Walters W.H.G. A comparative study of behavioral aspects in encopretic children. Psycotherapy, Psychosomatics, 24:86-97, 1974.

25. Fitzgerald J.F. Editorial: Encopresis, soiling, constipation: What's to be done? Pediatrics, 56(3):348-9, 1975.

26. Vaughn V.C., McKay R.J., Nelson W.E. Textbook of pediatrics (10th ed) Philadelphia: W.B. Saunders, 1975.

27. Prugh D.G. Toward an understanding of psychosomatic concepts in relation to illness in children. In Modern Perspectives in Child Development, ed. A Salnit and S Provinces NY: International Universities Press, 246-367, 1963.

28. Freud S. On the sexual theories of childhood. Collected Papers. London, Hogarth Press, 2:164, 1942.

29. Huschka M. The child's response to coercive bowel training. Psychosom. Med., 4:301-30, 1942.

30. Hoag J.M., Norris N.G., Himens E.T., Jacobs J. The encopretic child and his family. J Am Acad. Child Psychiatry 10:242-256, 1971.

31. Bemporad J.R., Pfeifer C.M., Gibbs L., Cortner R.H., Bloom W. Characteristics of encopretic patients and their families. J Am Acad. Child Psychia, 10:272-292, 1971.

32. Fenichel O. Psychoanalytic Theory of the Neurosis. NY: Norton, 1945.

33. Hilgard E.R., Bower G.H. Theories of Learning. NJ: Prentice Hall, 1975.

34. Davidson M., Kugler M.M., Baver C.H. Diagnosis and management in children with severe and protracted constipation and obstipation. J Pediatrician 62:261-275, 1963.

35. Coekin M., Gairdner D. Fecal incontinence in children, the physical factor. Br. Med. J, 2:1175, 1960.

36. Barr R.G., Levine M.D., Wilkinson R.H. Occult stool retention: A clinical tool for its evaluation in school-aged children. Clin Pediatr. 18:674, 1979.

37. Levine M.D., Bakow H. Children with encopresis: a study of treatment outcome. Pediatrics, 58:845, 1976.

38. Kisch E.H., Pfeffer C.R. Functional encopresis: a psychiatric inpatient treatment. Am J. Psychothera, 38 (2):264-71, Apr, 1984.

39. Geormaneanu M., Voiculescu V. Treatment of encopresis with imipramin. Neurol. Psychiatr. (Bucur) 18 (3):209-10, Jul-Sept., 1980.

40. Freud S. From the history of an infantile nuorosis. Standard Ed. 17:1-122. London: Hogarth Press, 1955.

41. Doley D.M., Arnold S.A. Treatment of childhood encopresis: Full cleanliness training. Mental Retardation, 13:14-16, 1975.

42. Wright L. Outcome of a standardized program for treating

psychogenic encopresis. Professional Psycho, 453-456, 1975.

43. Conger J. The treatment of encopresis by the management of social consequences. Beh. Ther., 1:386-390, 1970.

44. Crowley C.P., Armstrong P.M. Positive practice, over-correction and behavior rehearsal in the treatment of three cases of encopresis. J. Beh. Ther. and Exp. Psychiatr, 8:411-416, 1977.

45. Butler J.F. Treatment of encopresis by overcorrection. Psychol Rep., 40:639-646, 1977.

46. Epstein L.H., McCoy J.F. Bladder and bowel control in Hirschsprung's Disease. J Beh. Ther. and Exp. Psychiatr. 8:97-99, 1977.

47. Plachetta K.E. Encopresis: a case study utilizing contracting, scheduling, and selfcharting. J. Beh. Ther. and Exp. Psychiatr, 7:195-196, 1976.

48. Ferindon W., Van Handel D. Elimination of soiling behavior in an elementary school child through the application of aversive techniques: J. Sch. Psychol., 8:267-269, 1970.

49. Lehman E. Psychogenic incontinence of feces (encopresis) in children. Am J. Dis. Child, 68:190, 1944.

50. Levine M.D., Bakow H. Children with encopresis: A study of treatment outcome. Pediatrics, 58:845-852, 1976.

ENURESIS
REFERENCES

51. Glicklich, L. B. An Historical Account of Enuresis. Pediatrics. 8: 859-876. 1951.

52. Novello, A. C., and Novello, J. R. Enuresis. Pediatr. Clin. North Am. June 34(3): 719-733. 1987.

53. Kales, A., Soldatos, C. R., and Kales, J. D. Sleep disorders: Insomnia, Sleepwalking, Night Terrors, Nightmares, and Enuresis. Ann. Intern. Med. Apr. 106(4): 582-592. 1987.

54. Diagnostic and Statistical Manual III-R. Washington, D.C. American Psychiatric Association, 84-85. 1987.

55. Shaffer, D. "Nocturnal Enuresis: Its Investigation and Treatment" in The Clinical Guide to Child Psychiatry, Edited by D. Shaffer, A. Erhardt, and L. Greenhill, London: Collier MacMillan Publishers; New York: Free Press. 29-47. 1985.

56. Anders, T. F., and Freeman, E. D. "Enuresis" in Basic Handbook of Child Psychiatry, Edited by J. D. Noshpitz. New York: Basic Books, Inc., Vol. II: 546-555. 1979.

1262

57. Rutter, M. L., Yule, W., and Craham, P. J. 1973. Enuresis and Behavioral Deviance: Some Epidemiological Considerations. In **Bladder Control and Enuresis**, Ed. by I Kolvin, R. Mackeith, and S. R. Meadow, Clin. in Dev. 1973. Med., #48/49. London: Heinemann/SIMP: 137-147.

58. Meadow, R. and Berg, I. Controlled trial of Imipramine in Diurnal Enuresis. Archives of Diseases of the Child. Sept. 57(9): 714-716. 1982.

59. Hallgren B. Enuresis: a clinical and genetic study. Acta Psychiat. Neuro. Scand. (Suppl. 114) (32). 1957.

60. Shaffer, D. "Enuresis" in **Child and Adolescent Psychiatry**, Edited by M. Rutter and L. Hersov, Oxford: Blackwell Scientific Publications, 465-481. 1985.

61. Schmitt, B. D. Daytime wetting (Diurnal Enuresis). Pediat. Clin. North Am. Feb 29(1): 9-20. (a) 1982.

62. Gross, R. T. and Dornbusch, S. M. "Disordered Process of Elimination - Enuresis" in Developmental - Behavioral Pediatrics. Edited by M. D. Levine, W. B. Carey, A. C. Crocker, and R. T. Gross. Philadelphia: Saunders, 573-586. 1982.

63. Doleys, D. M. and Dolce, J. J. Toilet training and Enuresis. Pediat. Clin. North Am. April 29(2): 297-313. 1982.

64. O'Regan, S., Yazbeck, S., Hamberger, B., and Schick, E. Constipation: A Commonly Unrecognized Cause of Enuresis. Am. J. Dis. Child. Mar 140(3): 260-261. 1986.

65. Freud, A. Three Contributions to The Theory of Sexuality, London, Hogarth. 1962.

66. Sperling, M. "Dynamic Considerations and Treatment of Enuresis" J. Amer. Acad. Psych. 4: 19-31, 1965.

67. Gerard, M. "Enuresis in Childhood," Amer. J. Ortho. 9: 45-58. 1939.

68. Bakwin, H. Enuresis in Children. J. Pediatr. 58: 806-819. 1961.

69. Butler, R. J., Brewin, C. R., and Forsythe, W. I. Maternal Attributions and Tolerance for Nocturnal Enuresis. Behav. Res. Ther. 24(3) 307-312. 1986.

70. Bond, M. M. The Depth of Sleep in Enuretic School Children and in Non-Enuretic Controls. J. Psychosom. Res. 4: 274. 1960.

71. Friman, P. C. A Preventive Context for Enuresis. Pediatr. Clin. North Am. Aug 33(4): 871-886. 1986.

72. Troup, C. W., and Hodgson, N. B. Nocturnal Functional Bladder Capacity in Enuretic Children. J. Urol. 105: 129-132. 1971.

73. Bacopoulos, C., Karpathios, T., Panagiotou, J., Nicolaidou, P., Androulakakis, P., and Messaritakis, J. Primary Nocturnal Enuresis in Children with Vesicoureteric Reflex. Br. Med. J. [Clin Res] Mar 14; 294(6573): 678-679. 1987.

74. Hagglund, T.B. Enuretic Children Treated on Fluid Restriction or Forced Drinks. Ann. Paediat. Fenn. 11: 84-90. 1965.

75. Wagner, W., Johnson, S. B., Walker, D., Carter, R., and Wittner, J. A Controlled Comparison of Two Treatments for Nocturnal Enuresis. J. Pediatrics. Aug 101(2): 302-307. 1982.

76. Benjamin, L. S., Stover, D. O., Geppert, T. V. et al. The Relative Importance of Psychopathology, Training Procedure, and Urological Pathology in Nocturnal Enuresis. Child Psychiat. Hum. Develop. 1: 215-232. 1971.

77. Conchells, S. M., Johnson, S. B., and Carter, R. et al. Behavioral and Environmental Characteristics of Treated and Untreated Enuretic Children and Matched Nonenuretic Controls. Pediatrics. 99: 812-816. 1981.

78. Dimitriou, E., Koustas, K., and Logothetis, J. Relationship Between Parental Attitude Towards the Emotionally Disturbed Child in Nocturnal Enuresis. Behav. Neuropsychiatry 8: 76-77. 1977.

79. Fournier, J. P., Garfinkel, B. D., Bond, A., Beauchesne, H., and Shapiro, S. K. Pharmacological and Behavioral Management of Enuresis. J. Amer. Acad. Child. Adol. Psychiat. 26(6): 849-853. 1987.

80. Olness, K. The use of self-hypnosis in the treatment of childhood nocturnal enuresis. Clin. Ped. 14: 273-279. 1975.

81. Schmitt, B. D. Nocturnal Enuresis: An Update on Treatment. Pediat. Clin. North Am. Feb 29(1): 21-36. (b) 1982.

82. Azrin, N. H. and Foxx, R. M. Toilet Training in Less Than a Day. New York: Pocket Books, 1974.

83. Azrin, N. H. and Besalel, V. A. Parent's Guide to Bedwetting Control: A Step by Step Method. New York: Simon and Schuster, 1979.

84. Azrin, N. H., Sneed, T. J., and Foxx, R. M. Dry Bed Training: Rapid Elimination of Childhood Enuresis. Behav. Res. Ther. 12: 147-156. 1974.

85. May, H. J., Colligan, R. C., and Schwartz, M. S. Childhood Enuresis. Important Points in Assesment, Trends in Treatment. Postgrad. Med. Jul 74(1): 111-119. 1983.

86. Wille, S. Comparison of Desmopressin and Enuresis Alarm for Nocturnal Enuresis. Arch. Dis. Child. Jan 61(1): 30-33. 1986.

87. Rapaport, J. L., Mikkelson, E. J., Zavadil, A. et al. Childhood Enuresis II. Psychopathology Plasma Tricyclic Concentration, and Antienuretic Effect. Arch. Gen. Psychiatry 37: 1146-52. 1980.

88. Rapaport, J. L., Mikkelson, E. J., and Zavadel, A. P. Plasma Imipramine and Desmethylimipramine Concentration and Clinical Response in Childhood Enuresis Psychopharm. Bull. 14: 60-61. 1978.

89. Ambrosini, P. J. A Pharmacological Paradigm for Urinary Incontinence and Enuresis. J. Clin. Psychopharmacol. Oct 4(5): 247-253. 1984.

90. Mowrer, O. H., and Mowrer, W. M. Enuresis: A Method for Its Study and Treatment, in Behavior Therapy and Health Care, Edited by R. C. Katz, and S. Zlutnick, New York: Pergamon, 41-70. 1975.

91. Hansen, G. D. Enuresis control through fading, escape and avoidance training. J. of Applied Behav. Anal. 12: 303-307. 1979.

92. Turner, R. K. Conditioning Treatment of Nocturnal Enuresis: Present Studies in Bladder Control and Enuresis, Ed by I. Kolvin, R. Mackeith, and S. R. Meadow, Clin. in Dev. Med. No. 48/49. London: Heinemann/SIMP. 195-210. 1973.

93. Macaulay, A. J., Gupta, M., Crisp, A. H., and Bhat, A. V. The Relationship Between Nocturnal Motility and the Enuresis Alarm Device. J. Psychosom. Res. 30(1): 63-65. 1986.

94. Goel, K. M., Thomson, R. B., Gibb, E. M., and McAinsh, T. F. Evaluation of Nine Different Types of Enuresis Alarms. Arch. Dis. Child. Aug 59(8): 748-752. 1984.

95. Halliday, S., Meadow, S. R., and Berg, I. Successful Management of Daytime Enuresis Using Alarm Procedures: A Randomly Controlled Trial. Arch. Dis. Child. Feb 62(2): 132-137. 1987.

96. Miller, F. J. W., Court, S. D. M., Walton, W. S. and Knox, E. G. Growing Up in Newcastle - Upon Tyne London: Oxford University Press. 1960.

97. Lovibond, S. H. Conditioning and Enuresis. Oxford: Pergamon, 1964.

98. Oppel, W. C., Harper, P. A., and Rider, R. V. Social, Psychological and Neurological Factors Associated With Enuresis. Pediatr. 42: 627-641. 1968.

99. Douglas, J. W. B. Early Disturbing Events and Later Enuresis. In Bladder Control and Enuresis. Edited by I. Kolvin, R. Mackeith, & S. R. Meadows. Clinics in Developmental Medicine, #48/49. London: Heinemann/SIMP. 1973.

100. Miller, P. M. An Experimental Analysis in Retention Control Training in the Treatment of Nocturnal Enuresis in Two Institutionalized Adolescents. Behav. Therapy. 4: 288-294. 1973.

101. Fritz, G.K. and Armbrust, J. Enuresis and Encopresis. Psychiatric Clin. North Am. Aug 5(2): 283-296. 1982.

102. Diamond, J. M. and Stein, J. M. Enuresis: A New Look at Stimulant Therapy. Can. J. Psychiatry. Aug 28(5): 395-397. 1983.

103. Post, E. M., Richman, R. A., Blackett, P. R., Duncan, K. P., and Miller, K. Desmopressin Response of Enuretic Children. Effects of Age and Frequency of Enuresis. Am. J. Dis. Child. Oct 137(10): 962-963. 1983.

104. Foxman, B., Valdez, R.B., and Brook, R. H. Childhood Enuresis: Prevalence, Perceived Impact, and Prescribed Treatments. Pediatrics. April 77(4): 482-487. 1986.

105. Moffat, M. E., Kato, C., and Pless, I. B. Improvements in Self-Concept after Treatment of Nocturnal Enuresis: Randomized Controlled Trial. J. Pediatr. Apr 110(4): 647-652. 1987.

EVALUATING TREATMENTS IN MEDICAL PSYCHIATRY

M. Dhyanne Warner, Ph.D.[1]
Medical Student

Cecilia A. Peabody, M.D.[1]
Associate Professor of Psychiatry

Sue Thiemann[2]
Biostatistician

Helena C. Kraemer, Ph.D.[2]
Professor of Biostatistics in Psychiatry

[1]University of Texas Medical School at Houston
Department of Psychiatry
Houston, Texas   77030

and

[2]Stanford University School of Medicine
Department of Psychiatry and Behavioral Sciences
Stanford, California 94305

TABLE OF CONTENTS

INTRODUCTION

This paper discusses the basic considerations necessary for understanding and interpreting clinical drug trials. Many articles have been written for clinicians on statistical analysis, and most published studies use only the most elementary analytic procedures. One study (1) suggests that a reader of the New England Journal of Medicine who understands percentages, means, standard deviations, and t-tests has statistical access to 67 percent of the articles in the journal.

However, a basic knowledge of design issues is also necessary for evaluating clinical drug trials. Such knowledge is important both for clinicians making decisions in clinical practice and for researchers reviewing research proposals and reports. The importance of evaluating clinical drug trials is underscored by the recent development of a Trial Assessment Procedure Scale (TAPS) (2), which contains sections on design characteristics, as well as on data collection and analysis. The following key design issues will be discussed: 1) control and randomization techniques; 2) sample size, power, and statistical significance; 3) measurement considerations; 4) effect size and clinical significance; and 5) the use of parallel versus crossover designs.

CONTROLS

Studies with few subjects or without a control group should be considered pilot or preliminary studies. Such studies may indicate whether a well-controlled clinical drug trial is justified, and are also particularly valuable in assessing difficult or rare patient populations (3).

An "uncontrolled" design is one in which all subjects receive exactly the same protocol and treatments. An example is a study in which all subjects receive placebo for the first week, an active drug for the second week, and placebo again for the third week. If there are no significant differences between the responses to the drug and the two placebos, the researcher may conclude that the drug is not effective and that future study is not warranted. However, had there been a control group that deteriorated over the course of the study, the same results might have suggested a drug effect. Deterioration may occur because of hospitalization, a natural progression of a disease, or for other unknown reasons.

Alternatively, there might have been improvement during the drug period relative to both of the placebo periods. These results must still be interpreted cautiously. An improvement with the drug may simply be due to learning, acclimation, continued placebo effect, or a combination of these effects. In addition, a decrease in response in the last placebo period may be due to a negative carryover effect of the drug or simply to fatigue. Finally, there might have been a significant improvement with the drug that continues or plateaus during the second placebo period. The improvement could be explained by either learning or placebo effects rather than the drug's effectiveness.

Thus, whatever the outcome of an uncontrolled trial, no clear conclusions regarding drug efficacy can be drawn, since improvement cannot be unequivocally attributed to the drug. Such studies, however, can provide preliminary evidence as to the potential safety of the drug and give some indication of how effective it might be.

When uncontrolled studies are not specifically labelled as pilot studies, unwarranted conclusions are often made or implied. The clinician should regard the results of such studies as suggestive or promising, somewhat as one would regard a case history or a theoretical speculation.

A separate control group is necessary for a definitive drug trial. It has been suggested that an historical control group, one composed of patients seen in the past with the same disorder, may legitimately be used in some areas of research (4). The use of historical control groups is based on the premise that neither the disorder being treated nor the nature of the population change rapidly over time. These premises are questionable, however, since diagnostic and treatment procedures changes rapidly in all fields of medicine. Additionally, measurements, personnel, and environmental factors change over time and may themselves produce differences in the data. For all these reasons, if at all possible, a concurrent control group should be included.

The next question is what treatment the control group should receive: a placebo or a standard drug treatment. Miller and Perry (5) argue for a standard drug treatment on ethical grounds. If no such treatment exists, then placebo is the obvious and only choice. If there is a standard treatment available, the ideal strategy would be to have two randomized control groups, one receiving placebo and the other a known treatment. However, there is a recent report (6) describing an institutional review board that would not approve two studies with placebo control groups, since known treatments existed. Ironically, the Food and Drug Administration had insisted on the placebo controls.

Some investigators, particularly in cancer research (4), object to a randomized concurrent control group because of ethical and logistical considerations. But, if a control group is not randomly selected, any factors that are used in the assignment of subjects to groups cannot be separated from the drug's effects. For example, numerous studies purport to document the deleterious effects of drugs used during labor and delivery on newborn babies. In almost all of these studies, the obstetrician decided whether a drug was necessary, and if so, at what dosage, and at what point in the labor. As a result, the babies in the drug groups tended to be those resulting from a longer or more difficult labor. Any reported differences in the groups of babies may have been due to the length or difficulty of labor, and not to the long-lasting effects of the drugs (7). Randomization of the treatment and control groups is the safest way to identify a drug's effects.

RANDOMIZATION

Two major considerations in the assignment of subjects to groups are randomization and sample size. With a total sample size as small as 20-30 patients, the groups should be nearly equal in size (10-15 per group), both for purposes of credibility as well as for statistical power. Furthermore, there should be no major differences in those patient characteristics that influence response. Unfortunately, assignment of subjects to groups by a random number table or coinflip technique does not always produce groups equal in size. One strategy for balancing the groups has been to alternate assignments to each: however, research personnel may unintentionally manipulate the order and thereby bias the sample. Efron (8) has suggested a simple and useful solution to this problem. As long as group sizes are equal, subjects should be randomly assigned. If group sizes are unequal, a subject has a 1 in 3 chance of entry into the larger group and a 2 in 3 chance of entry into the smaller group. This procedure exerts constant pressure to balance the group sizes without risk of bias and is very easy to use in clinical trials.

The problem of assuring that each group is matched for the pertinent subject characteristics is more difficult, but randomization strategies have been proposed to deal with these problems as well (9,10). In general, if randomization is done correctly by someone not directly involved with study patients, it will help to insure that treatment will not be manipulated unintentionally by the investigator or the subject.

In summary, randomized concurrent control groups are vital to credible drug trials. Randomization methods that produce evenly balanced and matched groups, even within small sample studies, are recommended.

TYPE I and TYPE II ERRORS

An understanding of design issues such as measurement and power depends on an understanding of type I and type II statistical errors. A type I error (or a false positive) is the claim that a drug or treatment is effective when it is not. A type I error occurs when a researcher reports a result to be "statistically significant" when, in fact, it happened by chance. The probability of committing a type I error is reported as the significance level or p-value. Therefore, p-value represents the likelihood that the results occurred by chance.

A drug or treatment reported as significant at the 5 percent level is not necessarily less effective than one reported as significant at the .001 percent level. Both are being reported as effective, but there is more doubt about the truth of the first report than the second, perhaps only because the sample size is smaller. Traditionally, any p-value higher than 5 percent is not considered convincing. This convention affords protection against the proliferation of false positive findings.

In contrast, there is no convention as to what constitutes an acceptable level of type II error. A type II error (or a false negative) is the claim that a drug or treatment is ineffective when, in fact, it is effective to some degree. The probability of avoiding such an error is called power. Thus, power is a measure of the ability of a particular study to find a significant result that truly exists. For example, assuming a real difference exists, a power of 90 percent means there is a 90 percent chance of finding a statistically significant difference in the study samples.

When a nonsignificant finding is reported, clinicians should regard the result as they would a "hung jury" in a legal trial, not as an "innocent" verdict. It may well be that the drug or treatment is ineffective. However, it may also be that the drug is effective but is not found to be so because of insufficient sample size, inefficient design, unreliable measurements, or just bad luck. Since there is no convention as to what constitutes adequate power, there is little protection against proliferation of false negative reports except the reluctance of an editor to publish such results. Lavori et al. (11) surveyed 47 parallel studies in the New England Journal of Medicine and found that authors frequently misinterpreted non-significant differences between groups to mean that the groups were the same. In summary, if a significant result is found, it can be stated with a measure of doubt -- specifically, the reported significance level. However, if a result is reported as non-significant, no definite conclusions can be drawn.

SAMPLE SIZE

One of the most frequent concerns of investigators is adequate sample size. Agras and Berkowitz (12) found that the median number of subjects involved in behavioral research is 24, and Fletcher and Fletcher (13) found that the median number in general medical research is 30. However, of the 612 medical articles reviewed, 38 percent used a total of 10 subjects or less. When compared with the sample sizes that are recommended in textbooks on research design and analysis, these numbers are extraordinarily small (14). Ideally, sample size is determined by a power calculation based on the desired levels of type I and type II errors and the minimum effect size desired. In practice, however, the number of subjects is also a practical decision, based on the available resources of the researcher. Recruiting appropriate subjects, treating and evaluating them, and analyzing the data generated is often extremely costly and time-consuming. It is not unusual for a protocol with a total of 20 subjects to require one year simply to complete subject recruitment. After recruitment, many studies still require an extended period for evaluation. Seldom do clinical drug trials take less than a year to complete.

While statistical considerations dictate that a sample size be as large as possible, cost and feasibility considerations dictate that the sample size be rather limited. However, if a research protocol utilizes fewer than 10 subjects, one or two outliers can totally control the results of the study (15). An outlier is a subject whose measurements are markedly different from the others in the sample and represents either a very unusual subject or an error in measurement. Even without outliers, the power of such a small study is very low, although the drug may indeed be effective (14). For these reasons, researchers should make every effort to include a minimum of 10 to 15 subjects per group. If the response is carefully measured, this sample size frequently yields enough power to make a study worthwhile. Larger sample sizes, of course, will offer greater statistical power and more precise estimates of treatment effects, but small sample sizes (10-15 subjects per group) are often adequate to detect the differences that have clinical significance.

MEASUREMENT

The measurements chosen to test a drug's effectiveness are a crucial part of a design. The major issues concerning measurement are the validity, reliability, and sensitivity of a particular measure.

A measure is valid when it accurately measures what is intended to measure. For example, if a measure that is intended to measure intellectual function of a child depends more on visual and hearing ability than on cognitive functioning, the results of any study using this measurement can be misleading. If a test does not measure what it purports to, then the study is flawed because the hypothesis under consideration is not truly being tested.

Reliability refers to a measure that is precise, reproducible, and consistent. A measure may be highly reliable and totally invalid (i.e., it may be a very precise measurement of the wrong thing). A measure cannot be valid, however, unless it is also reliable. Thus, the reliability of a valid measurement is an important consideration.

The power of a study depends strongly on the reliability of the measurements involved, since in many studies, the power depends on the product of the sample size and the reliability coefficient (16). Thus, a study with 100 subjects and a coefficient of reliability of 20 percent can have the same power as one with 20 subjects and a coefficient of reliability of 100 percent. Therefore, when sample sizes are small, it is important to choose measures with high test-retest reliability in order to preserve power. A reliability coefficient above 60 percent is generally considered satisfactory. This level of reliability may sometimes be achieved by combining the repeated independent measures of each subject (17,18).

A third consideration in measurement is sensitivity, or the ability of a measurement to detect small changes in the clinical condition of the patient. It is possible to have valid and highly reliable measures that do not change with even the most effective treatment because they are insensitive. The problem of insensitivity often arises when valid and reliable quantitative responses are grouped into a few categories -- for example, when an observed continuum is recorded on a five-point scale. Because sensitivity is reduced when data are collapsed into larger, less specific groups, power is also reduced. The necessary sample size needed to detect true drug effects must then be increased to compensate for the decrease in sensitivity of the scale. Thus, a "yes/no" response (e.g. Has the patient improved?), may require sample sizes in the 100's, as in epidemiological studies, while a sample size of 20 might suffice with a continuous response.

To the clinician reading a study, the most important question is whether the response was validly measured. If the measure is valid and the results are significant, it is clear that the treatment is effective (with a degree of doubt as signaled by the reported significance level). However, if a measure is valid and the results are not significant, the clinician must consider whether the measurements of subjects' responses were possibly unreliable or insensitive, thereby concealing true drug or treatment differences, and whether the sample size was large enough to yield sufficient power to detect a true difference.

CLINICAL SIGNIFICANCE

Clinical significance and statistical significance are two separate issues. A statistically significant difference may or may not be clinically important. For example, in a study involving Alzheimer's patients, a statistically significant improvement (at $p < .05$) of 10 percent is found on a list-learning task for the experimental drug group. This 10 percent represents an average improvement of one additional word retained per subject. Is the retention of an additional word practically or clinically significant ? Often the answer to such questions is unclear.

The effect size, a measure of the difference between the treatment and control groups, may help in determining clinical significance (19). Glass et al. (20) defined effect size as the "mean difference between experimental control groups, divided by the within [control] group standard deviation." Thus, an effect size of "0" means there is no difference between the two groups, and effect size of "1" means the groups differ by one standard deviation. The greater the effect size, the greater the clinical significance of the difference between the groups. For a fixed sample size, the greater the true effect size, the greater the power of the test and the greater the chances of a statistically significant result as well. However, one may achieve statistical significance with any non-zero effect size simply by making the sample size large enough. The same is not true of clinical significance.

There have been attempts to set standards for "low," "medium," and "high" effect sizes (21). These have been unsuccessful because the importance of effect size usually depends upon the situation. In one situation, an effect size of 0.2 may be clinically significant, whereas in another, an effect size of 3.0 may not be. Only if past research in a particular area has consistently found an effect size of 0.6 to indicate clinical improvement can a current study with an effect size of 0.6 or greater legitimately claim clinical significance.

It should be emphasized that the first task is to establish statistical significance (Is there anything there?) and only then to consider clinical significance (Is it of real clinical importance?).

CROSSOVER DESIGN

There are two major designs used in clinical drug trials: crossover and parallel. A crossover design involves two or more groups that all receive identical treatments but not in the same order (figure 1). An example of a crossover design is one in which one group of subjects receives placebo or standard drug treatment for the first week (control phase) and the experimental drug for the second (treatment phase), perhaps following a "washout" period. The second group receives the treatment phase first, followed by the control phase.

The major assumption of the crossover design is that the drug has a negligible carryover effect, either positive or negative. If a drug changes some response of the patient (either therapeutically or by causing side effects), the effect may persist after the drug has been withdrawn. This is known as a "carryover effect." This effect may last far beyond the half life of the drug. For example, the treatment effect of phenytoin in binge eating was found to persist for six weeks after the drug was stopped (22), even though the half life of phenytoin is approximately 22 hours (23) and there was no detectable plasma level in any of the subjects.

If the trial drug has a positive carryover effect, the group that receives the drug first will retain some of the drug's effects, and the response during the control phase will be improved due to the lasting efficacy of the trial drug. This will result in less of a difference between the treatment and control phases. In this case, there is a greater chance of failing to show a statistically significant difference where a true difference exists (type II error). If, on the other hand, the drug has a negative carryover effect, then the group that receives the trial drug first will not perform as well in the control period. Thus, there will be a larger difference between phases due to this contamination and a statistically significant result where none exists (type I error).

Carryover effects of a drug cannot be assumed to be negligible unless this has been demonstrated in clinical drug trials. Brown (24) emphasizes that "there is no economical way to test the [carryover effect] adequately using the data from the crossover itself." Very rarely do studies even mention the potential carryover effects of a drug or attempt to assess them. In a review of 13 crossover studies in the New England Journal of Medicine (3), only one study reported results of calculated carryover effects. Therefore, unless carryover effects have been proven to be negligible, the simple crossover design has questionable validity.

PARALLEL DESIGN

A parallel design involves the use of two or more groups of subjects who follow the same protocol except that the treatment is different (figure 2). One of the treatments may be placebo, especially in studies that involve diseases for which there is no known treatment. In the "simple" parallel design, one group receives the trial drug and the other group receives a known treatment drug or placebo, and measurements are taken only at the end of the study. Individual baseline differences are not measured in this design and thus not taken into account. This design may be greatly improved by adding a pre-treatment measurement for both groups. Such a design is termed an "extended" parallel design (figure 3). The pre-treatment measurement could be used to control for individual differences and thus increase the power of the design (25).

A major strength of the parallel design is that it makes no assumption about the nature of the drug effects. Therefore, unlike the crossover design, there are very few reservations about its validity. On the other hand, subjects must be informed that they have only a 50 percent chance of receiving the experimental drug, which may decrease motivation to participate. One may compensate for this disadvantage by offering medication to all subjects at the end of the study if it proves to be effective (open-label follow-up). By including baseline measures and repeated measures over the treatment period, the extended parallel design can offer a powerful, and, more importantly, a valid alternative to crossover studies.

CONCLUSIONS

Ideal designs are rarely, if ever, implemented because of the practical considerations of finances and logistics. Nonetheless, the same principles that dictate an ideal design must be used in evaluating an actual research study. Major factors to be considered in evaluating clinical drug trials include: 1) the presence of a control group; 2) the use of randomization techniques for group assignments; 3) power and sample size; 4) validity, reliability and sensitivity of measures; 5) clinical significance; 6) the use of parallel vs. crossover design.

Sample size is one of the most important factors in evaluating a drug trial, as well as one of the most obvious. Studies with very few subjects not only suffer from low statistical power, but may provide poor estimates of treatment effects if there are outliers in the data. Therefore, well-controlled clinical trials need a minimum of 10-15 subjects per group.

Regardless of the sample size, the design itself may not yield valid data. This is the case with a crossover design. Quite frequently, carryover effects are not known and crossover studies assume there are none. It then becomes extremely difficult or impossible to interpret the results of the study.

There are many other situations that will jeopardize the validity of the results. No analytic procedure can salvage an invalid measure. While uncontrolled or non-randomized trials may be useful as pilot or preliminary studies, they should be interpreted very cautiously and no definite conclusions can be drawn regarding drug efficacy.

A valid study reporting a significant result may be taken as an indication of the efficacy of the drug or treatment with a degree of doubt indicated by the reported significance level. A non-significant result should be regarded as an equivocal finding, for it may be related to inadequacies of measurement, design, or sample size, rather than to the inefficiacy of the treatment. A statistically significant finding may or may not be clinically significant, depending on the magnitude of the response differences.

There is a certain basic bias in science: a new theory is considered false until researchers provide convincing evidence that it is true. Once the researchers have provided evidence that a new drug is effective, it is for the clinicians to determine that such evidence is, or is not, convincing enough to warrant application to their own patients.

SIMPLE CROSSOVER DESIGN

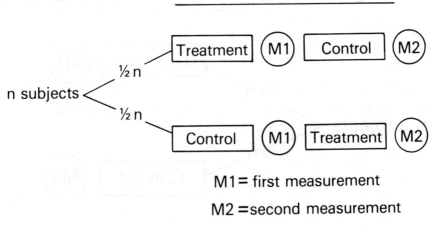

M1 = first measurement

M2 = second measurement

Figure 1: Simple crossover design

SIMPLE PARALLEL DESIGN

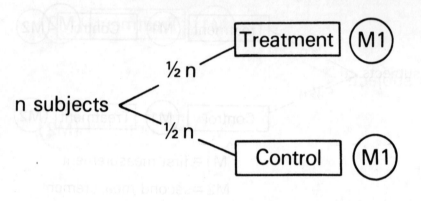

M1= only measurement

Figure 2: Simple parallel design

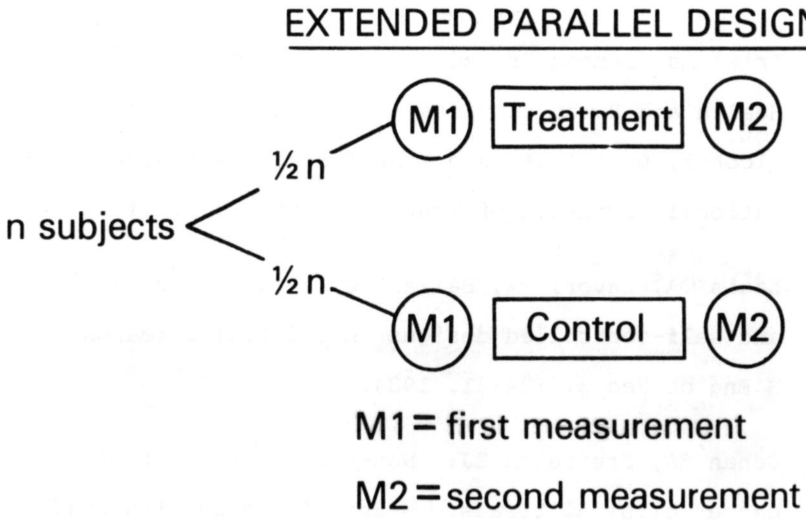

Figure 3: Extended parallel design

REFERENCES

1. Emerson JD, Golditz GA: Use of statistical analysis in
   New England Journal of Medicine. New Eng of Med 309:
   709-713, 1983.

2. Trial Assessment Procedure Scale (TAPS), Department of
   Health and Human Services, Public Health Service,
   Alcohol, Drug Abuse and Mental Health Administration,
   National Institute of Mental Health, 1980.

3. Louis TA, Lavori PW, Bailar JC, et al. Crossover
   and self-controlled designs in clinical research.
   N Eng of Med 310:24-31, 1984.

4. Gehan EA, Freireich EJ: Non-randomized controls in
   cancer clinical trials. N Eng of Med 290:198-203,
   1974.

5. Miller ST, Perry C: New lessons favoring physicians'
   support of clinical trials. The Am of Med 77:533-536,
   1984.

6. Way W: Placebo controls. N Eng of Med 311:413-414,
   1984.

7. Kraemer HC, Korner A, Anders T, et al. Obstetric drugs
   and infant behavior: A reevaluation.
   Journal of Pediatric Psychology 10:345-353, 1985.

8. Efron B: Forcing a sequential experiment to be balanced. Biometrics 58:403-417, 1971.

9. Pocock SJ, Simon R: Sequential treatment assignment with balancing for prognostic factors in the controlled clinical trial. Biometrics 31:103-115, 1975.

10. Taves DR: Minimization: A new method of assigning patients to treatment and control groups. Therapeutics 15:443-453, 1974.

11. Lavori PW, Louis TA, Bailar JC, et al. Designs for experiments - parallel comparisons of treatment. New England Journal of Medicine 309:1291-1299, 1983.

12. Agras WS, Berkowitz R: Clinical research in behavior therapy: Halfway there? Behavior Therapy 11:472-487, 1980.

13. Fletcher RH, Fletcher SW: Clinical research in general medicine journals: A thirty year perspective. N Eng of Med 301:180-183, 1979.

14. Kraemer HC, Theimann S. How many subjects? Statistical power analysis in research. Newbury Park, Sage Publications, 1987.

15. Kraemer HC: Coping strategies in psychiatric clinical research. Of Cons and Clin Psycho 49:309-319, 1981

16. Kraemer HC: Ramifications of a population model for K

as a coefficient of reliability. Psychometrika 44:461-472, 1979.

17. Spearman C: Correlation calculated from faulty data. Brit of Psycho 3:271-295, 1910.

18. Brown W: Some experimental results in the correlation of mental abilities. Brit of Psycho 3:296-322, 1910.

19. Hedges LV, Olkin I: Statistical Methods in Meta Analysis. Academic Press, New York, 1985.

20. Glass GV, McGraw B, Smith ML: Meta analysis in social research. Sage Publications, Beverly Hills, pp. 102-104, 1981.

21. Cohen J: Statistical Power Analysis for the Behavioral Sciences. New York, Academic Press, 1969.

22. Wermuth BM, Davis KL, Hollister LE, et al. Phenytoin treatment of the binge-eating syndrome. American Journal of Psychiatry 134:1249-1253, 1977.

23. Arnold K, Gerber N: The rate of decline of diphenylhyd-antoin in human plasma. Clin Pharm and Ther 11:121-134, 1970.

24. Brown BW: The crossover experiment for clinical trials. Biometrics 36:69-79, 1980.

25. Kraemer HC: Parallel or crossover designs in evalua-

25. Kraemer HC: Parallel or crossover designs in evaluation of antiarrythmic therapy. <u>The Evaluation of New Antiarrythmic Drugs.</u> Morganroth et al.(eds.), The Hague, Martinez Mighoff Publishers, pp. 149-157, 1981.

ACKNOWLEDGMENTS

This work was supported by a grant from the National Institute of Mental Health, MH-30854, to the Norris Mental Health Clinical Research Center at Stanford University (MHCRC). The authors thank Palmela J. Elliott for manuscript preparation and editorial advice.

LIST OF CONTRIBUTORS

ARTHUR J. BARSKY, M.D.
Warren 605
Fruit Street
Boston, MA. 02114
(617) 726-2989

Director, P.C.
and Acute Psychiatry
Service Unit;
Associate Prof.
Dept. of Psychiatry

Harvard Med.
School
Massachusetts
Gen. Hospital

ANN BRENNAN, M.D.
Univ. of Louisville
Dept. of Psychology
Rm. 103
Life Sciences Bldg.
Louis., KY 40292

Associate Prof. Psy.

Univ. of
Louisville
(Kentucky)

DENNIS J. BUCHHOLZ,PHD
Dept. of Psychiatry
Univ. of Louisville

Clin. Assc. Prof.
Psych. & Neurosurg.

Univ. of
Louisville
(Kentucky)

LAURIEANN CHUTIS, ACSW
4545 North Damen
Chicago, Ill.
(312) 878-4300 X1455

Director of
Consultation and
Education Services

Ravenwood Hosp.
Community
Mental Health

M. WAYNE COOPER, M.D.
1318 Broadway
Lubbock, TX. 79401
(806) 763-2161

Associate Professor
Internal Medicine
(Chief, Cardiology)

Tex Tech Univ.
Health Sci.
Ctr. at Lubbock

TERESA CORONA, M.D.
Ave. Cuauhtemoc No. 330
Mexico, DFCP. 06725

Assistant Professor
Neurology (UNAM)

Hospital Gen.
Centro Medico
Nacional, Inst.
Mexicano del
Seguro Social

CARROLL CRADDOCK, PH.D.
4550 North Winchester
Chicago, Ill. 60640

Director of Child
and Adolescent
Services

Ravenswood
Hosp. Comm.,
Mental Health
Center

JUAN RAMON DE LA FUENTE,
Calzada Mexico
Xochimilco
No. 101, Colonia San
Lorenzo Huipulco,
Tlalpan 14370
Mexico, D. F
(011525) 655-28-11 X141

Associate Professor
of Psychiatry
Director of Division
of Clinical Research

Instituto
Mexicano de
Psiquiatria

KRISHNA DASGUPTA, M.D.
Department of Psychiatry
Room B6210, Univ. of

Assistant Prof. of
Psychiatry

Univ. of
Wisconsin

Wisconsin Hospitals
600 Highland Ave.
Madison, Wisconsin
53792
(608) 263-6082
      263-8200

JOEL DIMSDALE, M.D.   Associate Professor   Univ. of Calif.
225 Dickinson St.   of Psychiatry   San Diego Med.
San Diego, CA.   Center
92103-9981

DOROTHY DINARDO-EKERY, M.D.
4800 Alberta   Associate Professor   Tex Tech Univ.
El Paso, TX.   79905   of Internal Med.   Regional Acad.
(915) 533-3020 X237   (Cardiology)   Health Center

JAVIER ESCOBAR, M.D.   Professor of   Univ. of
232 South Main St.   Psychiatry   Connecticut at
West Hartford, CT.   Vice-Chairman   West Hartford
06107   Dept. of Psychiatry

BRUNO ESTAÑOL, M.D.   Chief of Neurology   Hospital Gen.
B. Traven 180-604   Service, Associate   Centro Medico
Col. General Anaya   Professor of Neurology Nacional
Mexico 13, D. F.   Instituto del
6-88-77-02/ 5-84-46-35   Seguro Social
                                                     (UNAM)

FRANCISCO FERNANDEZ, M.D. Associate Professor   Baylor College
6720 Bertner   of Psychiatry, Chief,   of Medicine
Houston, TX.   77030   Consultation Service
(713)   791-2655

ENRIQUE S. GARZA-TREVIÑO, M.D.   Assistant   The Univ. of
2800 S. MCGregor Drive   Professor of   Tex Med. Sch.
P. O. Box 20249   Psychiatry   at Houston
Houston, TX.   77225-0249
(713) 772-5354 - Home
(713) 741-3843 - Work

MOISES GAVIRIA, M.D.   Associate Professor   Univ. of Ill.
912 South Wood St.,   of Psychiatry   at Chicago
P. O. Box 6998   Director: Affective
Chicago, ILL.   60680   Disorders Clinic
(312) 996-3581
(312) 996-6139 (Work)
            9162 (Work)

LESLIE H. GISE, M.D.   Associate Director   Mount Sinai
The Mount Sinai Med.   Beh. Med. & Cons. Psy   Schl. of Med.
1 Gustave L. Levy Place
New York, N.Y.   10029

EVARISTO GOMEZ, M.D. 230 N. Michigan, Ste. 2700 Chicago, Ill. 60601 (312) 346-9595	Clinical Professor of Psychiatry	Univ. of Ill. at Chicago
MADELINE GOMEZ, M.D. (312) 346-9595	Clinical Assistant Professor of Psychiatry	Univ. of Ill. at Chicago
MARTIN GUERRERO, M.D. 4800 Alberta El Paso, TX. 79905 (915) 533-3020 X303 (OPC) 533-2472	Assistant Professor of Psychiatry	Tex Tech Univ. Regional Academic Health Center, El Paso
LEO E. HOLLISTER 2800 S. MacGregor Houston, Texas 77021 (713) 741-7800	Professor, Director of Psychiatry, HCPC	The Univ. of Tex Med. Sch. at Houston
VALERIE HOLMES, M.D. Dept. of Psych. and Behavioral Science SUNY at Stoneybrook Health Science Center T-10 Stoneybrook, N.Y. 11794-8101	Assistant Professor of Medicine (Psych)	State Univ. of New York
JAMES W. JEFFERSON M.D. Dept. of Psychiatry Room B6210 Univ. of Wisconsin Hospitals 600 Highland Ave. Madison, Wisconsin 53792 (608) 263-6082 263-8200	Prof. of Psych. Director, Center for Affective Disorders	Univ. of Wisconsin
ROY JULIAN, M.D. V. A. Outpatient Clinic 5919 Brookhollow St. El Paso, TX. 79925	Clinical Assistant Professor of Psychiatry	Tex Tech Univ. Regional Acad. Health Center
BORIS KAIM, M.D. 1100 North Stanton El Paso, TX 79902 (915) 544-6400	Associate Clinical Prof. of Neurology and Psychiatry	Tex Tech Univ. Regional Acad. Health Center
EDWARD KAUFMAN, M.D. Dept. of Psych. & Human Behavior Univ. of Calif.	Professor, Psychiatry & Human Behavior Director, Psychiatric Education	Univ. of Calif.

Irvine Med. Ctr.
101 City Drive S.
Psychiatry Rt. 81,
Bldg. 53
Orange, Calif.   92668
(714) 634-6021

HELENA C. KRAEMER, PH.D.	Prof., Biostatistics	Stanford Univ.
Stanford University	in Psychiatry	School of Med.
School of Medicine		Dept. Psych. &
Dept. Psych. &		Beh. Science
Beh. Sciences		

WOLFGANG F. KUHN, M.D.	Clin. Asst. Prof. Psyc.	Univ. of
Dept. of Psychiatry		Louisville
Univ. of Louisville		
Louisville, KY.		

GWENDOLYN LEE-DUKES, M.D.		UT, Medical
UT, Med. Branch		Branch at
Div. of Child & Adol.		Galveston
Psychiatry		
Galveston, Tx. 77550		
(409) 761-2416		

JARY LESSER, M.D.	Assistant	Univ. of Texas
6431 Fannin	Prof. of Psychiatry	Health Science
Houston, TX. 77030		Center at
		Houston

JOEL K. LEVY, PH.D.	Assistant	Baylor College
St. Luke's Episcopal	Prof. of Psychiatry	of Medicine
Hospital		Psych. Consult.
Houston, Texas		Service

Z.J. LIPOWSKI, MD, FRCP	Prof. Psych.	U. of Toronto
Univ. of Toronto	Psych.-in-Chief	Psychosom. Med.
Psychosom. Med. Unit		Unit (Canada)
Clarke Institute of Psych.		
Toronto, Ontario		

DIANE MARTINEZ, M.D.	Assistant Professor	Univ. of Tex.
Box 189C, RT. 26	of Psychiatry	Health Science
San Antonio, TX 78249		Ctr. at San
		Antonio

MARY NEIDHART	AIDS Nurse Coord.	Univ. of New
Univ. New Mexico		Mexico
Albuquerque, New Mex.		Dept. Int. Med.

HECTOR ORTEGA SOTO, M.D.	Associate Professor	Universidad
Instituto Mexicano de	of Psychiatry	Nacional
Psiquiatria		Autonoma
Calzada Mexico		de Mexico

Xochimilco
No. 101, Colonia
San Lorenzo
Huipulco, Tlalpan,
14370 Mex. D. F
(011525) 655-2811 X141

CECILIA A. PEABODY, M.D. Assc. Prof. Psych.   UT, Med. Schl.
UT, Med. School
Dept. of Psych.

KENNETH REAMY, M.D.   Associate Professor   West Virginia
Morgantown, W. V. 26506 OB-GYN, Behavioral   Univ. Sch. of
                         Medicine and   Medicine
                         and Psychiatry

KAREN K. REDDING, LCSW   Irvine Medical
Irvine Medical Center   Center
Orange, California

ROBERT G. ROBINSON, M.D. Prof. Psychiatry   Johns Hopkins U
Dept. Psych. Beh. Sci.   Schl. of Med.
Johns Hopkins U
School of Medicine

DAVID SHEEHAN, M.D.   Professor of Psychiatry Univ. of South
12901 N. 30th St.   Director of Clinical   Florida, Sch.
P. O. Box 14   Research   of Medicine
Tampa, Fla. 33612
(813) 974-3374

SERGIO E. STARKSTEIN, MD Postdoctoral Fellow   Johns Hopkins U
Dept. Psych. Beh. Sci.   Schl. of Med.
Johsn Hopkins Univ.
School of Medicine

MICHAEL E. STEFANEK, M.D.Asst. Prof., Oncology
Johns Hopkins   Asst. Prof., Medical
Oncology Center   Psychology
Oncology B150
600 N. Wolfe St.
Baltimore, MD. 21205
(301) 955-3300

ALAN SWANN, M.D.   Associate Prof. of   Univ. of Texas
P.O. Box 20708   Psychiatry   Health Science
Houston, Tx. 77225   Center, Houston
(713) 792-5541

JOHN R. SWENSON, M.D.   Asst. Prof. Psych.   Univ. of Ottawa
University of Ottawa   (Canada)
Department of Psychiatry
Otawa, Canada

1300

SUE THIEMANN   Biostatistician   Stanford Univ.
Dept. Psych. Beh. Sci.   Schl. of Med.
Stanford University
School of Medicine

M. DHYANNE WARNER, PHD   Med. Student   UT, Med. Schl.
Dept. of Psychiatry   at Houston
UT, Med. School
at Houston

INDEX

major depressive illness. J Clin Endocrinol Metab 61:
429-438, 1985.

38. Rubin, R.T. & Polland, R.E. Pituitary-adreno-cortical and
pituitary-gonadal function in affective disorder. In
Neuroendocrinology and Psychiatric Disorders. (ed. G.M.Brown,
S.H. Kaslow & S. Reichlin) pp. 151-164. Raven Press, New
York, 1984.

39. de la Fuente, J.R., Salin-Pascual, R.J., Gutierrez, R.,
et al. Alterations in sleep in depressed patients.
Salud Mental 8:57-59, 1986.

40. Sachar, E.J., Hellman, L., Roffwarg, H.P., et al.
Disrupted 24-hour patterns of cortisol secretion in
psychotic depression. Arch Gen Psychiatry
28:19-24, 1973.

41. Kupfer, J.D., Foster, G., Coble, P., et al.
The application of EEG sleep for the differential diagnosis of
affective disorders. Am J Psychiatry 135:69-74, 1978.

42. Wehr. T.A., Gillin, J.C., Goodwin, F.K. Sleep
and circadian rhythms in depression: In Sleep
Disorders: Basic and clinical research. (eds M.
Chase, E.D., Weitzman) pp. 195-225. Spectrum
Publishers Inc., New York, 1983.

43. Baldessarini, R.S., Arana, G.W. Does the
dexamethasone suppression test have clinical utility in

psychiatry? J Clin Psychiatry 46(supl 2,sec 2):25-29, 1985.

44. Carroll, B. The dexamethasone suppression test for melancholia. Brit J Psychiatry 140:292-304, 1983.

45. de la Fuente, J.R. & Speulveda, A. Does ethnicity affect DST results? Am J Psychiatry 143:275-276, 1986.

46. Rubinow, D.R., Gold, P.W., Post, R.M., et al. The relationship between cortisol and clinical phenomenology of affective illness. In Neurobiology of Mood Disorders. (eds. R. M. Post, J.C. Ballenger) pp 664-672, Williams and Wilkins, 1984.

47. de la Fuente, J.R. & Ortega, H. Dexametasone suppression test in psychiatry. Salud Mental 10:23-30, 1987.

48. Amsterdam, J.D., Bryant, S., Larkin, J., et al. The dexamethasone suppression test as a predictor of antidepressant response. Psychopharmacol 80:43-45, 1983.

49. Holsboer, F., Gerken, A., von Bardeleben, U., et al. Human corticotropin-releasing hormone in depression correlation with thyrotropin secretion following thyrotropin-releasing hormone. Biol Psychiat 21:601-611, 1986.

50. Gold, P.W., Loriaux, L. Roy, A., et al. Responses to corticotropin-releasing hormone in the hypercortisolism of depression and Cushing's disease. NEJM 314:1329-1335, 1986.

51. Gold, P.W., Corticotropin-releasing factor stimulation in hypercortisolemic psychiatric states.

Ann of Intern Med 102:352-355, 1985.

52. Gormley, G.J., Lowy, M.T., Reder, A.T., et al. Glucocorticoid receptors in depression: relationship to the dexamethasone suppression test. Am J Psychiatry 143:1278-1284, 1986.

53. Whalley, L.S., Borthwick, H., Copolov, D., et al. Glucocorticoid receptors and depression. Brit Med J 292:859-861, 1986.

54. Angelucci, L., Patacchilo, R.R., Bohus, B., et al. Serotoninergic innervation and glucocorticoid binding in the hippocampus: relevance to depression. En: Typical and atypical antidepressants: molecular mechanism. (eds E. Costa y cols) pp. 365-370. Raven Press, New York, 1982.

55. Pitt, B. Depression and childbirth. In: Handbook of Affective Disorders. (ed E.S. Paykel) pp. 361-378. Guilford Press, New York, 1982.

56. Janowsky, D.S., Garney, R., Kelley, B. The course vicissitudes and variations of the female fertility cycle: I Psychiatric aspects. Psychosomatics 7:242-247, 1966.

57. Maggi, A., Perez, J. Role of female gonadal hormones in the CNS: Clinical and experimental aspects. Life Sci 37:893-906, 1985.

58. Halbreich, U., Endicott, J., Goldstein, S., et al. Premenstrual changes and changes in gonadal hormones. Acta Psychiat Scand 74:576-586, 1986.

59. Post, R.M., Uhde, T.W., Putnam, P.W., et al.

Kindling and carbamazepine in affective illness. J Nerv Ment Dis. 170:717-731, 1982.

60. Janowsky, D.S. & Rausch, J. Biochemical hypothesis of premenstrual tension syndrome. Psychol Med 15:2-8, 1985.

61. Wetzel, J.N., Reich, T., McClure, J.M., et al. Premenstrual affective syndrome and psychiatric disorder. Brit J Psychiatry 127:219-221, 1975.

62. Brambilla, F., et al. Deranged Anterior Pituitary Responsiveness to Hypothalamic Hormones in Depressed Patients, Arch Gen Psych 1231-1238, 1978.

63. Linnoila, M.,et al. Thyroid Hormones and TSH, Prolactin and LH Responses to Repeated TRH and LRH Injections in Depressed Patients, Acta Psych Scand 59:536-544, 1979.

64. Rubin, R.T., et al. Hypothalamo-Pituitary-Gonadal Function in Primary Endogenously Depressed Men; Preliminary Findings, in K. Fuxe et al., eds., Steroid Hormone Regulation of the brain. Oxford: Pergamon Press, pp.387-396, 1981.

65. Amsterdam, J.D., et al. Gonadotropin Release After Administration of GnRH in Depressed Patients and Healthy Volunteers, J Affec Dis, 3:367-380, 1981.

66. Beck-Friis, J., et al. Hormonal Changes in Acute Depression, in C. Perris et al., eds., Biological Psychiatry. Amsterdam: Elsevier North Holland Biomedical Press, pp. 1244-1248, 1981

67. Ettigi, P.G., Brown, G.M., and Seggie, J. A. TSH and LH Responses in Sub-types of Depression, Psychosomatic